BEATING CANCER

WITH NUTRITION

Harnessing the incredible healing power of nature and science

✻

A healthy human body is self-regulating and self-repairing.

✻

Optimal nutrition can improve outcome in medically-treated cancer patients.

PATRICK QUILLIN, PhD,RD,CNS

WITH NOREEN QUILLIN

Nutrition Times Press, Inc.

UNSOLICITED PRAISE FROM OUR READERS:

"...I love this book...Thank you for this book!!!" L.S.

"Your book has been my guideline for the past 16 months. A recent visit to my urologist revealed a PSA of 0.4 (125% reduction). Also, he was unable to feel any tumor. Beating prostate cancer in 16 months is a tribute to your nutritional approach." L.A.

"I've used your book like a bible. I've learned many things since my original diagnosis, but your book has been one of the greatest helps." S.R.

"I have purchased and read your book with great interest and gratitude, as it is impeccably researched and written." B.P.

" Just wanted to let you know that my wife is doing great. She was diagnosed in August with invasive ductal carcinoma, with node involvement. After 4 rounds of chemo her lymph nodes were clean -- 100%! We're pretty sure that the supplements you recommended had a lot to do with her positive outcome. Just wanted to say thank you for all of your books -- they've really been the foundation for her treatment program, and, we feel anyway, the reason for her positive response." G.W.

"Thank you for all your help in your terrific book." M.O.

"Your book is great. I have survived 6 1/2 years (ovarian cancer stage III) and, with the help of a naturopath, have been taking supplements and taking care with my diet. Your strategies have now been added to my arsenal of defense tools." C.L.

"Your book became our nutritional bible in fighting multiple myeloma. The dragon-slayer drink into which we add nutritional supplements has made pill-taking much easier. I am a survivor." R.F.

"Your recipes in the book are delicious!" H.M.

"Your book was outstanding. I thought I knew a lot, but I learned a lot more from you. I don't expect to "hear" from my own cancer again." E.H.

"In August 98 I was diagnosed with testicular cancer. After reading your book I started up a series of changes in my life style. After orchiectomy was done I decided not to go under chemo and followed instead a natural approach. I am doing pretty well. I already had a metastasis in the retroperitoneal area and this tumor has been decreased drastically." J.S.

"My husband was diagnosed this year with eye malignant melanoma that has now metastasized on his liver. We have purchased your book and it has helped us more than any other means of information. We have devoured your book (good fiber) and refer to it all the time." C.F.

"First of all your book is the best on the subject. We know, we've read them all. My wife was diagnosed with Stage 3 breast cancer in December 1999. She feels fantastic and super charged." K.S.

"I read your book and credit it with helping my 37 year old husband overcome non-hodgkins lymphoma which was misdiagnosed for over 6 months." M.K.

"...helping me to eat better to prevent a recurrence. Now in my 6th year." S.O.

Other books & products by Patrick Quillin, PhD,RD,CNS
available at your local bookstore or health food store, or www.amazon.com
-DIABETES IMPROVEMENT PROGRAM, Leader Co., N.Canton,OH, 1999
-HEALING POWER OF CAYENNE, Leader Co., N.Canton,OH, 1998
-IMMUNOPOWER, Nutrition Times Press, Tulsa, 1998
-HEALING SECRETS FROM THE BIBLE, Nutrition Times Press, Tulsa, 1996
-HONEY, GARLIC & VINEGAR, Leader Co., N. Canton, OH, 1996
-ADJUVANT NUTRITION IN CANCER TREATMENT, Cancer Treatment Research
Foundation, Arlington Heights, IL, 1994
-AMISH FOLK MEDICINE, Leader Co., N.Canton, OH, 1993
-SAFE EATING, M.Evans, NY, 1990
-LA COSTA BOOK OF NUTRITION, Pharos Books, New York, 1988
-HEALING NUTRIENTS, Random House, NY, 1988
-THE LA COSTA PRESCRIPTION FOR LONGER LIFE, Ballantine Books, NY,
1985

Printed in the United States of America

How to order this book:
BOOKMASTERS 1-800-247-6553
BOOKWORLD 1-800-444-2524

Nutrition Times Press, Inc., Box 130789, Carlsbad, CA 92013
ph.760-804-5703, fax 760-804-5704, NutritionCancer.com

About the cover: Cancer cells have abnormal DNA, which is the
"blueprint" for making healthy cells. Healthy foods contain substances that
help prevent and possibly reverse cancer. The power of nature that is
within a lightning bolt is also within us to heal. Design by Oxana Gusak.

TELL US YOUR STORY
We want to hear about your experiences using nutrition as part of your cancer
treatment. Please send us your personal experience with an address or phone
number on how to contact you. Your story may provide hope for others
suffering from the same condition. Thank you. email: pq@patrickquillin.com

---

CONTENTS

Dedication

To the many cancer patients whom I have worked with. You have taught me more about living than I have taught you about healing.

Acknowledgements

To Ignaz Semmelweis, MD, Max Gerson, MD, Hugh Riordan, MD, Linus Pauling, PhD, Weston Price, DDS, Donald Kelly, DDS, John Prudden, MD, PhD, Jonathan Wright, MD, Julian Whitaker, MD, Jeffrey Bland, PhD, Joseph Pizzorno, ND, and Abram Hoffer, MD, PhD. All are/were geniuses who cared more about helping patients than peer approval, profit, or license revocation. Nobody ever said that being an ice breaker is an easy job. But the world is better off because you assumed the task.

NO ADVERTISERS. In this book there are thousands of services and doctors along with hundreds of products listed. No one paid to be listed in this book. I have included products and services that I believe may help you in your quest for wellness.

IMPORTANT NOTICE!!! PLEASE READ!!!

CAUTION!! Cancer is a life-threatening disease. The program outlined in this book is for educational purposes and not to be considered a substitute for medical care. Information provided in this book is to be used in conjunction with, not instead of, your doctor's program. All of the foods and supplements described in this book will work synergistically with your oncologist's program. Do not use this information as your sole therapy against cancer. Patient profiles listed in this book are not typical. Your results may vary. No results are guaranteed. If you cannot agree to these terms, then you may return this book in new condition for a full refund. This information has not been evaluated by the Food and Drug Administration.

SHORTCUT: EXECUTIVE SUMMARY
✴
IF YOU ARE TOO SICK TO READ MUCH, THEN READ THIS SECTION
✴
21 days to a healthier cancer patient

"Dance as if no one is watching. Work as if you don't need the money." Anonymous

BEATING CANCER THROUGH:

DAY 1: HOPE, OPTIMISM, AND A FIGHTING SPIRIT

Focus on the parts of your body that are working properly, not on the cancer. Since you are alive enough to read this book, then something and perhaps quite a bit are working in your body. Give thanks for everything that you can think of. Thanksgiving is a healing balm on the body and soul.

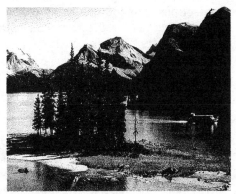

What are your priorities in life? Have they changed since finding out about your cancer diagnosis? Have they changed for the better? Is it possible that cancer has become a life-threatening, yet valuable wakeup call for you?

We are all going to die. The question is not "if", but rather "when". For cancer patients, sometimes this "when" becomes a more immediate issue. But our finite lives should be an issue for all of us, all of the time. Life is precious. Not to be wasted. Many of us cram our days with minutia, trivial details. We spend too much time worrying about insignificant events and lose sight of the real issues in life:

↪ be here now
↪ value your mission
↪ cherish your friends and family
↪ savor sunsets and sunrises
↪ soak up the beauty and music and laughter and play that is all around you, but drowned out by the cacophony of crass commercialism
↪ be at peace with your Creator, however you conceive that Higher Power

People beat cancer all the time. But fear of death is not a reason to live. What do you want them to say at your funeral? "Look, I think she's moving!!" Not going to happen. Begin today with a renewed sense of purpose and proper perspective for the truly memorable things in life. Build a fighting "can-do" spirit that will serve you well for the coming journey of treating your cancer. Find a "co-patient", a loved one, or family member who is so supportive that they will keep you motivated when you have run out of steam.

Be enthusiastic. The word "enthusiasm" comes from the Greek words meaning "God within". With joy, enthusiasm, appreciation, and altruism, we literally become a conduit for God's life itself.

DAY 2: KNOWLEDGE, OPTIONS, DATA GATHERING

While your doctor who made the cancer diagnosis may have a plan for you, it is probably not the only therapy that is appropriate for your cancer and may not even be the best therapy. You need to explore your options. In today's society, getting information is easier than ever before. Get on the Internet and spend a few hours gathering data and phone numbers on who can help you with your particular cancer. The more knowledge that you have on the treatment and curing of your cancer, the more likely you are to make the right decision on which "wagon master" to choose for your vital treatment ahead.

Consider hyperthermia as primary or adjunctive therapy for your cancer. The following can provide a detailed report on doctors around the world who have a successful track record in treating your cancer:
↪ Janice Guthrie, Health Resource, ph.800-949-0090
↪ Greg Anderson, CancerRecovery.org, ph.800-238-6479
↪ Frank Wiewel, People Against Cancer, ph.515-972-4444
↪ Susan Silberstein, PhD, Cancer Education, ph.610-642-4810
↪ Steven Ross, PhD, World Research Foundation ph.520-284-3300

DAY 3: THE POWER OF NUTRITIONAL SYNERGISM

Synergism means that $1 + 1 = 3$ or 500, but a whole lot more than 2. Synergism tells us that the combined efforts of certain factors yield more than what would have been expected. Do not rely on any "magic bullet" nutrient to beat your cancer. There are no such things. Your body needs the 50 recognized essential nutrients plus a couple of hundred other valuable nutrients that can only be found in a wholesome diet that is supplemented with the right nutrients.

"What is the most important part of a car?" Some people answer: "The engine." Fine. Then I will give you an engine and let's see you drive it home. A car, like a healthy human body, is composed of many essential parts. The most important part of the car is the one that is not working. In building a house, all of the raw materials must arrive in the proper ratio at the proper time, otherwise you cannot build a sturdy home. Same thing with the human body. Nutritional synergism says that when you gather the right nutrients together at the right time in the right ratio, the body becomes a lean, mean, disease-fighting machine. Nothing less will do in your quest to beat cancer.

DAY 4: STARVE THE CANCER

Cancer is a sugar-feeder. The scientists call it an "obligate glucose metabolizer". You can slow cancer growth by lowering the amount of fuel available to the tumor cells. Americans have become humming birds in our constant consumption of sweet fluids and foods. The resulting constant high blood glucose levels yield many diseases, including cancer, diabetes, heart disease, hypertension, and yeast infections. Trying to beat cancer while eating a diet that constantly raises blood glucose is like trying to put out a forest fire while someone nearby is throwing gasoline on the trees.

Stop eating sugar. Eat very few sweet foods, including high glycemic fruits. Begin an exercise program to burn blood glucose down to a manageable level. Your cancer is not going to be happy as you begin to starve it. You will develop sugar cravings worse than you currently have. Ignore them and push through the discomfort.

Make fish and colorful vegetables the staples in your diet. Eat small amounts of fresh fruits at a mixed meal, which will blunt the rises in blood glucose. Use cinnamon liberally, since it helps to stabilize blood glucose. Take supplements of chromium and magnesium. I have yet to see a cancer patient beat the disease who continued to load up on the average amounts of sugar in our diet, which is 140 pounds per year per person.

DAY 5: AVOID MALNUTRITION

Cancer is a wasting disease. Over 40% of cancer patients actually die from malnutrition, not from the cancer. Cancer generates chemicals that lower appetite while increasing calorie needs. The net effect is that many cancer patients begin to lose weight. You cannot fight a life-threatening disease while malnourished. You need all the proper nutrition you can get to feed your immune system, which is your army assigned to killing the cancer cells. The backbone of the immune system is protein.

If you cannot eat solid foods, then try the Dragon-slayer shake mentioned later in this book.

DAY 6: NUTRITION + MEDICINE= IMPROVED RESULTS

While chemotherapy and radiation can kill cancer cells, these therapies are general toxins against your body cells also. A well-nourished cancer patient can protect healthy cells against the toxic effects of chemo and radiation, thus making the cancer cells more vulnerable to the medicine. Proper nutrition can make chemo and radiation more of a selective toxin against the cancer and less damaging to the patient.

DAY 7: TURBOCHARGE YOUR IMMUNE SYSTEM

Your immune system consists of 20 trillion cells that compose your police force and garbage collectors. The immune system is responsible for killing the bad guys, any cells that are not participating in the processes of your body, including cancer, yeast, bacteria, virus, and dead cells. "Kill the bad guys and take out the trash." That is what your immune system is supposed to do. But since you have cancer, something is wrong with your immune system: usually either stress, toxic burden, or malnutrition.

Eat well and take professionally designed nutrition supplements. Lower your stress levels. Use guided imagery to imagine your immune cells like sharks gobbling up the cancer cells. This technique really works!! Detoxify your body. The average American body has 1,000 times more heavy toxic metals than our primitive ancestors before the dawning of the industrial age. Toxins shut down the ability of the immune system to mount a good battle against the cancer cells.

As your cells divide billions of times daily, mistake cells are the inevitable consequence. These mistake cells sometimes grow into cancer cells, which your immune system recognizes as being defective and then gobbles them up like Pac Man. The average adult gets 6 bouts of cancer in a lifetime, yet only 42% of Americans will end up in a cancer hospital. The other 58% had a respectable immune system, which protected the person against defective cells rising up to become palpable life-threatening cancer. Get your immune system working and the end of your cancer is in sight. Nutrition products that have demonstrated an ability to bolster immune functions include: colostrum extracts (lactoferrin, transfer factor), whey extracts, aloe extracts, mushroom extracts (Maitake, AHCC), yeast cell wall extracts (1,3 beta glucan), IP-6 (phytic acid), ImmKine (Aidan 480-446-8181), and Essiac tea.

DAY 8: THE HEALING POWER OF WHOLE FOODS

It is amazing how simple the answer to cancer can be. Our brilliant researchers have spent 33 years and $50 billion of your tax dollars wrestling with the complex issue of curing cancer. Yet Nature has been solving the dilemma for thousands of years. All of us get cancer all of the time, yet magical ingredients in a whole food diet are there to help the body beat cancer. Ellagic acid from berries induces "suicide" in the cancer cells. Lycopenes from tomatoes help to suppress cancer growth. Genistein in soy, glutathione in green leafy vegetables, and S-allyl cysteine in garlic are examples of the new scientifically-validated cancer fighters of the 21st century.

You don't have to wait for 7 years while some drug company goes through the $800 million drug approval process, nor for FDA approval, nor for a doctor's prescription for some drug that has many toxic side effects and costs thousands of dollars each month. These miracle anti-cancer agents are waiting patiently at your nearby grocery store and health food store.

↳ Eat foods in as close to their natural state as is possible.

↳ Eat as much colorful vegetables as your colon can tolerate.

↳ If a food will not rot or sprout, then throw it out.

↳ Shop the perimeter (outside aisles) of the grocery store.

DAY 9: NUTRITIOUS AND DELICIOUS RECIPES

Now that you understand the importance of eating wholesome foods to beat your cancer, you will need some tips on making this food palatable. See Noreen's chapter on "Nutritious & Delicious" for many great tasting recipes. I have hosted many a class with hundreds of cancer patients where we would tell them what foods might help them to beat their cancer. Women, in general, seem more receptive to these new cooking ideas. Men, in general, seem less interested in changing 50 years of eating habits. Gravy is not a beverage, contrary to popular belief in America. Those same men who turned their nose up at our recipe suggestions are now dead.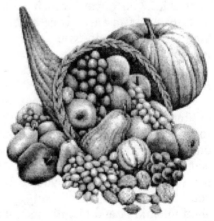

You are trying to take simple food straight from Nature and use healthy seasonings to make a quick and tasty meal. Crock pot, pressure cooker, steaming, and grilling are all wonderful means of cooking nourishing foods. Some produce is most nutritious when eaten raw, such as many vegetables and all fruit. A high speed blender can take any leftovers or foods that are not appealing and blend them in to a smoothie drink or a nice soup.

Try a couple of boiled eggs with a bowl of oatmeal and a half cup of cantaloupe for breakfast. Move on to a lunch with grilled chicken breast sandwich with spinach and onions, wild rice, a bowl of deep-colored fresh vegetables with homemade Italian dressing, and a half cup of raspberries for dessert. A sample dinner might be grilled halibut with lemon, baked sweet potatoes, fresh tomato slices with onions and homemade Italian dressing, and a dessert of a half cup of fresh papaya.

This is all nourishing food that you can learn to savor, easy to prepare, and easy to find at your local grocery store. And it will help you to beat your cancer.

DAY 10: HERBAL MEDICINE

There are thousands of herbs that have been used for thousands of years to treat cancer. None are guaranteed cures for all cancers, but many are non-toxic boosters of immune function and detoxification pathways. If you want just the basic herb that all cancer patients should be using daily, then start with garlic--as a food, seasoning, and/or pill supplement.

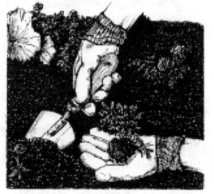

Many other herbs merit attention, as you will see in the chapter on herbs. Astragalus, echinacea, goldenseal, licorice, ginseng, ginkgo, ginger, Rhodiola rosea, and cat's claw are on the golden hit parade of herbs to help you toward recovery from cancer. Work with a professional who can help guide you toward which herb is best for your disease, your therapy, your wallet, and your stomach tolerances.

DAY 11: HEALTHY FATS

While too much fat and the wrong kind of fat have been killing millions of Americans for the past 50 years, we are now finding a new form of fat malnutrition: deficiencies of the essential fats. Fish oil, borage or primrose oil, flax oil, conjugated linoleic acid (from the meat and milk of ruminants like cows and sheep), and shark liver oil are all fats that can help you to beat your cancer. For a simple starter, begin taking a few capsules of fish oil daily, preferably basic cod liver oil with all the good vitamin A and D still intact. You can also make a delicious, healthy Italian salad dressing by using flax oil, olive oil, water, vinegar, and some seasonings.

The right fats in your diet will feed the precious pathways for beneficial prostaglandins, which are crucial to beating cancer. Healthy fats line the cell membranes and help to lower blood glucose by making insulin more effective. Healthy fats make the immune cells more likely to recognize and destroy cancer cells.

DAY 12: MINERALS

Before modern agriculture, farmers would use manure and compost to nourish the soil before planting the crops. Today, we use only nitrogen, phosphorus, and potassium (N:P:K) as the basic fertilizer. With each passing harvest, the American soils and our bodies become more deficient in essential minerals for health. For instance, scientists have found that a dust speck of selenium (200 micrograms daily) can lower cancer incidence by 60% and raise immune functions dramatically. Deprive animals of magnesium and they spontaneously develop lymphoma. Some of our cancer epidemic in America is due to our serious and widespread deficiency in essential minerals.

Buy a basic mineral supplement, containing decent amounts of calcium, magnesium, chromium, and selenium. Add some kelp, which is rich in the trace minerals that are found both in the ocean and supposed to be found in your body fluid.

DAY 13: VITAMINS

Vitamins are the factory workers that get things done. Calories are the fuel for energy, and minerals are part of the structure or help vitamins to get things done. Most Americans are deficient in vitamins, even on the basic survival Recommended Dietary Allowance level. For a starter package, buy a quality broad spectrum vitamin supplement; then add extra vitamin C (1-4 grams per day), E (200-800 mg/d), green tea capsules, curcumin, and fish oil. If your stomach and wallet can tolerate it, take ImmunoPower (ImmunoPower.com or 800-247-6553), a convenient and cost-effective mixture of 87 nutrition ingredients or ImmunoPower EZ with 44 ingredients (GettingHealthier.com).

DAY 14: PROBIOTICS--FRIENDLY BACTERIA

Professor Elie Metchnikoff won a Nobel prize in 1908 for his work on the immune system. He later discovered the bacteria that makes yogurt (lactobacillus) and declared "Death begins in the colon." Indeed, it may. And the colon and gut of most Americans are under siege by unfriendly organisms and free radicals.

When we eat nourishing food, our well-established colony of friendly bacteria in the colon eats yeast like a bird munches on insects. Many Americans eat too much fat, too much sugar, not enough fiber, and very little probiotic food (like yogurt and tempeh); take antibiotics (which wipe out all bacteria in the body, including the friendly bacteria); and subject ourselves to stress-- all of which affects the balance of power between good and bad microorganisms in the gut. The net effect is an overgrowth of yeast, along with a deficiency of friendly bacteria that feed the immune system via the lining of the intestines. The yeast, which are there to degrade feces upon elimination, become hateful dictators in the gut. Many health problems result from what is called "dysbiosis" of the gut, or not having the right kind of microorganisms in charge.

Eat more fiber and no white sugar. Drink plenty of clean water. Eat yogurt daily or take a probiotic supplement. Make sure that you have a daily bowel movement. Use gentle herbal laxatives, like senna, if necessary. After 40 years of poor diet and chronic constipation, some people need colon flushing. Find a qualified expert to help on this issue.

At least 40% of our immune system surrounds the gastro-intestinal tract. For better or for worse, the status of our gut will begin the healing or the deterioration of a cancer patient.

DAY 15: WATER

Only one substance is found in all forms of life: water. Our bodies and the earth's surface are composed of 2/3 water. Water is the most amazing substance on earth, providing the fluid of life in your body and the bathing solution for all cells in your body. Yet, most Americans do not get enough water and are drinking contaminated water.

Our water pollution situation in this country has been called "a ticking time bomb." by the Environmental Protection Agency. We have used our rivers, lakes, and oceans as if they were sewers to dump unconscionable amounts of toxins. And we end up drinking that stuff. Pollution in our water supply is part of the reason for our growing cancer epidemic in this country.

Buy yourself a good water filter system and install it on your kitchen tap. Dual stage carbon filtration may cost $100-$200, with reverse osmosis costing two or three times that much. If need be, buy bottled water from a respectable vendor. Some bottled water is merely bottled city tap water with sugar added to make it taste better. Drink enough water to dilute your urine so that it is nearly clear in color and inoffensive in odor. Chronic dehydration first shows up in wrinkled skin, poor concentration, constipation, frequent infections, and eventually may appear as cancer. Water is your friend. Drink lots of clean water.

DAY 16: BREATHING

Cancer is an anaerobic growth. Healthy cells in your body are aerobic, meaning that they need oxygen. Cancer hates well-oxygenated tissues of the body. Lung tissue, which is well oxygenated, develops cancer as the result of smoking carcinogens and excessive "rusting" of tissue in the absence of antioxidants to protect the lung tissue. I have found lung cancer in non-smokers to be quite reversible if the person is willing to follow the guidelines in this book.

Of all nutrients required by the human body, oxygen is the most essential. We can go weeks and even months without food, days without water, but only a few minutes without oxygen. We are aerobic creatures by design. Cancer is the opposite. Unfortunately, many Americans breathe shallowly, thinking that sucking in our stomach is more important than diaphragm breathing to fully oxygenate our tissues.

Get some exercise. Do some yoga. Start breathing properly all the time. Lay on the floor with a book on your stomach. Begin breathing by pushing the book up and sucking in air to the bottom of your lungs. Continue breathing by filling the lungs fully and expanding your chest. Reverse the process on exhaling. This "belly breathing" will fully oxygenate your body to help make it less friendly to cancer cells, like shining sunlight on a vampire.

DAY 17: CHANGE THE UNDERLYING CAUSE

No one with a headache is suffering from a deficiency of aspirin. And no one with cancer has a deficiency of chemo or radiation. While these therapies might temporarily reduce tumor burden, they do not change the underlying cause of the disease.

Mrs. Jones might be suffering from metastatic breast cancer because, in her case, she is still hurting from a hateful divorce of 2 years ago, which drives her catecholamines into a stress mode and depresses her immune system; she goes to bed on a box of high sugar cookies each night; she has a deficiency of fish oil, zinc, and vitamin E; and she has an imbalance of estrogen and progesterone in her body. Her oncologist may remove the breasts, give her Tamoxifen to bind up estrogen, and administer chemo and radiation; but none of these therapies deals with the underlying causes of the disease. And it will come back unless these driving forces for the disease are reversed.

Find a nutritionally-oriented doctor (listed in the back of this book) and determine what got you into this condition, which will provide a detailed map on how to get you out of this situation.

DAY 18: IS CANCER AN INFECTION?

There is compelling evidence that some or many cancers are advanced infections. Medline literature shows us that stomach cancer is often from the bacteria Helicobacter pylori, liver cancer from the infection hepatitis, cervical cancer from the infection human papilloma virus, and more. Hence, the need to address the infection is crucial in reversing the cancer. Yeast (fungi), virus, bacteria, mycoplasma, and parasites are among the critters that dwell within us and can create life-threatening diseases, like cancer. There are over 400,000 different strains of yeast, of which 400 can cause diseases in humans. Yeast is the "undertaker and the ecologist", decomposing all of life back to mother earth. Unfortunately, due to lowered vitality we are becoming premature victims of yeast and other infections. Just like wolves attack the weakest of the herd, opportunistic pathogens attack the weakest of cells within our body. Your mission is to make your body so full of wellness that there is no room for illness.

Take a simple urine test to see if you have a yeast overgrowth (Great Plains Labs 913-341-8949) or blood test (ImmmunoSciences 310-657-1077) to see if you have other infections. Your doctor will then:

↳ kill the infectious organism with prescription medication and/or nutrition supplements

↳ starve the yeast, by eating a diet that lowers simple carbohydrate intake

↳ make the environment uncomfortable for the infectious agent, by bolstering your body's defense mechanisms

DAY 19: BEATING CANCER SYMPTOMS

"If the heat don't kill you then the humidity will." "And if the cancer don't kill you then the side effects will." Actually, both are worthy of your attention. Nausea, depression, insomnia, constipation, diarrhea, anemia, weakness, fatigue, pain, and more can be common side effects of cancer. Depending on how advanced your cancer is, your medical therapies being given, your general health, etc., you can reduce symptoms to a tolerable level. See chapter 27 in this book. This is crucial because some cancer patients just give up, after suffering too much for too long. Much of this suffering can be reduced by allopathic and naturopathic treatments. Pain and discomfort induce stress, which lowers immune functions, which can be a real show-stopper for cancer patients. Pain management is crucial for many cancer patients. Get help.

DAY 20: SELECTIVELY REDUCE TUMOR BURDEN

It is very likely that your body needs some help in removing 10 or 20 trillion cancer cells, in order to reduce tumor burden enough to get your own anti-cancer defenses up and running. Working with the information that you gathered on day 2 (know your options of treatment), begin the process of debulking your tumor. Surgery, chemo, radiation, immune therapies, and hyperthermia are all common options. The key here is "restrained" tumor debulking. Anyone can kill all the cancer cells in your body. A thimble full of arsenic will do the job. No more cancer cells. No more you.

Surgeons used to take the aggressive cowboy approach and remove all surrounding tissue near the tumor. Then they found that by removing too many lymph nodes, that lymphedema, or pooling of lymph fluid, could create such pain that amputation of limbs became necessary. "Remove the target organ" was the battle cry of many an oncology surgeon. The hemi-ectomy was the pinnacle of aggressive surgery, where the cancer patient with a sarcoma below the waist had the body removed from the waist down. The survival statistics of these poor victims were no different than sarcoma patients who did nothing. Pelvic exenteration, taking out all internal organs near the tumor, yielded no improvement in survival curves and a serious reduction in quality of life for the remaining months. "Maximum sub-lethal chemo" has been the mantra of many oncologists. Bring the patient to the therapeutic brink of death, and then salvage the patient if possible.

Find a doctor who will work with you on RESTRAINED tumor debulking. Just like the childhood fable of Goldilocks, you want a doctor to remove--not too much, not too little, but just the right amount of tumor mass. Your oncologist can be the beginning of your demise or can give your body some breathing room so that your natural host defense mechanisms can take over. Choose your doctor "wagon master" wisely.

DAY 21: ILLNESS AS A TEACHING TOOL

What have you learned since being diagnosed with cancer? How have your priorities changed? Do you see life differently? Do you appreciate sunsets and friends more? If so, then you are heading in the right direction toward healing. If not, then wake up.

In working with over 3,000 cancer patients individually and speaking to many thousands of cancer patients, there is a clear message in the appearance of a serious disease in anyone's life. Illness can be an unavoidable teaching tool. You can ignore advice from friends and loved ones. But you cannot ignore a terminal diagnosis.

I have had my own health challenges and each has taught me much. We are here on this earth for a very limited amount of time. What are we doing with our precious time and talents? Are you a human being or a human doing? Do you hate more than you love? Take more than you give? See the glass as half empty rather than half full? Spend more time contemplating regrets than your dreams? Treat people with respect or victimize them? Understand your unique skills that the world needs?

Cancer is more than just a physical systemic disease. And it requires more than just good nutrition and medicine to cure. It is a wake up call of the highest magnitude. Cancer patients who heed the call become better people having experienced this acid bath, this gauntlet, this baptism of fire. Many a cancer patient has stood in front of an audience and said: "Cancer is the best thing that ever happened to me." If you are nodding in agreement with this statement, then you are moving toward healing.

In Oriental language, "crisis" is written with two characters: one meaning "danger", the other character meaning "opportunity". Cancer is truly a dangerous disease. Nearly 600,000 Americans die from this disease annually. Yet, for thousands of cancer patients, the disease has forced them into rearranging their priorities and lifestyle. Respect your body, your "temple of the Holy Spirit". Fill your mind and your hours so full of joy, passion, helpfulness, music, laughter, play, worship, thanksgiving, friends, family, and your work that there is no room left for cancer in your life. A diamond is nothing more than a piece of coal that was put under a lot of pressure. You can become a diamond through the healing of your cancer.

PATIENT PROFILE: BEAT ENDSTAGE TUBERCULOSIS

True story. The number one cause of death throughout most of the 19th century was tuberculosis. Galen Clark went to Yosemite Valley to die of endstage tuberculosis at age 42 in the fall of 1856. His doctor told him that coughing up chunks of his lungs meant he had up to 2-6 months to live. There was no cure for this disease. Clark reasoned that "If I'm going to die soon, then I'm going to die in Yosemite, the prettiest place I've ever seen." He got happy. Scientists now tell us that happiness brings on the flow of endorphins, which supercharge our immune system and may slow down cancer.

Next, Galen Clark carved his own tombstone, thus accepting his mortality, a ritual that would give us all a better appreciation of our finite time on earth. He then started eating what was available in Yosemite in those days; clean and lean wild game, mountain trout, nuts, berries, vegetables, and lots of clean water. No sugar and no dairy products. He then began doing what he wanted to do, hiking and creating trails, in the place he treasured the most, Yosemite Valley. He didn't die 6 months later, but rather 54 years later, just shy of his 96th birthday. He bolstered his "non-specific host defense mechanisms" with good thoughts and good nutrition.

Our bodies want to be well. There is an innate wisdom within all of life that knows how to fix disease. No one has to tell the scab on your hand how to heal properly. Your body knows what to do. We just have to give our body the proper physical and metaphysical resources to do its job right while purging our systems of toxins that inhibit healing.

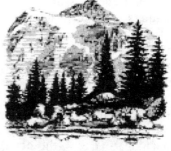

Feed your mind the good thoughts of music, beauty, laughter, play, art, and friends; share a glass of wine or a cup of tea at sunset, and discuss the events of the day with a loved one. Feed your heart the good feelings of love, forgiveness, confidence in your abilities, a sense of purpose in your life, and a trusting relationship with your Creator. And feed your body good nutrients through diet and supplements, thus providing your body the raw materials that it needs to rebuild itself. You can recover from your cancer.

PREFACE

✴

YOUR BODY WANTS TO BE WELL

TAKE TIME

Take time to think, it is the source of power. Take time to play, it is the source of perpetual youth. Take time to read, it is the fountain of wisdom. Take time to pray, it is the greatest power on earth. Take time to love and be loved, it is a God-given privilege. Take time to be friendly, it is the road to happiness. Take time to laugh, it is the music of the soul. Take time to give, it is too short a day to be selfish. Take time to work, it is the price of success. Take time to do charity, it is the key to heaven.

–Salesian Missions, New Rochelle, NY

There is a mysterious yet irreplacable force in all of life that "knows" how to heal itself. The broken bone, the scab on your arm, the baby being made in that woman's uterus, the ability of children to regenerate a severed fingertip--all tell us that Nature has an incredible plan for good health and long life. But only if those same natural forces within us have been given the raw building blocks of physical nutrients and metaphysical thoughts and feelings, plus relative freedom from toxic blockages.

PARADIGM SHIFTS TAKE TIME
the world is flat
what you can't see can't hurt you
cancer is irreversible; therapies must be highly toxic
antioxidants neutralize the tumor killing of chemo and radiation

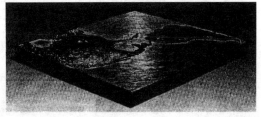

A couple of years ago, I tore a calf muscle while exercising. Didn't do enough stretching exercises before starting. The sound of the muscle snapping was like a giant rubber band breaking. It really hurt. My gastrocnemius bunched up in a ball in my leg. I considered surgery to repair the torn muscle. A veterinarian friend told me that if any part of the muscle or tendon was still connected to the bone, then the muscle will repair itself. I waited. The muscle crawled back into place. Slowly but surely it healed itself. Occasionally, I would feel electrical firings in my muscle as a muscle fiber was reconnected with its nerve ending. No outside intervention was necessary. Within certain limits, the body knows exactly how to repair itself.

Cancer patients may need some outside intervention to reduce tumor burden. At a certain point, say 10 trillion cancer cells in the human body, our recuperative powers are overwhelmed and possibly unable to heal without outside assistance. However, while your doctor is using restrained therapies to debulk your tumor, you need to pursue everything in your power to feed your body's repair mechanisms.

Some doctors today look at the human body as a defective mechanism that requires constant outside intervention to keep it running. Not true. Pregnancy is not a 9 month illness to be cured by a doctor. Heart disease is not caused by a deficiency of statin drugs. Cancer is not caused by a deficiency of chemo drugs. Heart disease, cancer, wounds, infections, arthritis, and other conditions are abnormalities. If the body is so defective and fragile, then how did the human species survive a couple of million years without modern medicine? Restore your body's ability to regulate itself, and these common ailments oftentimes will disappear. Reverse the obesity and the diabetes goes away. Eliminate the offending food and allergies clear up. Fix the underlying cause of cancer, and the cancer can clear up.

> A WELL-NOURISHED CANCER PATIENT CAN BETTER MANAGE AND BEAT THE DISEASE.
> 1) Less cachexia.
> 2) Fewer side effects from medical therapy.
> 3) Nourish host defenses for internal recuperative powers.
> 4) Reduce risk for future cancers--prevention.
> 5) Improve quality & quantity of life.
> 6) Improve chances for complete remission.
>
> "WELL-NOURISHED" comes from:
> 1) Food. Whole food omnivorous plant-based diet. Minimal processing & cooking. Rich in colorful vegetables. No sugar.
> 2) Supplements. Vitamins, minerals, herbs, fatty acids, probiotics, glandulars, food extracts, etc. become BRM.

CANCER ATTACKS THE SICKER CELLS.

In the Disney movie, "Never Cry Wolf", a biologist was assigned the task of observing wolves in the Arctic north to see if wolves were killing the elk, and whether the wolves must be killed. The biologist found that wolves primarily eat rodents, such as mice and rats. When the wolf pack ran down a herd of elk, the wolves caught and ate the slowest and sickest of the elk herd. The biologist ran out to the elk carcass that the wolves had finished feasting on, broke off a piece of ribbing, and found that the elk had been suffering from leukemia. In other words, the wolves pruned the sick and feeble in the elk herd. Similarly, cancer and infections attack a feeble and compromised host. Cancer cannot invade a healthy body. Make your body healthy, and the cancer simply goes away. Improve the health of the elk herd, and the wolves cannot catch the healthy ones. Only the sick elk (or body cells) are vulnerable to the wolves (or cancer).

This book will show you how to get your body so healthy that cancer is unwelcome in your body. You will probably need some outside help, both a doctor who uses restraint in removing cancer cells, and a health care professional who can help you to detect and change the underlying causes of your disease. Why are your body cells not healthy? This is a simple question involving a complex quest to find and eliminate the cause of the disease.

CANCER IN A HOST AS A SEED IN THE SOIL

If you drop a watermelon seed on the concrete, then the seed will not grow, because the conditions required for growth (warm temperature, fertile soil and moisture) have not been met. For decades, American doctors have spent 100% of their time trying to kill the "seed", or the cancer cell. Yet Antoine Bechamp (1816-1908), a French biologist, was the first to notice that the "soil" or the environment on which the yeast or bacteria fell was crucial in germinating the disease. Dr.

CANCER IN A HOST AS A "SEED IN THE SOIL"

"Cancer metastasis involves a complicated biochemical 'conversation' between the seed and the soil."
Stephen Paget, MD, Lancet, 1889

"Deficiency of vitamins or minerals appear to mimic radiation in damaging DNA." Bruce Ames, PhD, Toxicology Letters, 102,1998,5

cancer "seed"

"conversation"
cytokines, cell/cell comm
signal cell transduction

Host patient "the soil"

"The time has come to put major emphasis on the soil."
Isaiah Fidler, MD, 2004   MD Anderson Cancer Center

Stephen Paget wrote in *Lancet* in 1889 "Cancer metastasis involves a complicated biochemical 'conversation' between the seed and the soil." Professor Bruce Ames at the University of California Berkeley has shown that cancer can be generated in animals simply by depriving the animal of certain nutrients, which results in "biochemical chaos" and cancer. Oncologist Isaiah Fidler at the MD Anderson Cancer Center in Houston has recently added his endorsement of this "seed and soil" theory in cancer: "The time has come to put major emphasis on the soil."

KILLING CANCER IS EASY

It is simple to kill all the cancer cells in your body. A thimbleful of arsenic will do the job. The cancer cells have been killed--and so has the cancer patient. Not much of a victory. If you had mice in your garage and you used a hand grenade to blow up the garage, then you no longer have a mouse problem--nor do you have a garage. Cancer treatment hovers on these comparisons. Maximum sub-lethal chemotherapy, remove the target organ, and prophylactic radiation to the brain are among the more invasive and unsuccessful of techniques used by modern oncologists to "cure" the cancer patient. But is the treatment worse than the condition? Never mind the fact that these highly toxic strategies rarely cure advanced cancer!

WHAT IS YOUR VITALITY RATING?

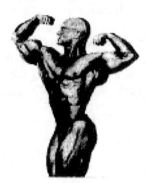

Your body is composed of 60 trillion well-orchestrated cells that perform miracles each and every second. Your body is built from food that you have consumed over your lifetime, plus the inevitable toxins that come with living in 21st century developed nations. When you are young, well-nourished, rested, well-exercised, free of toxins and negative emotions, excited about life, trusting of your surroundings, with something to do, someone to love, and something to look forward to--then your vitality rating is high. It is unlikely that you will get cancer or any other disease. You can be around infected people and not get an infection. You can live in an invisible sea of allergenic substances (pollen, dust, mold) and not get an allergic sneezing attack.

When we live on highly refined junk food that is full of toxins and does not provide our body with the necessary nutrients for optimal health, when we feel imprisoned, when we consume more toxins than our body can neutralize or eliminate, when we do not get the prerequisite of exercise-- then our bodies lose that magical self-regenerating ability. Heart disease, diabetes, or cancer may be the result. If you have cancer, then your vitality rating is low. This book has information that will help you boost your vitality rating. You will at least become a healthier cancer patient. Ideally, you will become cancer-free.

A clam has two pieces to its protective shell. Imagine if one piece of that shell is your physical protection: proper nutrient intake, exercise, avoidance of chemical toxins, and proper alignment of your body structure and energy meridians. The second half of that clam shell is represented by your metaphysical protection: love, connection to others, sense of purpose in life, fun things to do, pleasure, and relying on a Higher Power. Put the two shell halves together and the clam is well protected. If either side is missing, the fragile clam body becomes vulnerable to infections and predators. If either side of your "non-specific host defense mechanisms" (physical or metaphysical) is missing, then you become vulnerable to cancer and other ailments. Through the information provided in this book, we are going to restore the protective and recuperative powers that are yours. To finish the clam metaphor, a pearl is a beautiful and valuable item that starts out as an irritation in the clam, which is covered by multiple layers of calcium that only the clam can make. My hope is that the irritation of cancer will be covered over by your miraculous healing abilities so that when the cancer is gone, all that is left is a "pearl" that improves your life.

The bad news about all of this "vitality rating" and personal involvement in cancer recovery is that we will never develop a magic bullet drug for all cancer patients. The good news is that you can become actively involved in your healing process.

CRISIS=DANGER + OPPORTUNITY

"Cancer is the best thing that ever happened to me." The words almost knocked me over. I was listening to the testimonials from several cancer survivors who had gathered in a class reunion to celebrate life. These people later went on to explain this strange statement. "My life wasn't working. I didn't take care of my body. I didn't eat right. I didn't get enough rest. I didn't like my job, or myself, or those around me. I didn't appreciate life. I rarely stopped to smell the roses along the way. I asked too much of myself. I was too busy. Cancer was a great big red light flashing on the dashboard of my car saying 'pull this vehicle over and fix it now'".

These cancer victors had shown the ultimate courage by turning adversity into a major victory. In Oriental language, "crisis" is written by two characters, one meaning "danger" and the other meaning "opportunity". Cancer is a crisis of unparalleled proportions, both for the individual and for humanity. For a minority of cancer patients, cancer has become an extraordinary opportunity to convert their lives into a masterpiece.

Since the original version of this book was first published in January 1994, much water has passed underneath the bridge of nutritional oncology. There have been significant changes in the critical mass of data that endorses the use of nutrition for cancer patients. The internet has connected the world into one giant nervous system, whereby anyone anywhere can access almost any piece of information. A well-informed cancer patient is more likely to beat the disease.

The 1998 revised version of this book became the bestseller in its category on Amazon.com, the world's largest bookstore. I have organized three international scientific symposia, complete with continuing medical education (CME) units offered, on the subject of "Adjuvant Nutrition in Cancer Treatment". A textbook by the same title sprang from the seminal work reported in those conferences. More oncologists are receptive to the theory that nutrition may be valuable for their patients.

WHAT'S NEW IN THIS REVISED VERSION

This book contains improvements based on your feedback. As information continues to gather on the subject of beating cancer with natural methods of healing, it was mandatory to add many new studies that support the notion: "A well-nourished cancer patient can better manage and beat the disease." The sections on cancer as an infection, sugar and cancer, and antioxidant nutrients affecting pro-oxidant chemo and radiation have all been significantly expanded and updated with current information. Micronutrients have been given their own expanded chapter, rather than being bundled together.

You asked me for short written summaries and an audio version for those of you too sick to read much. You got it. You also sent me many emails (pq@patrickquillin.com) regarding your progress reports in your cancer. Some of those splendid "report cards" are featured in the "patient profile" section at the end of each chapter to provide hope and inspiration to others, who, like you, needed a reason to believe in the methods presented in this book. Thanks for your feedback. Keep it coming.

THE BIG CANCER PICTURE

Cancer is now the number one cause of death in America, surpassing heart disease as of January 2005. Over 4 million Americans are currently being treated for cancer, with another 4 million "in remission", and possibly awaiting a recurrence of the cancer. Each year, over 1.4 million more Americans are newly diagnosed with cancer with another 1 million skin cancers that are treated on an outpatient basis at the doctor's office. Half of all cancer patients in general are alive after five years. 42% of Americans living today can expect to develop cancer in his or her lifetime. Today, 24% of Americans die from cancer--a sharp contrast to the 3% who died from cancer in the year 1900. Europe has an even higher incidence of cancer. For the past four decades, both the incidence and age-adjusted death rate from cancer in America have been steadily climbing. Some people claim that the recent very modest improvements in cancer survival are explained by earlier diagnosis from more cancer screening procedures such as PSA, colonoscopy, breast exam, etc. Ironically, amidst the high-tech wizardry of modern medicine, at least 40% of cancer patients will die from malnutrition, not the cancer itself. This book highlights proven scientific methods that use nutrition to:

⇒Prevent or reverse the common malnutrition that plagues cancer patients.

⇒Make the medical therapies of chemotherapy and radiation more of a selective toxin to the cancer while protecting the patient from damage.

⇒Bolster the cancer patient's immune system to provide a microscopic army of warriors to fight the cancer throughout the body, because when the doctor says: "We think we got it all" that's when we are relying on a well-nourished immune system to locate, recognize, and destroy the inevitable remaining cancer cells.

⇒Help to selectively starve sugar-feeding tumor cells by altering intake of sugar, blood glucose levels, and circulating insulin.

⇒Slow down cancer with high doses of nutrients that make the body more resistant to invasion from tumor cells.

All of this good news means that cancer patients who use the comprehensive therapies described in this book may expect significant improvement in quality and quantity of life, and chances for a complete remission--by changing the underlying conditions that brought about the cancer. No cancer patient is suffering from a deficiency of adriamycin, a common chemotherapy drug! Cancer is an abnormal growth, not just a regionalized lump or bump. Chemo, radiation, and surgery will reduce tumor burden, but do nothing to change the underlying conditions that allowed this abnormal growth to thrive. In a nutshell, this book is designed to change the conditions in the body that favor tumor growth and return the cancer

Change the conditions that encourage abnormal growth

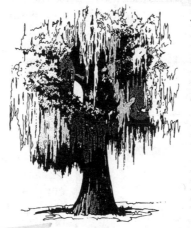

Fungus grows:
Heat
Moisture
Darkness
Sugar fuel
Low resistance

Cancer grows:
Low host resistance
High blood sugar
Low immunity
Altered pH
Toxic burden
Aging
Hormone imbalance
Stress
Malnutrition
Maldigestion
Yeast infection

victor to a healthier status. More wellness in the body means less illness, which depends on creating unfavorable conditions for cancer to thrive.

Fungus grows on a tree because of warmth, moisture, and darkness. You can cut, burn, and poison fungus off the tree, but the fungus will return as long as the conditions are favorable. Similarly, there are conditions that favor the growth of cancer. My extensive work with cancer patients shows that the cancer patient will thrive or wither, live or die based upon the ability to change the conditions that favor cancer growth.

CHOOSE YOUR WAGON MASTER WISELY

From around 1800 to 1900, the US West was settled by wagon trains crossing the Louisiana Purchase. Easterners would carry their precious few belongings to the launch point at St. Louis, where they would hire a "wagon master", or someone to lead them across the 2,000 miles of treacherous travel before reaching the west coast. Death from starvation, heat, dehydration, hostile Native Americans, and wild animals was a distinct possibility. People chose their wagon master based on track record of success. So should the cancer patient choose his/her cancer doctor, or wagon master, to help you through the treacherous terrain of cancer treatment. 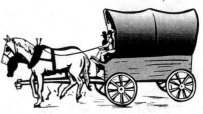 Too many cancer patients spend little time in selecting a wagon master. All too often, I speak with cancer patients who have had 30 rounds of radiation, 24 rounds of chemo, no nutrition, are badly starved, immune suppressed, anemic, and marginally salvageable. Then, the patient realizes, sometimes too late, that selecting your cancer doctor is at least as important as the early American pioneers selecting their wagon master. Ask your cancer doctor how often he/she has tackled your particular condition and, more importantly, how many patients are cured from his/her therapy. If your "wagon master" has a poor track record for bringing cancer patients, or "pioneers", safely through the hostile terrain, then you might consider seeking out another wagon master.

SHIFTING PARADIGMS

You never get the right answer if you are asking the wrong question.

How can we kill more cancer cells?

Why does cancer grow here?
How can we change the environment in the patient to discourage cancer growth?
How can we make the patient healthier?

Once Louis Pasteur discovered how to kill bacteria by heat processing (pasteurization), he embarked upon an energetic but ultimately frustrating career to eliminate all bacteria from the planet earth. Didn't work. And a century later, after the development of numerous "super drugs" to kill bacteria, Americans now have infections as the third leading cause of death, right after heart disease and cancer. Many bacteria are now drug resistant and virtually unstoppable. Similarly, after spending the last half century trying to poison the insects out of our fields with potent pesticides, we now have "super bugs" that are chemically resistant to all poisons and a net INCREASE in crop loss to insects. Same goes for cancer. We thought that we could poison the cancer out of the patient. But many cancers develop drug resistance or hormone independence, while the toxic drugs compromise our immune systems and leave us "naked" in the battle with the cancer.

There is a new philosophy emerging in science and medicine. According to several articles in major cancer journals, oncologists are asking the question: "Must we kill to cure?" In the prestigious *Journal of Clinical Oncology* (April 1995, p.801), Drs. Schipper, Goh, and Wang provide a compelling argument that curing the cancer patient need not include killing the cancer cells with potent cytotoxic therapies. In many ways, from our fields

---

SHIFTING THE CANCER PARADIGM
MUST WE KILL TO CURE?

Journal of Clinical Oncology (ASCO), vol.13, no.4, p.801, Apr.1995
H. Schipper, CR Goh, TL Wang

"the limits of the [cancer killing] model seem to have been reached"
"consider cancer as potentially reversible"
"killing strategies may be counterproductive because they impair host response and drive the already defective regulatory process [of the cancer cell] toward further aberrancy."
"[chemotherapy] treatment strategies have been based on the log-cell-kill hypothesis, derived from leukemia cells in culture...but is rarely seen in nature and only sustained under stringent conditions"
"remission does not predict cure...the failure of adjuvant therapies to flatten disease-free survival curves"
"conventional antineoplastic approaches will play a role as debulkers, ...the strategy will change to one of reregulation."

---

to our bacterial infection patients to our cancer patients, we need to re-examine Dr. Pasteur's grand deathbed epiphany: "The terrain is everything." The terrain is your human body. Nourish it properly with nutrients, oxygen, good thoughts, and exercise, and it will perform miraculous feats of disease recovery. We don't fully understand these "non-specific host defense mechanisms", but we need to respect and utilize them. That is how we will win the "war on cancer."

WHY ME AND WHY NOW?

You may ask, "What qualifies Patrick Quillin to write such a book on nutrition and cancer?" I have earned my bachelor's, master's, and doctorate degrees in nutrition, taught college nutrition for 9 years, have been a consultant to the Office of Alternative Medicine of the National Institutes of Health, the U.S. Army Breast Cancer research project, Scripps Clinic and La Costa Spa in southern California, am a registered and licensed dietitian, am one of only a thousand people in America who have earned my Certified Nutrition Specialist (CNS) status with the American College of Nutrition, have written 15 books, organized the first three international symposia on the subject of "Adjuvant (helpful) nutrition in cancer treatment", edited the textbook by the same name, written numerous articles, and contributed a chapter to a medical textbook. I am a member of the American College of Nutrition and New York Academy of Sciences.

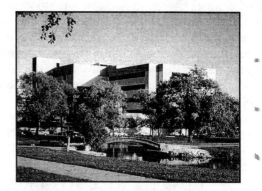

More importantly, I have studied the subject of nutrition in cancer as intensively as anyone. Even more critical, in my role as Vice President of Nutrition

CANCER TREATMENT CENTERS OF AMERICA, ZION, IL

from 1990 to 2000 for Cancer Treatment Centers of America, I was privileged to use nutrition in formal hospital settings for 10 years with over 3,000 cancer patients. The scientific studies are important, but even more crucial is what is happening to the patients in front of me. This stuff works. Since the first version of BEATING CANCER WITH NUTRITION was published in 1994, I have received hundreds of e-mails, letters, and face-to-face testimonials from patients who have said: "Thank you!! The information in this book saved my life." You will read a few profiles from patients whom I have worked with.

Some critics might say,"The evidence is very preliminary for you to be making any recommendations." I disagree. The evidence is substantial and points toward an inexpensive and low-risk method for extending the quality and quantity of life for cancer patients, many of whom have no options left. It can be an absurdly long wait for this or any field to become "politically correct", which requires people overcoming their reluctance to change. Traditional cancer therapies alone offer almost no hope for many cancer patients, especially lung, pancreas, liver, bone,

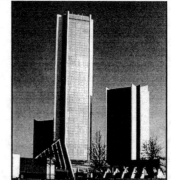

CANCER TREATMENT CENTERS OF AMERICA, TULSA, OK

and advanced colon and breast cancer. These people need supportive therapies to dovetail with traditional therapies. They need options and hope. There are too many lives at stake and nothing to lose in implementing the nutrition program presented in this book.

In the 1970s, amidst heavy criticism, two Canadian physicians, the Shute brothers, began writing about their clinical success using vitamin E supplements to reverse heart disease and relieve the symptoms of angina and leg pain. A multi-nation study was begun in Europe to examine this issue. As reported at the University of California, Berkeley conference on Antioxidants and Free Radicals in 1989 by Dr. Fred Gey, the best predictor of developing heart disease was low vitamin E levels in the blood. The Shute brothers were right. Since then, other work has shown that a low intake of vitamin E can also lead to suppressed immune functions, cancer, Alzheimer's disease and cataracts. How many people suffered and died needlessly while the authorities tried to make up their minds about whether to endorse non-toxic and inexpensive nutrients? Where is the downside to this equation?

In the early 1980s, I would ask scientists at professional meetings "how many of you are taking supplements?". The answer was about 5%, with the remainder being sarcastic about the subject. At a recent meeting, 90% of the scientists polled admitted to taking therapeutic levels of supplements to protect their health. Free radicals were discovered to be the cause of degenerative diseases by Denom Harmon, MD, PhD, of the University of Nebraska in the 1940s. This crucial area was then popularized by Dirk Pearson and Sandy Shaw in their 1982 book, LIFE EXTENSION, and fully supported by the world's most prestigious group of nutrition scientists in the American Journal of Clinical Nutrition conference held in 1990. A half century had produced more evidence and explanations, but had wasted many lives in the process.

America is a consumer-driven society. You will create the momentum for change. Don't wait for some government organization, or new law, or general endorsement from one of the major health care organizations to implement nutrition as part of comprehensive cancer treatment.

HOW IS THIS BOOK DIFFERENT?

Attacking cancer on many levels. A hammer, pliers, and screwdriver belong in any good tool box, just as chemo, radiation, and surgery have their place in cancer treatment. But that tool box is far from complete. There are many alternative cancer therapies that can be valuable assets in cancer treatment. This book offers other "tools" to support the basic, but incomplete, toolbox that we currently use against cancer.

There are a number of books on the market that offer alternative advice for cancer patients. Many of these books have served a valuable purpose and have helped cancer patients to be aware of cancer treatment options. This book offers a unique multi-disciplinary approach to treating cancer that is based on both scientific studies and actual clinical experience. My basic strategy is a three-pronged attack on cancer:

1) **Change the cause of the cancer**. Use nutrition, exercise, attitude, and detoxification to elevate the body's own internal healing abilities.

2) **Restrained tumor debulking**. Reduce cancer burden with chemo, radiation, hyperthermia, and other appropriate therapies.

3) **Symptom management**. Cancer can bring many symptoms that

COMPREHENSIVE CANCER TREATMENT INCLUDES:		
1↓	2↓	3↓
change underlying cause(s) of disease	restrained tumor debulking	symptom management
NUTRITION	CHEMO?	PAIN**
DETOXIFICATION	RADIATION	NAUSEA
DYSBIOSIS	SURGERY	ANOREXIA
HORMONE BAL.	BURZYNSKI	ANEMIA
HYPERGLYCEMIA	HYPERTHERM	LEUKOPENIA
INFECTIONS	PHOTO-CYTO	DEPRESSION
STRESS	HERBALS	CACHEXIA
EXERCISE	APHERESIS	HAIR LOSS
ENERGY PATHWAYS	LYMPH.INFUS.	
ETC.		

make life a purgatory. There are many allopathic and naturopathic therapies to manage the symptoms and make the disease and medical treatments more tolerable.

Avoid tunnel vision. It is important to avoid the mistake of the past, which is to focus on one aspect of cancer treatment and forget the other potentially valuable therapies. Avoid monomania, or obsession with one "magic bullet" idea. This book pays homage to the complexities of the human body and mind and draws on many fields to provide maximum firepower against cancer. We need all the weapons we can muster, for cancer is no simple beast to kill.

Individualize treatment plans. I recognize the diversity of the human population. There are nearly 6 billion people on the planet earth. We are as different as we are alike. There is no one perfect diet. The macrobiotic diet is truly a major improvement over the typical American diet, yet was developed by a Japanese physician who was drawing heavily on his ancestral Oriental diet. Eskimos eat 60% of their calories from high fat animal food, with very little vitamin C, fiber, fruit, or vegetables in their diet, yet they have a very low incidence of cancer and heart disease. There are groups of people in Africa and Asia that rely on their dairy herds for dietary staples and others that are vegans, or pure vegetarians. Each of these groups has adapted to a unique diet that strongly influences their health. Rather than give you one set diet to follow, I am going to work with you to find a diet that reflects your ancestral heritage and your unique biochemical needs.

Also, we need to fix the problem(s) that may have triggered the cancer. If low thyroid and milk allergies were the initial problems, then you will never really resolve the cancer until the problems have been fixed. I will present a logical flow later in the book that will help you to detect common problems that can be the original insult that triggered the cancer.

RE-ENGINEERING CANCER TREATMENT

American health care is nearing a financial "meltdown". Millions of jobs are lost to other countries because the cost of doing business in America is so high. One of the primary business costs in America is health care insurance. General Motors spends as much on health care insurance for its workers as it does for the metal on its cars. Medicare expenses threaten the financial stability of the world's greatest superpower. We spent $2 trillion in 2004 on disease maintenance, which is 14% of our gross national product--twice the expense per capita of any other health care system on earth. Notice that I said "disease maintenance", because we certainly do not support health care in America, and "health insurance" is neither related to health nor solid actuarial insurance.

The most expensive disease in America is cancer. These opulent expenses would be easier to swallow if we were obtaining impressive results. But many experts argue that we have made limited progress in the costly and lengthy "war on cancer". Annually in America, there are more than 50 million cancer-related visits to the doctor, one million cancer operations, and 750,000 radiation treatments.

By 1971, cancer had become enough of a nuisance that President Richard Nixon launched the long-awaited "war on cancer", confidently proclaiming that we would have a cure within 5 years, before the Bicentennial celebration in 1976. With over $50 billion spent on research in the past 33 years, $1 trillion spent on therapy, 7 million casualties, and no relief in sight from traditional therapies--it is blindingly obvious that we must re-examine some options in cancer prevention and treatment.

As of 2002, experts estimate that 45% of males and 39% of females living in America will develop cancer in their lifetime. Breast cancer has increased from one out of 20 women in the year 1950 to one out of eight women in 1995. With some cancers, notably liver, lung, pancreas, bone, and advanced breast cancer, our five-year survival rate from traditional therapy alone is virtually the same as it was 30 years ago. In 2000, there were 570,000 deaths in America from cancer, which is 1,560 people per day, which is the equivalent of six loaded 747 airplanes killing all occupants on board.

This book is about options. If our current results from traditional cancer treatment were encouraging, then there would be no need for alternative therapies against cancer. Unfortunately, traditional cancer therapies have plateaued--some might say that they hit a dead-end brick wall. In many instances, the treatment is worse than the disease, with chronic nausea and vomiting, hair loss, painful mouth sores, extreme fatigue, and depression as common side effects of therapy and minimal improvements in lifespan. Long-term complications include toxicity to the heart, kidneys, and bone marrow. While many children may recover from cancer, they are placed at much higher risk for getting cancer later in life from their cancer therapy. And if the cancer patient recovers from the disease, which is no small task, then recovering from the therapy may be even more challenging. Many patients come to me suffering from peripheral neuropathy (tingling numbness and pain in the hands and feet), after too much chemo with no nutrients to protect the delicate nerves.

Obviously, if what we are doing isn't working, then we need to look at some sensible, scientific, non-toxic, and cost-effective options that can amplify the tumor-killing abilities of traditional therapies. Nutrition is at the top of that list.

The best selling cancer drug in the world is a mushroom extract, PSK, manufactured in Japan and sold throughout Europe and Japan. Only 30% of cancer therapy in Japan is from the "big three" of radiation, chemo, and surgery. The bark of the yew tree, Taxol, holds promise as a potent cancer drug. Digestive enzymes and mistletoe (Iscador) are government-approved prescription cancer drugs in Germany. Evening primrose oil is an accepted cancer therapy in England. Do not discount any possibilities in this "war on cancer". While America is considered one of the world's heavy-weight champions at developing new industrial technologies and patents, we are lagging well behind the rest of the world in cancer treatment.

The recommendations provided in this book are scientifically-backed, time-tested, logical, and supported by my clinical observations in working with hundreds of cancer patients over the course of 15 years. Follow the program outlined in this book and you, the cancer patient, can surpass the recovery predictions of your oncologist.

PATIENT PROFILE: BEAT PANCREATIC CANCER. RM was diagnosed with advanced adenocarcinoma of the pancreas in August 1996 at the age of 53. His lifestyle was unhealthy. He was obese and on cholesterol lowering drugs. His doctors admitted that this cancer was a "poor prognostic" cancer, meaning very few people beat the condition. RM underwent surgery (Whipple), chemo, and radiation. He felt sorry for himself briefly, then realized that he was going to do everything in his power to beat this cancer, including a fighting spirit. RM followed the advice in BEATING CANCER WITH NUTRITION, including food, supplements, and eating your way through the nausea of intra-arterial infusion chemo. He kept the port (medical device that allows doctors to inject chemo into the vein near the neck) in place for another 7 years to remind himself of his newfound healthier lifestyle. As of February 2005, and at 61 years of age, RM is in complete remission, travels the world, feels great, and doesn't worry anymore. Cancer has brought RM a newfound sense of "life is short and precious, savor it, and do not worry your way through it." His doctors were very pleased and surprised at RM's admirable outcome.

CHAPTER 1

YOU HAVE ALREADY BEATEN CANCER

✴

...and you can do it again!

How your body stops cancer in its tracks

What a piece of work is man! how noble in reason! how infinite in faculty! in form and moving how express and admirable! in action how like an angel! in apprehension how like a god! the beauty of the world, the paragon of animals!   *—William Shakespeare*

WHAT'S AHEAD?

Nutrients from food and supplements change the way your body works, making it less receptive to cancer cells and more supportive of healthy cells. Nutrients affect:

⤷ immune functions
⤷ DNA, or genetic expression of cancer
⤷ cell membrane interactions, how your cells
    float and communicate
⤷ detoxification, and other vital ways of beating cancer.

Although our 33 year $60 billion "war on cancer" has not produced an unqualified cure for any type of cancer, we do know much more about cancer now than when we started this quest in 1972. One of the more well-accepted theories is the "surveillance theory" of cancer, which says that cancer is popping up in all of us all the time, but is checked early in its growth by our own host defense mechanisms. Drugs that prevent rejection of a kidney after a transplantation operation (cyclosporine) also increase the risk for cancer.[1] There is a substantial increase in skin cancers[2] and benign breast disease[3] (which can turn into breast cancer) in patients who have received transplants. Shut down the immune system and the smoldering embers of cancer become a raging fire. Professor Bruce Ames at the University of California, Berkeley has shown that the average human cell

---

SURVEILLANCE THEORY OF CANCER

innate mechanisms protect us against the inevitable cancers

Immunosuppressive drugs increase cancer after kidney transpl.
Lutz, J., Curr.Opin.Urol. 2003, Mar.13, (2): 105-9

"Enormous increase in skin cancers" after transpl.
Wu,JJ, Dermatol.OnlineJ., 2002, Oct.8(2):4

"Far greater incidence of benign breast dis" after transplant.
ANZ J.Surg.2002 Mar.72(3):222-5

DNA adducts (potential cancer)/cell/day is 1000 to 10,000
Ames, BN, Ann.NY Acad.Sci. 1992 Nov.21,663:85-96

Nutritional status influences non-specific host defense mechanisms that keep 2/3 of humans out of cancer hospital. Once cancer diagnosed, need to debulk tumor while resuscitating these defense mechanisms with optimal nutrition.

immune system + cell commun + apoptosis + angiogenesis + encapsulation + detoxif + DNA repair + et al= host defenses

---

(and there are about 60 trillion cells in an adult body) is subjected to 1,000 to 10,000 potentially cancer-causing "hits" each and every day.[4]

Your body survives endless assaults on the integrity of the DNA and is able to repair most of this damage. If the defective cells still exist, then the telegraph system within the healthy cell colony tells the cancer cell to revert back to normal functioning, called cell-to-cell communication. If the defective cell with bad DNA continues to grow, then the body instructs the cancer cell to commit suicide, aka apoptosis. If this doesn't work, then the body shuts down the making of blood vessels to the tumor, call anti-angiogenesis. If the tumor continues to grow, then the body begins to wall off the cancer cells with a tough envelope made of collagen and calcium, called tumor encapsulation. This is good news indeed. All of these anti-cancer mechanisms are fed by the nutrients in your diet. That's why an aggressive nutrition program is essential, but may not be sufficient for all cancer patients. The fact is, your body has the internal means of beating cancer if given the right collection of precursors (nutrients) and the proper toxin-free and restful environment.

The task of the immune system is to recognize "self from non-self", meaning whatever cells have your unique DNA can stay and everything else must be killed and escorted out of the body.

Your immune system is the "cops and army" that finds and destroys cells that are unfriendly to your body. Cancer certainly qualifies as "unfriendly". In 58% of Americans, these cancers will sprout up and immediately be squashed by the mechanisms that you will read about in this chapter. In 42% of Americans, the cancer gets a foothold and must be treated. You have already beaten cancer. At least once. And you can do it again. If you bolster your own internal cancer fighting squad while finding medical therapies that are proven to help debulk your tumor with reasonable safety, then you are well en route to "beating cancer".

For nearly 30 years, experts at the National Cancer Institute have labored brilliantly in the quest for a "biological response modifier", or

---

NUTRIENTS AS BIOLOGICAL RESPONSE MODIFIERS
changing the way the body works to reverse cancer

→IMMUNE REGULATORS, ELIMINATE INFECTIONS?
→ALTER GENETIC EXPRESSION OF CANCER
→CELL MEMBRANE DYNAMICS
→DETOXIFICATION
→PH MAINTENANCE, BALANCING PROTONS
→PROOXIDANTS & AOX, BALANCING ELECTRONS
→CELLULAR COMMUNICATIONS (signal cell transduction)
→PROSTAGLANDIN REGULATION
→STEROID HORMONE CONTROL
→ENERGY METABOLISM: AEROBIC VS ANAEROBIC
→PROBIOTICS VS DYSBIOSIS
→ANTI-PROLIFERATIVE AGENTS
→ALTER TUMOR PROTECTIVE MECHANISMS
→APOPTOSIS, PROGRAMMED CELL DEATH

BRM, which would cure cancer with the effectiveness that penicillin used to cure many bacterial infections. Among the candidates in this quest were interferon, interleukin, tumor derived activated killer cells (TDAK), and various vaccines. None of these BRMs have lived up to their media hype of being a cure for cancer. However, scientists can now prove that everything you put in your mouth is a "biological response modifier" in the sense that nutrients change the way the body works. Amino acids (which form proteins), fats, carbohydrates, fiber, vitamins, minerals, food extracts, and minor dietary constituents are among the new heroes in the quest for a cancer cure. While none of these nutrients by themselves will ever cure all cancer, we do know that nutrients alter "non-specific host defense" mechanisms, which means "how we get well". Fats in the diet become fats in the cell membrane, which must have unique properties in order for the immune cells to recognize and destroy cancer cells.

As a blatant example of a nutrient as a cure for a life-threatening disease, think of water as the cure for heat stroke. Around 30 young American men die each autumn in football practice due to heat exhaustion and dehydration. Nothing else but water will help the person. And water works like a BRM, like magic. When a cancer patient adds nutrients to the diet that have been missing, it is amazing how well the body can suddenly begin to defend itself against cancer. This chapter is a brief overview of some of the ways that nutrients can become BRMs to slow and reverse cancer.

IMMUNE STIMULANTS

A healthy adult body includes around 60 trillion cells, of which nearly a third, or 20 trillion cells, are immune factors. Immune cells are given the responsibility of killing unfriendly cells--including bacteria, virus, yeast, tumor cells, dead cells, and toxins. This is no small task. Some nutrients boost immune cell numbers. Some nutrients provide the immune warriors with a protective coating, like an asbestos suit, so that the immune cell is not destroyed in the process of killing a cancer cell with some "napalm". Some nutrients provide the immune cells with more "napalm" or "bullets" in the form of granulocytes and nitric oxide.

Many nutrition factors affect the ability of the immune system to recognize and destroy cancer cells and invading bacteria.

ALTER GENETIC EXPRESSION OF CANCER

Cancer involves DNA that has "gone mad" or lost its ability to properly replicate and then die at the appropriate time. There are numerous checks and balances in the control of abnormal DNA. Nutrients, like folate and B-12, help to provide correct duplication of DNA. Nutrients, like vitamin D, help to squelch the growth of abnormal genetic fragments, or episomes. Nutrients, like vitamin A, actually have a receptor site on the DNA, without which cancer is likely to happen. Nutrition factors, like genistein from soy and oligomeric proanthocyanidins from bioflavonoids, can actually help a cancer cell to revert back to a normal healthy cell in the process of cell differentiation.

Your 60 trillion cells possess a thread of material that holds all the "blue print" information to make another you. This thread, called DNA, is truly the essence of life itself. DNA looks like a spiral staircase that is so long and flexible, it begins to wind around and wrap into "X" shapes. Stored on 23 pairs of chromosomes are 50,000 to 100,000 genes, collectively called the human genome.[5]

This long spiral staircase is constantly under attack. Dr. Bruce Ames and his colleagues at the University of California at Berkeley have shown that each cell in the human body takes an average of 1,000 to 10,000 "hits" or DNA breaks each day. Imagine sitting on your roof in the middle of a hurricane while shingles are constantly being ripped off and you have to continuously repair this damage. Make a mistake, and cancer could be the consequence. Geneticists have estimated that each DNA molecule contains about the same amount of information as would be typed on 500,000 pages of manuscript. Imagine if trillions of times daily, you had to type a half million pages error-free. A mistake can lead to cancer.

Fortunately, the body is well prepared to keep the inevitable DNA errors from turning into cancer. DNA polymerase is a repair enzyme system that moves along this spiral staircase, like a railcar on railroad tracks, finding and fixing broken rail ties, or base pairs. This crucial repair system is fueled by folacin, zinc, and other nutrients. A low intake of folacin increases the likelihood that cancer will become metastatic. One of the earlier drugs used against cancer, methotrexate, is a folacin inhibitor that limits new cell growth in both healthy and cancer cells. Giving folacin to a patient on methotrexate does not inhibit the effectiveness of the drug, since it is folinic acid, a more metabolically-active form of folacin, that is required to rescue a patient from methotrexate therapy.

Repeated mechanical injury can turn into cancer. I worked with a young patient who developed a cancerous growth in the exact same area where he had experienced a mechanical injury. This 32 year old male had been in a snow skiing accident, in which he fell and accidentally stabbed himself in his thigh muscle with his ski pole. He was a smoker and ate a typical American diet, which is low in zinc and folacin. His wound seemed to heal well within the expected few months; then one year later he developed a massive metastatic sarcoma exactly where he had injured himself and died soon thereafter. The injury created the stress, the tobacco provided generous amounts of a carcinogen to interrupt the repair process, and his typical American diet lacked the growth nutrients required for accurate DNA synthesis. Another patient that I worked with was a typical 20 year old college male, who had crowded dentition, with wisdom teeth constantly gnashing at the insides of his cheeks--which is where he developed cancer. He started a wise nutrition program, used restrained medical therapies, and survived his brush with cancer.

This continuous repair process of DNA is like a high-speed bullet train that is easily derailed. Cancer is the resulting train wreck. We need to get these DNA repair mechanisms working properly in the cancer patient.

CELL MEMBRANE DYNAMICS

Most of the 60 trillion cells in an adult body are like "water balloons" floating in an ocean of extracellular fluid, in the sense that they are full of fluid and have a barrier that keeps them intact. This barrier, or cell membrane, has a three-layered look, with water-soluble molecules on the outside and fatty tails toward the inside. This lipid bilayer gives rise to the ability of the cell to accept the proper nutrients along with oxygen, to eliminate the hazardous toxins produced within the cell, and to reject the circulating toxins and cancer cells that try to penetrate the cell membrane barrier. A healthy cell membrane is built from the essential fatty acids from fish oil (eicosapentaenoic acid), flax oil (alpha linolenic acid), evening primrose oil (gamma linolenic acid), lecithin (phosphatidylcholine), cholesterol, and other nutrients. A defective cell membrane is built from hydrogenated fats (trans fatty acids) and too much saturated fats, and has been "tanned" by exposure to excess sugar floating through the bloodstream and various nutritional deficiencies. A healthy cell membrane allows the cell to "breathe" aerobically and to expel waste products. Otherwise, cancer can be the result.

The ratio of minerals in the "electrolyte soup" that drives cell membrane potential also influences cell membrane dynamics. The ratio of sodium to potassium to calcium to magnesium is crucial. We also probably have a need for the ultra-trace minerals that are found in the ocean at about 1% concentration, which need to be in our diet but are missing in standard commercial salt.

Potassium is found primarily in unprocessed plant food, like vegetables, fruit, whole grains, and legumes. There is some sodium in all foods, with higher concentrations in animal foods, and much more of it in processed foods. Americans eat 10 times the sodium that our ancestors consumed. An ideal ratio of sodium to potassium would be 1 to 4, but ours is 4 to 1. By drastically changing this ratio, we have changed the "electrolyte soup" that bathes all cells and creates the electrical battery of life. This electrical charge influences the gatekeeper. High sodium diets increase both cancer incidence and metastasis.

DETOXIFICATION

America's increasing incidence of cancer has closely paralleled our increasing exposure to cancer-causing substances in our environment. We consume toxins:

⇒ voluntarily through alcohol, drugs, and tobacco

⇒ involuntarily through industrial and agricultural pollutants that end up in the food, air, and water supply

⇒ internally (endogenously) produced toxins from energy metabolism in the cell and from bacterial fermentation in the gut.

We detoxify by eliminating waste products through urine, feces, sweat, and liver detoxification. Nutrients assist each of these processes. The liver is a chemical detoxification "factory" in its ability to bind toxins (conjugate), split toxins (hydrolyze), and neutralize toxins through Phase I and Phase II enzyme pathways. These pathways are augmented with nutrients, like garlic, calcium D-glucarate, selenium, vitamin E, and glutathione.

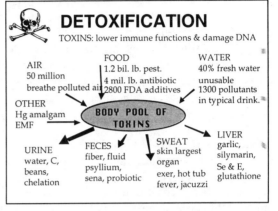

DETOXIFICATION

TOXINS: lower immune functions & damage DNA

AIR
50 million
breathe polluted air

FOOD
1.2 bil. lb. pest.
4 mil. lb. antibiotic
2800 FDA additives

WATER
40% fresh water
unusable
1300 pollutants
in typical drink.

OTHER
Hg amalgam
EMF

BODY POOL OF TOXINS

URINE
water, C,
beans,
chelation

FECES
fiber, fluid
psyllium,
sena, probiotic

SWEAT
skin largest
organ
exer, hot tub
fever, jacuzzi

LIVER
garlic,
silymarin,
Se & E,
glutathione

ACID & BASE BALANCE

Humans have a very specific need to maintain a proper pH balance. pH refers to "potential hydrogens" and is measured on a scale from 1 (very acidic) to 7 (neutral) to 14 (very alkaline, base). Foods that encourage a healthy pH are vegetables and other plant foods. Foods that encourage an unhealthy pH include excess protein, dairy, and sugar. Proper breathing, exercise, and adequate water intake further improve pH to discourage cancer growth. Cancer cells give off lactic acid in anaerobic fermentation of foodstuffs. This Cori cycle generates a lower pH, which then further compromises the cells' ability to fight off the cancer. Infections in the body will generate lactic acid and other acids which lower the pH and make the body less effective. Acid foods (such as tomatoes, citrus, and vinegar) help to create an "alkaline tide" which helps to discourage cancer and fungus growth.

You can tell if you have an abnormal pH by some of the following characteristics: your jewelry, rings, and metal watch bands turn color (oxidize) quickly; insects like mosquitoes are not attracted to you; you frequently develop yeast infections like toenail fungus. Acid/base is best tested by having your blood checked for pH in the veins. A quicker and cheaper method of testing your pH is using pH litmus paper from your pharmacy store or pH-Ion.com (888-744-8589) or HealthTreasures.com (800-586-0947). If your saliva pH is too acidic, this can be a clue to abnormal internal chemistry, or an infection, or a marker for cancer. Abnormal pH values compromise "host defense" mechanisms and complicate the ability to get rid of cancer.

A diet rich in beef, milk, and sugar plus poor breathing habits and no exercise will create a disease-prone pH. Infections (especially fungal) or cancer generate acidic pH. Proper deep diaphragm breathing, exercise, lots of clean water, and a diet including more vegetables and legumes will help to rectify most pH problems. Some people who are supposed to be omnivores (including meat) will become ardent vegetarians and end up with abnormally high pH. These people may need meats like lean chicken, fish, and turkey to bring their pH value down to normal healthy levels.

CELLULAR COMMUNICATION

Cells communicate between one another, a.k.a. intercellular or "gap junction" communication, through ions that float in and out of pores in the cell membranes. Vitamins A, D, and beta-carotene are among the crucial nutrients that encourage this "telegraph" system that keeps cells healthy and non-cancerous. Communication also exists within a cell (intracellular communication, signal cell transduction) through glycoproteins from aloe vera and other essential carbohydrate foods.

PROSTAGLANDIN SYNTHESIS

Prostaglandins (aka eicosanoids) are hormone-like substances that are produced regionally within most cells and have an incredible influence on the functions that help us to beat cancer. Essentially, when our blood glucose is high and our intake of fish oil and primrose oil is low, then emergency prostaglandins (PGE-2) are generated to augment cancer growth.

When our blood sugar levels are kept low (around 60 to 90 milligrams per deciliter), and when we eat enough fish oil and evening primrose oil, then the favorable prostaglandin of PGE-1 will:

⇒ stimulate immune activity

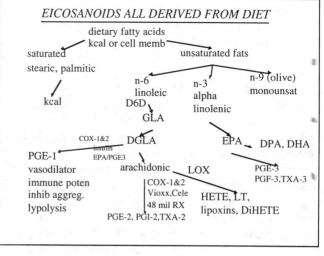

EICOSANOIDS ALL DERIVED FROM DIET

⇒ improve circulation through vasodilation

⇒ reduce the stickiness of cells, which inhibits metastasis through platelet aggregation

⇒ help to produce estrogen receptors to dull the potential damage from circulating estrogen

Only a concerted effort of dietary regulation and proper supplements can produce healthy prostaglandins to suppress cancer.

STEROID HORMONE ACTIVITY

Certain cancers are very dependent on testosterone (prostate cancer) or estrogen (breast, ovarian, and cervical cancer). These hormones are not only produced by the gonads (testosterone) and ovaries (estrogen), but are also produced by fat cells. Hence, the more body fat a person has, the higher the likelihood of generating more tumor-enhancing hormones. A calculated program to gradually reduce excess body fat is crucial in the treatment of hormone-dependent tumors.

Also, a number of nutrition factors help to reduce the tumor-enhancing capacity of hormones, including fish oil, evening primrose oil, cruciferous sulforaphane, calcium D-glucarate, and others.

BIOENERGETICS: AEROBIC VS ANAEROBIC

Cancer cells are anaerobic sugar feeders, while healthy cells are aerobic (oxygen-requiring) cells that can burn sugar, protein, or fats. Professor Otto Warburg was awarded the Nobel prize in medicine in 1931 for his work in cell respiration and received a second Nobel prize in 1944 for his work in electron transfer. This brilliant researcher spent considerable time investigating the differences between healthy cells and cancer cells: "...the prime cause of cancer is the replacement of the respiration of oxygen in normal body cells by a fermentation of sugar."[6] It was Professor Warburg's work that led to the development of the $1.5 million PET (positron emission tomography) scan device, which finds cancer by injecting radioactively labeled sugar into the veins of the cancer patient, then tracking the labeled sugar. Cancer cells will absorb more than their fair share of this radioactive sugar, which tells the doctor where the cancer is concentrated.

The more dense and anaerobic the mass of cancer, the more resistant it is to treatment, medical or otherwise. In order to beat cancer, one must make the body a well-oxygenated aerobic organism. Proper breathing and exercise are crucial to generate an aerobic environment.

Also, there are nutrients, including coenzyme Q-10, chromium GTF (glucose tolerance factor), thiamin, niacin, riboflavin, lipoic acid, and others, that enhance aerobic metabolism.

BACTERIA IN THE GUT

According to Nobel prize winner, Eli Metchnikoff, PhD, "death begins in the colon". There are more bacteria in our lower intestines than cells in our body. The bacteria in our gut either enhance or detract from immune functions and general health. Healthy bacteria (probiotics) help to:

⇨ produce essential vitamins (such as K and biotin)
⇨ generate a critical immune factor (IgA)
⇨ protect the gut mucosa against translocation of bacteria into the bloodstream
⇨ improve the pH in the colon
⇨ aid in digestion and absorption of essential nutrients
⇨ reduce the carcinogenic by-products that are produced in the colon from putrefaction of fecal matter.

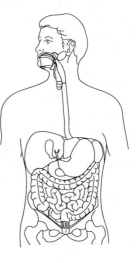

Healthy bacteria are encouraged by a diet low in sugar and meat and high in vegetables, whole grains, and active-cultured foods (like yogurt or soy tempeh). High fiber and fluid intake help this crucial balance of friendly bacteria. Fructo-oligosaccharides are special starches found in whole grains and onions that help to nourish the friendly bacteria.

PRO-OXIDANTS VS ANTIOXIDANTS

Our greatest enemy is oxygen, since it generates free radicals (a.k.a. pro-oxidants, reactive oxygen species), which can damage the delicate DNA, immune factors, and cell membranes. Yet our greatest ally is a well-oxygenated system. How, then, to balance this seeming paradox? A well-oxygenated (aerobic) system along with optimal protection from free radicals via antioxidants is the ideal combination for good health. Free radicals cannot be eliminated in the human body, but must be controlled, or they turn into "forest fires" that devastate the cells.

A strategic blend of antioxidants can provide broad-spectrum protection against damage from chemotherapy and radiation therapy, protecting the immune cells from their own poisons and improving vigor in the cancer patient undergoing treatment. Vitamins C, E, beta-carotene, selenium, lipoic acid, lycopene, glutathione, tocotrienols, quercetin, coenzyme Q, oligomeric proanthocyanidins from grape seed, curcumin, ginkgo biloba, and green tea provide antioxidant protection.

ANTI-PROLIFERATIVE AGENTS

While most nutritionists agree on the importance of growth (proliferative) nutrients, few nutritionists respect the importance for anti-proliferative nutrients. Various nutrients and substances in the body stimulate or subdue angiogenesis (making of new blood vessels), including the powerful vascular endothelial growth factor (VEGF).

Selenium, fish oil, garlic, cat's claw, Maitake D-fraction, vitamin E succinate, vitamin K, quercetin, genistein, bindweed, and bovine cartilage all may assist the cancer patient in this manner.

ALTER TUMOR PROTECTIVE MECHANISMS

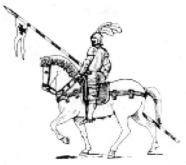

The tumor is a well-adapted parasite that hides from the body's immune system by generating a "stealth" coating of human chorionic gonadotropin (HCG), which provides regional immune suppression. The cancer pretends to be a fetus and, in doing so, stops the attack by the immune system. High doses of niacin (B-3) as inositol hexanicotinate and digestive enzymes work to dissolve this "stealth" coating of the tumor. Your body's immune system is then free to do its job of ridding the body of "non-self" cells, such as cancer. Your immune "knights" are now back in action.

PATIENT PROFILE: S.R. was diagnosed at age 48 with stage 4 non-Hodgkins B-cell lymphoma. Tumor was the size of a potato and choking off blood to the intestines. Underwent chemo regimen. S.R. used nutrition supplements in spite of oncologist's hostility to the subject. S.R. was able to work throughout chemo, travelling to trade shows, though he did lose his hair. As of 2005, S.R. is in complete remission and has learned the value of good nutrition, living more joyfully, and faith in God.

ENDNOTES

[1] . Lutz, J., Curr.Opin.Urol., vol.2, p.105, Mar.13, 2003
[2] . Wu,JJ, Dermatol.Online J., vol.2, p.4, Oct.8, 2002
[3] . ANZ J.Surg., vol.72, no.3, p.222, Mar.2002
[4] . Ames, BN, Ann.NY Acad.Sci., vol.663, p.85, Nov.21, 1992
[5] . Naisbitt, J., et al., MEGATRENDS 2000, p.257, Morrow, NY, 1990
[6] . Levine, SA, et al., ANTIOXIDANT ADAPTATION, p.209, Biocurrents, San Leandro, CA 1986

CHAPTER 2

WHAT CAUSES CANCER?

★

"Nature, to be commanded, must be obeyed." Francis Bacon

WHAT'S AHEAD?

In order to defeat cancer, it helps to better understand how cancer starts and progresses in the human body. Cancer is a mistake cell that is growing wildly out of control and may consume the patient through
malnutrition, organ failure, or infections, unless the tumor is debulked (get rid of some of it) and then the whole body is re-regulated (change the underlying causes of the cancer). Primary causes of cancer include:

→ poor nutrition; an excess, deficiency, or imbalance of any nutrients

→ stress; the mind generates chemicals that can lower protective mechanisms against cancer

→ sedentary lifestyle; exercise helps to oxygenate and regulate the entire body

→ toxic burden, hence detoxification becomes crucial

In the terrifying film, "The Predator", a chameleon-like beast from outer space descends upon the sweltering jungles of Central America to hunt humans, including Arnold Schwarzenegger. If you sweated through this film, then you have an idea of how hard it is to kill cancer. The Predator wore a shield that allowed it to blend into the surrounding environment, making it almost invisible. Cancer mimics the chemistry of a fetus, and hence becomes invisible to the human immune system. Cancer also mutates by changing its DNA (deoxyribose nucleic acid) composition almost weekly, which is a major reason why many cancers develop a drug resistance that often limits the value of chemotherapy. Cancer also weakens its host by installing its own abnormal biochemistry, including:

    -changes in the pH, or acid/base balance

-creation of anaerobic (oxygen-deprived) pockets of tissue that resist radiation therapy like someone hunkered into a bomb shelter

-blunting the immune system

-elevating metabolism and calorie needs, while simultaneously lowering appetite and food intake to slowly starve the host

-ejecting by-products that create weakness, apathy, pain, and depression in the host

-siphoning nutrients out of the bloodstream like a parasite.

With its invisible, predatory, and every-changing nature, cancer is truly a tough condition to treat. Cancer is essentially an abnormal cell growth. Its unchecked growth tends to overwhelm other functions in the body until death comes from:

1) organ failure, e.g., the kidneys shut down

2) infection, e.g., pneumonia, because the immune system has been blunted

3) malnutrition, because the parasitic cancer shifts the host's metabolism into high gear through inefficient use of fuel, while also inducing a loss of appetite.

SUBDUE SYMPTOMS OR DEAL WITH THE UNDERLYING CAUSE OF DISEASE?

There is a basic flaw in our thinking about health care in this country. We treat symptoms, not the underlying cause of the disease. Yet, the only way to provide long-lasting relief in any degenerative disease, like cancer, arthritis, and heart disease, is to reverse the basic cause of the disease. For example, let's say that you developed a headache because your neighbor's teenager is playing drums too loudly. You take an aspirin to subdue the headache, then your stomach starts churning. So you take some antacids to ease the stomach nausea, then your blood pressure goes up. And on it goes. We shift symptoms with medication, as if in a bizarre "shell game", when we really need to deal with the fundamental cause of the disease.

Let me give you another example. What if the first thing I do every morning when I arrive at my office is to slam my thumb in the desk drawer. Boy, that hurt! Yet I keep doing the same masochistic act of slamming my thumb in the desk drawer every morning for a week. And by then, my thumb is swollen, painful, discolored, and bleeding. So I go to Dr. A who recommends analgesics to better tolerate the pain. Dr. B suggests an injection of cortisone to reduce the swelling in my thumb. And Dr. C recommends surgery to cut off the finger because it looks defective. Of course, the real answer is to stop slamming my thumb in the desk drawer.

What's that? You say that my example has no relevance in American health care? Let's look at the millions of Americans with rheumatoid arthritis, such as Mrs. Smith, whose condition is caused by eating too much sugar, plus an allergy to milk protein, and a deficiency of fish oil, vitamin C, and zinc. Mrs. Smith goes to Dr. A, who recommends analgesics to better tolerate the pain. Dr. B suggests cortisone to reduce the swelling. And Dr. C recommends hip replacement surgery to cut off the defective parts. The real answer is to change the underlying cause of the disease.

A more common example is heart disease. There are over 60,000 miles of blood vessels in the average adult body. When a person develops blockage in the arteries near the heart, open-heart bypass surgery will probably be recommended. In this procedure, a short section of vein from the leg is used to replace the plugged-up vessels near the heart. But what has been done to improve the other 59,999 miles left that are probably equally obstructed? A Harvard professor, Dr. E. Braunwald, investigated the records from thousands of bypass patients in the Veteran's Administration Hospitals and found no improvement in lifespan after this expensive and risky surgery.[1] Why? Because the underlying cause, which could be a complex array of diet, exercise, stress, and toxins, has not been resolved. Bypass surgery treats the symptoms of heart disease in the same way that chemo and radiation treat the symptoms of cancer. Each provide temporary relief, but no long-term cure.

Meanwhile, Dr. Dean Ornish was working as a physician doing bypass surgery in the early 1970s and watching some patients come back for their second bypass operation. Ornish reasoned: "Obviously, this procedure is not a cure for heart disease." At the time, there was convincing data that a low-fat diet, coupled with exercise and stress reduction, could lower the incidence of heart disease. Ornish wondered if we took that same program and cranked it up a notch or two, making it more therapeutic, might it reverse heart disease? And it did. His program recently was found effective in a clinical study. While the American Cancer Society was violently opposed to Dr. Max Gerson's nutritional program to treat cancer patients in the 1950s, the ACS then released in the 1980s its dietary guidelines for the prevention of cancer, which was very similar to the Gerson program.

When you deal with the underlying causes of a degenerative disease, you are more likely to get long-term favorable benefits. When you allow the fundamental causes to continue and merely treat the symptoms that surface, then the outlook for the patient is dismal. In dozens of diseases and millions of patients, this obvious law holds true.

The crucial missing link in most cancer therapy is stimulating the patient's own healing abilities, because the best medical equipment cannot detect one billion cancer cells. Imagine leaving behind only one billion dandelion seeds on your lawn after you thought you got them all.

The "war on cancer" is an internal microscopic war that can only be won by working within the laws of nature: stimulating the patient's own abilities to fight cancer while changing the abnormal conditions that allow cancer to grow. All other therapies are doomed to disappointing results. Combined together, these treatments of restrained external medicine coupled with stimulating the cancer patient's internal healing abilities hold great promise for dramatically improving your chances of success against cancer.

WHAT CAUSES CANCER?

Most degenerative diseases, including cancer, do not have a readily identifiable enemy. In a bacterial infection, you can attack the "cause" of the disease with an antibiotic. Cancer seems to be caused by a collection of lifestyle and environmental factors that accumulate over the years. Since success against any degenerative disease requires getting to the root of the problem, let's examine the accepted causes of cancer.

-**Toxic overload.** Of the 5 million registered chemicals in the world, mankind comes in contact with 70,000, of which at least 20,000 are known carcinogens, or cancer-causing agents. Each year, America alone sprays 1.2 billion pounds of pesticides on our food crops, dumps 90 billion pounds of toxic waste in our 55,000 toxic waste sites, feeds 9 million pounds of antibiotics to our farm animals to help them gain weight faster, and generally bombards the landscape with questionable amounts of electromagnetic radiation.

Bruce Ames, PhD, of the University of California at Berkeley, has estimated that each of the 60 trillion cells in your body undergoes from 1,000 to 10,000 DNA "hits" or potentially cancer-causing breaks every day. Newer studies examining the role of the immune system in protecting us against cancer show that the average adult has one cancer cell appear each day. Yet somehow, for most of us, our DNA repair mechanisms and immune system surveillance are able to keep this storm of genetic damage under control. Wallowing in our own high-tech waste products is a major cause of cancer in modern society, since carcinogens add to the fury of the continuous assault on the DNA. Noted authority Samuel Epstein, MD, of the University of Illinois, says that a major thrust of cancer prevention must be detoxifying our earth. Toxins not only cause DNA breakage, which can trigger cancer, but also subdue the immune system, which then allows cancer to become the "fox in the chicken coop", with no controlling force.

Early research indicated that once cancer has been upregulated, or " the lion is out of the cage", then no amount of detoxification is going to matter. Newer evidence says otherwise. Cancer growth can be both slowed and even reversed, under the right conditions. According to the National Cancer Institute, there are 7 million Americans alive today who have lived 5 or more years after their cancer diagnosis. Cancer is reversible. If toxins caused the problem, then detoxification is the solution. For more on detoxification, see the chapter on changing the underlying causes of cancer.

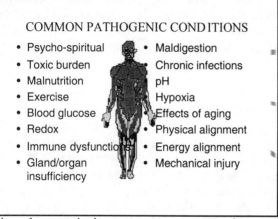

COMMON PATHOGENIC CONDITIONS

- Psycho-spiritual
- Toxic burden
- Malnutrition
- Exercise
- Blood glucose
- Redox
- Immune dysfunction
- Gland/organ insufficiency

- Maldigestion
- Chronic infections
- pH
- Hypoxia
- Effects of aging
- Physical alignment
- Energy alignment
- Mechanical injury

-Distress. It was the Canadian physician and researcher, Hans Selye, MD, who coined the term "the stress of life", so he could document the physiological changes that took place in lab animals when exposed to noise, bright lights, confinement, and electric shocks. The thymus gland is a pivotal organ in immune system protection against infections and cancer. Dr. Selye noted that stress induces thymus gland shrinkage, increases fats in the blood (for the beginnings of heart disease), and erodes the stomach lining (ulcers).

Since the 1920s, scientific evidence has been advancing the theory that emotional stress can depress the immune system and make that individual more vulnerable to infections and cancer. It was Norman Cousins' book, ANATOMY OF AN ILLNESS, that thrust this mind-body principle in front of the public. After 10 years of lecturing and researching at the University of California at Los Angeles, Cousins' theories held valid under scientific scrutiny.

Carl Simonton, MD, a radiation oncologist, found that his mental imagery techniques seemed to produce better results with fewer side effects for his cancer patients. In a study published in the British Medical Journal, scientists found that women who had experienced a "severe" stressful life event had a 1,500% increase in the risk of developing breast cancer.[2] Bernie Siegel, MD, a Yale surgeon, found that certain mental characteristics helped his cancer patients to recover. Candace Pert, PhD, a celebrated researcher at the National Institutes of Health, discovered endorphins in human brains and led the charge toward unravelling the chemical mysteries of the mind. Dr. Pert says that the mind is a pharmacy and is continuously producing potent substances that either improve or worsen health. Since the mind can create cancer, it should seem a logical leap that the mind can help to prevent and even subdue cancer. Noted physician and researcher at the University of California San Francisco, Kenneth Pelletier, MD, PhD, wrote his ground-breaking book, MIND AS HEALER, MIND AS SLAYER, to show that certain personalities are more prone to certain diseases. Many alternative therapists use a wide variety of psychological approaches to help rid the body of cancer.

Clearly, there is some mental link in the development of cancer for many patients.[3] I have worked with many cancer patients whose major hurdle was spiritual healing. While dietary changes are difficult for many people, it is far easier to change the diet or take some nutrient pills than change the way we think. Pulling emotional splinters is a painful but essential experience. Not only is there a metaphysical link to cancer, but the site of the cancer may provide clues regarding how to fix the problem. Many breast cancer patients have experienced a recent divorce, which results in the loss of a feminine organ. One patient of mine suffered from cancer of the larynx, which began one year after his wife left him with the thought "there's nothing you can say that will make me stay." If spiritual wounds started the cancer, then spiritual healing is an essential element for a cure.

-**Nutrition**. The human body is built from, repaired by, and fueled by substances found in the diet. In the most literal sense, "we are what we eat...and think, and breathe, and do." Nutrition therapy merely tries to re-establish "metabolic balance" in the cancer patients. Medical doctors Gerson, Moerman, and Livingston have each provided their own nutrition 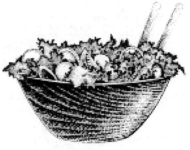 programs to treat cancer. Other schools of thought include macrobiotics, vegetarianism, acid/alkaline balancing, fasting, fruit and vegetable juicing, and others. I will assess all of these therapies in more detail later. After decades of living outside the accepted realm of cancer therapies, nutrition therapy has found a new level of scientific acceptance with the 1990 report from the Office of Technology Assessment, an advisory branch of Congress, whose expert scientific panel wrote in UNCONVENTIONAL CANCER TREATMENTS:

"It is our collective professional judgment that nutritional interventions are going to follow psychosocial interventions up the ladder into clinical respectability as adjunctive and complementary approaches to the treatment of cancer."[4]

-**Exercise**. While 40% of Americans will eventually develop cancer, only 14% of active Americans will get cancer. A half hour of exercise every other day cuts the risk for breast cancer by 75%. Exercise imparts many benefits, including oxygenation of the tissues to thwart the anaerobic needs of cancer cells. Exercise also helps to stabilize blood glucose levels, which can restrict the amount of fuel available for cancer cells to grow. Exercise improves immune function, lymph flow, and detoxification systems. Exercise helps us better tolerate stressful situations. For cancer patients who are able to participate, exercise improves tolerance to chemotherapy. Some therapists use hydrogen peroxide or ozone to oxygenate the tissue. Humans evolved as active creatures. Inactivity is an abnormal, under-oxygenated metabolic state--so is cancer.

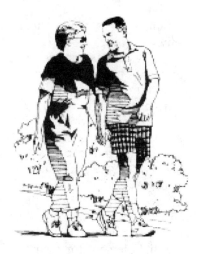

PATIENT PROFILE: STAGE 4 LUNG CANCER STABILIZED

S.D. was 40 years old when diagnosed in January of 2004 with stage 4 lung cancer. Used advice in this book to gather an aggressive food and supplement program to buttress chemo regimen. Did not have the common neuropathy or nausea found in carboplatin users. Oncologists were amazed at the patient's ability to tolerate chemotherapy and agreed to write prescription for nutrition supplements in hopes of insurance reimbursement. As of December 2004, disease is stable, patient has excellent quality of life, no shortness of breath. S.D. realizes how much she took for granted and how this disease has allowed her to grow spiritually. Her kids provided motivation to keep trying.

ENDNOTES

[1]. Braunwald, E., New England Journal Medicine, vol.309, p.1181, Nov.10, 1983
[2] .Chen, CC, et al., Brit.Med.J., vol.311, no.7019, p.1527, Dec.9,1995
[3]. Newell, GR, Primary Care in Cancer, p.29, May 1991
[4]. Office of Technology Assessment, UNCONVENTIONAL CANCER TREATMENTS, p.14, IBID

CHAPTER 3

PROGRESS REPORT IN THE WAR ON CANCER

★

"Cancer is one of the most curable chronic diseases in this country today." Vincent DeVita, Jr., MD, former Director of the National Cancer Institute from 1980-1988

WHAT'S AHEAD?
Your tax dollars have spent $60 billion on the 33-year "war on cancer" at the National Cancer Institute, with continuing increases in the incidence and death rate from cancer. Since we cannot buy a "magic bullet" cure for cancer, we need to consider logical, scientifically validated, non-toxic, inexpensive, and effective therapies to improve outcome in cancer treatment, such as nutrition. Results from chemo, radiation, and surgery have either plateaued or been disappointing. The risk-to-benefit ratio is heavily in favor of using nutrition as part of every cancer patient's comprehensive treatment program.

Cancer is not a new phenomenon. Archeologists have discovered tumors on dinosaur skeletons and Egyptian mummies. From 1600 B.C. on, historians find records of attempts to treat cancer. In the naturalist Disney film, "Never Cry Wolf", the biologist sent to the Arctic to observe the behavior of wolves found that the wolves would kill off the easiest prey, which were sometimes animals suffering from leukemia. Cancer is an abnormal and rapidly growing tissue, which, if unchecked, will eventually smother the body's normal processes. Cancer may have been with us from the beginning of time, but the fervor with which it attacks modern civilization is unprecedented. While this chapter's beginning quote from Dr. DeVita, former Director of the National Cancer Institute, is noble in optimism, it does not appease the 563,700 Americans who died in 2004 of cancer, or roughly 1,544 people per day.

CANCER CASES & DEATHS, US 2000

SOURCE: CA Cancer Journal for Clinicians, vol.50, no.1, p.16, Jan.2000

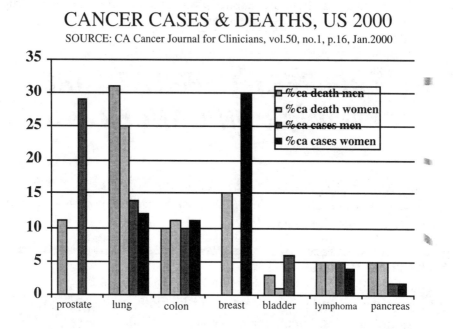

President Richard Nixon declared "war on cancer" on December 23, 1971. Nixon confidently proclaimed that we would have a cure for cancer within 5 years, by the 1976 Bicentennial. However, by 1991, a group of 60 noted physicians and scientists gathered a press conference to tell the public "The cancer establishment confuses the public with repeated claims that we are winning the war on cancer... Our ability to treat and cure most cancers has not materially improved."[1] The unsettling bad news is irrefutable:
⇒ newly-diagnosed cancer incidence continues to escalate, from 1.1 million Americans in 1991 to 1.6 million in 1998
⇒ deaths from cancer in 1992 were 547,000, up from 514,000 in 1991
⇒ since 1950, the overall cancer incidence has increased by 44%, with breast cancer and male colon cancer up by 60% and prostate cancer by 100%
⇒ for decades, the 5 year survival has remained constant, for non-localized breast cancer at 18% and lung cancer at 13%
⇒ only 5% of the $1.8-3 billion annual budget for the National Cancer Institute is spent on prevention

⇒ grouped together, the average cancer patient has a 50/50 chance of living another 5 years, which are the same odds he or she had in 1971

⇒ claims for cancer drugs are generally based on tumor response rather than prolongation of life. Many tumors will initially shrink when chemo and radiation are applied, yet tumors often develop drug-resistance and are then unaffected by therapy.

⇒ within the next few years, cancer is expected to eclipse heart disease as the number one cause of death in America. It is already the number one fear.

⇒ 42% of Americans living today can expect to develop cancer

HAVE WE MADE ANY PROGRESS?

PROGRESS REPORT IN THE WAR ON CANCER

"Many medical oncologists recommend chemotherapy for virtually any tumor, with a hopefulness undiscouraged by almost invariable failure."
Albert Braverman, MD, oncologist, *Lancet, vol.337, p.901,Apr.1991*

Chemotherapy is unsatisfactory; responses are rarely complete, five year survival rates [for metastatic melanoma] are less than 5%, and chemotherapeutic agents are toxic and expensive."
Morton, DL, et al, CA Cancer Journal Clinicians (ACS), vol.49,p.101,Mar.1999

"Chemotherapy is effective in about 3% of advanced epithelial cancers. A sober analysis of the literature has rarely revealed any therapeutic success by the chemotherapeutic regimens in question." *Abel,Hippocrates Verlag,1990*

IN SPITE OF THIS DATA, CHEMO, RAD TX, & SURGERY ARE ONLY ACCEPTED REIMBURSABLE CANCER TX IN US
"Nutrition reduces the effectiveness of chemo & rad tx???"

Depending on which expert you subscribe to, the war on cancer has been either "a qualified failure" or "is progressing slowly". No one is willing to spread the propaganda that it has been a victory. According to the National Cancer Institute (NCI), five year survival rates (definition of a cure) have increased from 20% of cancer patients in 1930 to 53% of adults and 70% of children today.[2] Critics of the NCI claim that living 5 years after diagnosis has nothing to do with being cured, and that earlier diagnosis alone could account for the improvement in survival.

There are 7 million Americans living today who have been cured of cancer. Twenty years ago, surgery for breast cancer routinely removed the entire breast, lymph nodes, and chest muscles in a procedure called radical mastectomy. New methods favor a "lumpectomy" or removal of merely the lump, followed by radiation and/or chemotherapy. In other words, surgeons are becoming more rational and restrained in their efforts to surgically remove the cancer.

Richard Adamson, PhD, Chief of Cancer Etiology at the National Cancer Institute, says that progress has been made against cancer, as death rates from colon and rectal cancer have fallen 15-20% in the last 20 years, and other death rates have dropped, including 20% for ovarian, 30% for bladder, and 40% for cervical cancer.

TIME FOR EXAMINING OPTIONS

The purpose of this section is not to blast the National Cancer Institute, but rather to make it blatantly obvious that our current cancer treatment methods are inadequate and incomplete and that we need to examine some options--like nutrition. Also, we need to address the urgent question: "Does nutrition reduce the effectiveness of chemotherapy?" There are two parts to this debate.

1) Does nutrition interfere with chemotherapy? "No."

2) Is chemotherapy effective? The answer is "sometimes".

A growing body of dissidents cite data to refute the NCI's confident numbers. Among the skeptics is John Bailar, MD, PhD, of Harvard University, whose outspoken article in the prestigious *New England Journal of Medicine* ushered in a champion for

---

HEALTH STATE OF THE UNION

US #1 WORLD HEALTH EXPENSES $2 trillion/year

US #37 HEALTH CARE SYSTEM, according to World Health Org.

HEART DISEASE: 50% of deaths, more ER, RX, disability

CANCER: #1 cause death in US; from 3% of deaths in 1900 to 24% in 1999; 42% of Americans will develop cancer in lifetime, 8 mil treated, another 7 mil "in remission", 250%^ br.ca. 1950

DIABETES: 20 million inUS, 120 mil around world

MIND DRUGS: 131 mil RX psychoactive 1988 to 233 mil 1998

MEDICATION: 3rd-5th cause death US; 140,000/yr, 9.6 mil rxn/yr

OBESITY: 60% US, 300% ^ morbid OB since 1980, 90% type 2 DB

ASPIRIN: 55 billion per year in US

ALZHEIMER'S: 4 mil US, 14 mil 2050, 4th leading cause death US

HYPERTENSION: 60 million in US, RX increases risk for heart att.

INFECTIONS: from obscure to 3rd cause death, drug resistant strains

---

the many strident critics of the National Cancer Institute[3]. Bailar, as a member of the National Academy of Sciences and former editor of the *Journal of the National Cancer Institute*, cannot be ignored. Dr. Bailar confronts the NCI's unfounded enthusiasm with "We are losing the war against cancer" and has shown that the death rate, age-adjusted death rate, and both crude and age-adjusted incidence rate of cancer continue to climb in spite of efforts by the NCI. Non-whites are excluded from the NCI statistics for vague reasons. Blacks, urban poor, and the 11 million workers exposed to toxic substances have all experienced a dramatic increase in cancer incidence and mortality. Less than 10% of patients with cancer of the pancreas, liver, stomach, and esophagus will be alive in five years.[4] Bailar wrote a followup article "Cancer Undefeated" published in the May 1997 edition of the New England Journal of Medicine with similar news. The exception and thin shaft of sunlight in this article indicated a 1% decline in age-adjusted mortality from all cancers from 1991 to 1994. Bailar felt that this almost insignificant improvement may have been due to earlier detection of cancer, not better treatment techniques.

As a percentage of total annual deaths in America, cancer has escalated from 3% in 1900 to 24% of today's deaths. Many experts have been quick to explain away this frightening trend by claiming that our aging population is responsible for the increase in cancer incidence--older people are more likely to get cancer. But aging does not entirely explain our epidemic proportions of cancer in America.

INCREASING INCIDENCE OF CANCER IN AMERICA

not totally due to our aging population

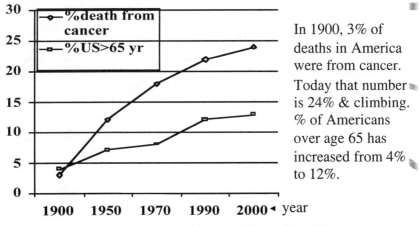

In 1900, 3% of deaths in America were from cancer. Today that number is 24% & climbing. % of Americans over age 65 has increased from 4% to 12%.

Source: Universal Almanac, p.225, Andrews, Kansas City, 1989
also:CA, Cancer Journal for Clinicians, vol.50, no.1, Jan.2000

Perhaps the most tragic "pawns" in this game are the children. The NCI admits to a 28% rise in the incidence of childhood cancers from 1950 through 1987, much of which is due to the ubiquitous presence of environmental pollutants.[5] On the other side of the coin, progress in pediatric oncology has produced cure rates in some forms of childhood cancer of up to 90%, which makes chemotherapy for childhood cancers an NCI victory, of sorts. However, while these patients do survive longer, they have a much higher risk for developing bone cancer later in life as a result of the chemo and/or radiation therapy.[6]

Not that money should be a top priority when health and life are at stake, but our health costs are out of control. We spend about $2 trillion per year or 14% of our gross national product on health care, compared to Sweden at 8%, a socialistic country with free health care for all, and compared to our former American level of 3% in the year 1900. Even after adjusting for inflation, we spend twice as much money on health care for the elderly as we did prior to the inauguration of Medicare.[7] Cancer care is the most expensive of all diseases, costing Americans about $110 billion annually.

Ulrich Abel, PhD, of the Heidelberg Tumor Center in Germany, has brought the issue to a fever pitch. Abel, a well-respected biostatistics expert, published a controversial 92-page review of the world's literature on survival of chemotherapy-treated cancer patients, showing that chemotherapy alone can help only about 3% of the patients with epithelial cancer (such as breast, lung, colon, and prostate), which kills 80% of total cancer patients. "...a sober and unprejudiced analysis of the literature has rarely revealed any therapeutic success by the regimens in question."[8]

A prominent scientist from the University of Wisconsin, Johan Bjorksten, PhD, has shown that chemotherapy alone destroys the immune system beyond a point of return, which increases the risk for early death from infections and other cancers in these immunologically-naked people.[9] Ralph Moss, PhD, former assistant director of public affairs at Sloan Kettering cancer hospital in New York, has written a thoroughly documented analysis of the history of chemotherapy, showing its troublesome beginning as mustard gas for warfare and its current questionable status as the prevailing treatment for the majority of cancer patients.[10] Critics of American cancer treatment point out that the therapy may sometimes be worse than the condition. Researchers reported in the *New England Journal of Medicine* that the risk of developing leukemia from chemotherapy treatment of ovarian cancer outweighs the benefits of the therapy.[11]

Breast and prostate cancers have recently surfaced in the press as "forgotten cancers", due to their intimate nature. While one out of 20 women in 1950 were hit with breast cancer, today that number is one in eight. Even with early detection and proper treatment, a "cured" breast cancer patient will lose an average of 19 years of lifespan. Breast cancer kills about 45,000 women each year.[12] Lack of faith in cancer treatment has led a few physicians to recommend that some women with a high incidence of breast or ovarian cancer in their family undergo "preventive surgery" to remove these high-risk body parts.[13] Life and health insurance companies now refer to healthy intact women as "with organs" and at high risk, therefore forced to pay higher health insurance premiums.

While Tamoxifen is an estrogen binder that can be of benefit in short-term use for breast cancer patients and it has been touted as a chemo-preventive agent for millions of high-risk breast cancer patients, other data show that long-term tamoxifen use elevates the risk for heart attack,[14] eye,[15] and liver damage[16] and INCREASES the risk of endometrial cancer.[17]

And while breast cancer is tragic, prostate cancer is equally prevalent in men and even more lethal. The NCI spends one fourth the amount on prostate cancer research as on breast cancer research. The prostate specific antigen (PSA) and digital rectal exam are the early screening procedures for prostate cancer. In the majority of the prostate cancers found, the cancer has spread beyond the prostate gland and is difficult to treat. Comparing the outcome of 223 patients with untreated prostate cancer to 58 patients who underwent radical prostatectomy, the 10-year disease-specific survival was 86.8% and 87.9%, respectively. There was essentially no difference in survival between the treated and untreated groups.[18]

According to an extensive review of the literature, there has been no improvement in cancer mortality from 1952 through 1985.[19] These authors state: "Evidence has steadily accrued that [cancer therapy] is essentially a failure." Meanwhile, we spend millions researching molecular biology in a futile quest for a "magic bullet" against cancer.[20] A London physician and researcher has provided statistical backing for his contention that breast cancer screenings in women under age 50 provide no benefit in 99.85% of the premenopausal women tested.[21] The average cancer patient has only a 60% chance of surviving the next five years—slightly better than survival rates from 30 years ago. A gathering chorus of scientists and clinicians proclaim that success from chemo and radiation therapy has plateaued, and that we need to examine alternative therapies.[22]

A 1971 textbook jointly published by the American Cancer Society and the University of Rochester stated that biopsy of cancer tissue may lead to the spread of cancer.[23] Although encapsulated cancer can be effectively treated with surgery, and 22% of all cancer can be "cured" through surgery[24], 30% or more of surgery patients with favorable prognosis still have cancer recurrences.[25] A study of 440,000 cancer patients who received chemotherapy or radiation showed that those treated with radiation had a significantly increased risk for a type of leukemia involving cells other than the lymphocytes.[26] Long-term effects of radiation include birth defects and infertility. Short-term effects include mouth sores and ulcers, which can interfere with the ability to eat, rectal ulcers, fistulas, bladder ulcers, diarrhea, and colitis.

In a survey of 79 Canadian oncologists, all of them would encourage patients with non-small cell lung cancer to participate in a chemotherapy protocol, yet 58% said that they themselves would not participate in such a therapy and 81% said they would not take cisplatin (a chemo drug) under any circumstances.[27]

Analysis of over 100 clinical trials using chemotherapy as sole treatment in breast cancer patients found no benefits and significant damage from the chemotherapy in post-menopausal patients.[28] Dr. Rose Kushner pointed out that toxic drugs are "literally making healthy people sick" and are "only of marginal benefit to the vast majority of women who develop breast cancer."[29] Some evidence indicates that chemotherapy actually shortens the life of breast cancer patients.[30]

According to a psychologist writing in the American Cancer Society Journal, "the side effects of cancer chemotherapy can cause more anxiety and distress than the disease itself."[31] A well-recognized side effect of chemotherapy is suppression of bone marrow, which produces the white blood cells that fight infection. This common immune suppression leads to the all-too-common death from infection.[32]

According to the literature that comes with each chemotherapeutic agent, methotrexate may be "hepatotoxic" (damaging to the liver) and suppresses immune function. Adriamycin can cause "serious irreversible myocardial toxicity (damage to heart) with delayed congestive heart failure often unresponsive to any cardiac supportive therapy." Cytoxan can cause "secondary malignancies" (cancer from its use). It is widely known among health care professionals that just working around chemotherapy agents can cause birth defects.[33]

In spite of $50 billion in research at the NCI and billions more spent in private industry, there have been few new chemotherapy drugs discovered in the past 20 years.[34] Not even NCI official Dr. Daniel Ihde can conjure up any enthusiasm for the failure of chemotherapy drugs against lung cancer.[35] Given the limited successes in traditional cancer treatment, it is not surprising that over 60% of all American cancer patients seek "alternative therapies".

Biological therapies, such as interferon and interleukin, are extremely toxic, with treatment requiring weeks of hospitalization, usually in intensive therapy, with multiple transfusions, severe bleeding, shock, and confusion as common side effects.[36] Interferon causes rapid onset of fever, chills, and severe muscle contractions that may require morphine.[37]

FINANCIAL MELTDOWN OF MODERN MEDICINE
"No good deed goes unpunished." Anonymous

In the dark days of World War II, America was struggling to climb out of the decade of financial depression while fighting a war on two continents. Most able-bodied young men went to war. Women, like my grandmother, worked in the factories to provide supplies to the war movement. In order to prevent inflation, the federal government mandated wage freezes. Yet manufacturers had contracts with the government to produce airplanes, ships, and all the other needs of war. So employers started offering "free health care" as an incentive to bring capable workers to their factories. Seemed like an innocent idea at the time, but it has become a Frankenstein in America that threatens to bring the world's greatest government to its knees. Once the war was over, the concept of free health care as a "perk" (perquisite) grew in popularity, especially among union jobs. Once Mom and Dad had free healthcare, the next step was getting free health care for Grandma and Grandpa, which began with the passage of the Medicare Act in 1965. We need to take care of our senior citizens. Yet America has lost the concept of "personal accountability" that founded this country and put us at the top of the world's caste system. Health care in general and cancer treatment in specific threaten our way of life unless we can get a handle on more cost effective and humane ways to treat cancer.

In a decade, Social Security becomes an "unsecured liability", meaning "we have no clue where the money will come from to support it". Medicare is even more immediately perched on the brink of financial ruin. We currently spend a billion dollars a day on Medicare, of which 60% goes to treat patients in their last 6 months of life, with questionable results in either quality or quantity of life. Our $2 trillion per year health care system, including $120 billion for cancer treatment, is added on to the cost of producing goods and services in America and has made America far less competitive in the global economy,

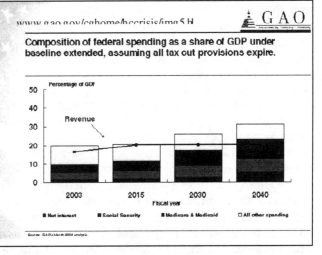

costing us millions of jobs, which are "outsourced" overseas.

As you can see from the accompanying graphs found at the Government Accountability Office (GAO.gov), Social Security and Medicare are already the largest expenses in the federal budget and, with the aging of the 75 million baby boomers, threaten the solvency of the American government. We need more effective and more economical ways of dealing with disease. Nutrition tops that list.

WHERE DID WE GO WRONG?

There is a lot of finger-pointing since the war on cancer has been so heavily criticized. For starters, it would be easy to blame bread mold, from which springs penicillin, which was discovered by Alexander Fleming in 1928 and gave us hope that there was a "magic bullet" against every disease. We could rest equal blame on Jonas Salk, inventor of the polio vaccine in 1952, for such a tremendous show from his medicine bag. With a simple vaccine, one of the most tragic pandemic plagues of history was felled. Again, more reasons to believe that a "magic bullet" against every disease must exist.

Another scapegoat is good old patriotic pride. After all, it was the Americans who rode in to World Wars I and II to rescue the world. Americans stepped in to finish the Panama Canal after the French had failed. Americans threw enough money at the Manhattan Project to develop a war-ending nuclear bomb and again bought our way to the moon in a massive and expensive effort from NASA scientists. Americans have more patents and Nobel laureates than any other nation on earth. We had good reasons to be confident of buying a cure for cancer.

Some of our problems lie in scientific research models. Using animals with induced leukemia, a non-localized disease of the blood-forming organs, is not a realistic representation of how well a cancer drug will work against a solid human tumor. We have also made the erroneous assumption that "no detectable cancer" means no cancer. A million cancer cells are undetectable by even the most sensitive medical equipment. A billion cancer cells become a tiny and nearly undetectable "lump".[38] When the surgeon says,"We think we got it all."--that is when the war on cancer must become an invisible battle involving the patient's well-nourished immune system.

We also have wrongly guessed that "response rate", or shrinkage of the tumor, is synonymous with cure. As mentioned, chemotherapy works on cancer cells like pesticides work on insects. Spraying pesticides on a field of plants may kill 99% of the bugs in the field, but the few insects that survive this baptism of poison have a unique genetic advantage to resist the toxicity of the pesticide. These "super bugs" then reproduce even more rapidly without competition, since the pesticides killed off biological predators in the field and reduced the fertility of the soil for an overall drop in plant health. Similarly, blasting a typically malnourished cancer patient with bolus (high dose once per week) injections of chemotherapy alone may elicit an initial shrinkage of the tumor, but the few tumor cells that survive this poison become resistant to therapy and may even accelerate the course of the disease in the now immune-suppressed patient. Meanwhile, the once marginally malnourished patient becomes clinically malnourished, since nausea becomes a prominent symptom in bolus chemo usage. An expert in cancer at Duke University, Dr. John Grant, has estimated that 40% or more of cancer patients actually die from malnutrition.[39]

We also made the mistake of becoming enamored with a few tools that we thought could eradicate cancer. We focused all of our energies in these three areas and ridiculed or even outlawed any new ideas. The real reason for our failure lies in our error in thinking. The wellness and illness of our bodies are almost entirely dependent on what we eat, think, drink, breathe, and how we move. These forces shape our general metabolism, which is the sum total of bodily processes. Our metabolism then either favors or discourages the growth of both infectious and degenerative diseases. Cancer is a degenerative disease of abnormal metabolism throughout the body--not just a regionalized lump or bump.

Our health is composed of a delicate interplay of nutrients consumed and toxins expelled, coupled with mental and spiritual forces that influence metabolism. We are a product of our genes, lifestyle, and environment. We are not dumb automobiles to be taken to the mechanic and fixed. We are physical and metaphysical beings who must become part of the cure, just as surely as we are a part of the disease process. Healing is a joint effort between patient, clinician, and that mysterious and wonderful force which most of us take for granted. The days of "magic bullet" cures are over. The days of cooperative efforts between patient and clinician are here to stay.

ONLY TEAMWORK WILL BEAT CANCER

Cancer is now the number one cause of death in America. Cancer is a cruel disease that infiltrates the body with abnormal tissue growth and finally strangles its victims with malnutrition, infections, or multiple organ failure. We need teamwork in cancer treatment because of the formidable "Predator" that we face. We cannot discard any cancer therapy, no matter how strange or perpendicular to medical theories, unless that therapy does not work. There are no "magic bullets" against cancer, nor can we anticipate such a development within our lifetime. We need to use restrained chemo, radiation, hyperthermia, and surgery to debulk the tumors, which can remove 10 or 20 trillion cancer cells and give the cancer patient's system a fighting chance. At the same time, we need to re-regulate the cancer back toward healthy cooperation in the body with agents like protease enzymes.[40] Then we need to apply nutrition and other naturopathic fields to bolster "non-specific host defense mechanisms" in the cancer patient to reverse the underlying cause of the disease. This threefold approach, reduction of tumor burden without harming the patient, re-regulating the cancer to convert to normal healthy tissue, and nourishing the patient's recuperative powers, will be the humane and clinically effective cancer treatment of the new millennium.

HOW DO WE HEAL?

•"NATURE alone cures."
•Florence Nightingale, founder of modern nursing, 1900 AD
•"Natural forces within us are the true healers."
•Hippocrates, father of modern medicine, 400 BC
•Germs do not cause disease in the real sense. Something happens in the body to allow the germs to become invasive." Antoine Bechamp, MD, PhD 1900
•"Each patient carries his own doctor inside him."
•Albert Schweitzer, MD, Nobel laureate, 1940
•"The germ is nothing. The 'terrain' is everything."
•Louis Pasteur, founder of microbiology, 1895
•"The doctor of the future will give no medicine, but will involve the patient in the proper use of food, fresh air & exercise."
•Thomas Edison, inventor with over 1000 patents

Chemotherapy can be useful, especially for certain types of cancer and when administered in fractionated dose or via intra-arterial infusion to a therapeutically-nourished patient. Radiation therapy has its place, especially as the highly-targeted brachytherapy or intensity modulated radiation therapy (IMRT). Surgery has its place, especially when the tumor has been encapsulated and can be removed without bursting the collagen envelope. Hyperthermia can be extremely valuable. Combinations of these traditional therapies are becoming better accepted in medical circles. Later in this book, you will see the synergism in creative combinations of conventional and unconventional cancer therapies, such as quercetin (a bioflavonoid) with heat therapy, or niacin with radiation therapy. The take-home lesson here is: "Just because traditional medicine has failed to develop an unconditional cure for cancer doesn't mean that we should categorically reject all traditional approaches."

Comprehensive cancer treatment uses traditional cancer therapies to reduce the tumor burden, while concurrently building up the "terrain" of the cancer patient to fight the cancer on a microscopic level. That is the "one-two punch" that will eventually bring the predator of cancer to its knees.

PATIENT PROFILE: Surviving asbestos cancer. K.F. was diagnosed with mesothelioma, having spent some time in his youth working with asbestos. His original oncologist gave him an optimistic 6 months to live. He and his wife began using an aggressive diet and supplement program in conjunction with his chemotherapy. Three years later, K.F. still has the cancer, but has had an excellent quality of life, looks better than his neighbors, and has received a handsome legal settlement for his cancer from asbestos exposure. Once again, nutrition doesn't cure every cancer patient, but it usually provides a dramatic extension of quality and quantity of life.

ENDNOTES

[1]. Ingram, B., Medical Tribune, vol.33, no.4, p.1, Feb.1992

[2]. Mayo Clinic Health Letter, vol.10, no.2, , p.1, Feb.1992

[3]. Bailar, JC, New England Journal of Medicine, vol.314, p.1226, May 1986

[4]. Squires, S, Washington Post, p.Z19, Dec.3, 1991

[5]. Epstein, SS, and Moss, RW, The Cancer Chronicles, p.5, Autumn 1991

[6]. Weiss, R., Science News, p.165, Sept.12, 1987

[7]. Stout, H, Wall Street Journal, p.B5, Feb.26, 1992

[8]. Abel, U., CHEMOTHERAPY OF ADVANCED EPITHELIAL CANCER: A Critical Survey, Hippokrates Verlag Stuttgart, 1990

[9]. Bjorksten, J, LONGEVITY, p.22, JAB Publ., Charleston, SC, 1987

[10]. Moss, RW, QUESTIONING CHEMOTHERAPY, Equinox Press, NYC, 1995

[11]. Kaldor, JM, et al., New England Journal of Medicine, vol.322, no.1, p.1, Jan.1990

[12]. Neuman, E, New York Times, Insight, p.7, Feb.9, 1992

[13]. Bartimus, T., Tulsa World, p.B3, Dec.22, 1991

[14]. Nakagawa, T., et al., Angiology, vol.45, p.333, May 1994

[15]. Pavlidis, NA, et al., Cancer, vol.69, p.2961, 1992

[16]. Catherino, WH, et al., Drug Safety, vol.8, p.381, 1993

[17]. Seoud, MAF, et al., Obstetrics & Gynecology, vol.82, p.165, Aug.1993

[18]. Johansson, JE, et al., Journal American Medical Association, vol.267, p.2191, Apr.22, 1992

[19]. Temple, NJ, et al., Journal Royal Society Medicine, vol.84, p.95, 1991

[20]. Temple, NJ, et al., Journal Royal Society of Medicine, vol.84, p.95, Feb.1991

[21]. Shaffer, M., Medical Tribune, p.4, Mar.26, 1992

[22]. Hollander, S., et al., Journal of Medicine, vol.21, p.143, 1990

[23]. Rubin, P., (ed), CLINICAL ONCOLOGY FOR MEDICAL STUDENTS AND PHYSICIANS: A MULTI-DISCIPLINARY APPROACH, 3rd edition, Univ. Rochester, 1971

[24]. American Cancer Society, "Modern cancer treatment" in CANCER BOOK, Doubleday, NY, 1986

[25]. National Cancer Institute, Update: Primary treatment is not enough for early stage breast cancer, Office of Cancer Communications, May 18, 1988

[26]. Curtis, RE, et al., Journal National Cancer Institute, p.72, Mar.1984

[27]. Ginsberg, RJ, et al., Cancer of the lung, in: DeVita, CANCER PRINCIPLES AND PRACTICES OF ONCOLOGY, Lippincott, Philadelphia, p.673, 1993

[28]. New England Journal Medicine, Feb.18, 1988; see also Boffey, PM, New York Times, Sept.13, 1985

[29]. Kushner, R., CA-Cancer Journal for Clinicians, p.34, Nov.1984

[30]. Powles, TJ, et al., Lancet, p.580, Mar.15, 1980

[31]. Redd, WH, CA-Cancer Journal for Clinicians, p.138, May1988

[32]. Whitley, RJ, et al., Pediatric Annals, vol.12, p.6, June 1983; see also Cancer Book, ibid.

[33]. Jones, RB, et al., California Journal of American Cancer Society, vol.33, no.5, p.262, 1983

[34]. Hollander, S., and Gordon, M., Journal of Medicine, vol.21, no.3, p.143, 1990

[35]. Ihde, DC, Annals of Internal Medicine, vol.115, no.9, p.737, Nov.1991

[36]. Moertel, CG, Journal American Medical Association, vol.256, p.3141, Dec.12, 1986

[37]. Hood, LE, American Journal of Nursing, p.459, Apr.1987

[38]. Dollinger, M., EVERYONE'S GUIDE TO CANCER THERAPY, p.2, Somerville, Kansas City, 1990

[39]. Grant, JP, Nutrition, vol.6, no.4, p.6S, July 1990 supl

[40]. Hoffman, EJ, CANCER AND THE SEARCH FOR SELECTIVE BIOCHEMICAL INHIBITORS, CRC Press, Boca Raton, FL, 1999

CHAPTER 4

UNDERSTANDING YOUR CANCER

✶

knowing what questions to ask your doctor

"Be thankful we are not getting all the government that we are paying for."   *Will Rogers (1879-1935) American humorist*

WHAT'S AHEAD?

Cancer is a collection of abnormal cells. This chapter will help you to understand your oncologist:
- ✓ how cancer is diagnosed and classified
- ✓ how to ask your doctor the right questions
- ✓ how to understand your doctor's discussions with you.

The diagnosis of cancer can be a scary thing. To maintain some sense of control in your treatment process, it helps to understand how doctors diagnose, classify, and treat cancers. This chapter is a very basic, but extremely valuable, guide to putting you in charge of your cancer treatment team. For more information, see EVERYONE'S GUIDE TO CANCER THERAPY by Dollinger, et al., Andrews McMeel Publishing, 2002.

HOW DOES CANCER START IN YOUR BODY?

Your body contains about 60 trillion cells working in harmony to keep you well. These amazing "non-specific host defense mechanisms" function smoothly in most of us for most of our lives. Part of this process of living involves cell replication, or the "copying" of a cell

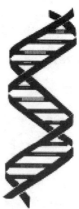

to make two new cells. The cell tears its DNA in half, copies the DNA for both sides of the torn halves, then creates new cells that can continue the work of life. This cell replication process can create defective new cells, which can eventually become cancer, or tumor. Researchers find that each of us carries the seeds of our own destruction in our DNA, called oncogenes, or genetic messages that can turn on and trigger a cancer. Of the 50,000 to 100,000 genes in the average human DNA, maybe 100 of these genes regulate new cell growth and have the potential to trigger a cancer. Think of genes as "loading the gun" and lifestyle, such as nutrition, "pulling the trigger" on this gun. Meaning, just because your family has a tendency toward cancer, does not mean that you are doomed to get cancer. Lifestyle is at least 90% responsible for cancer, while genes play a 5-10% role. This is good news, because it means that you can do something about "silencing" these oncogenes through lifestyle.

BENIGN VS MALIGNANT TUMORS

Tumors do not always threaten our lives. Some tumors, such as freckles, moles, and fatty lumps in the skin, do not invade the rest of the body, and hence do not cause death.

Malignant tumors differ in at least two respects:
1) they put down roots and begin to burrow into the tissue of your body
2) they spread through the body by generating enzymes that break down your tissue and also send out "seed" cells to start a new colony somewhere else in your body.

Rarely does anyone die from a lump or a bump tumor. It is the spreading, or metastasizing, that does the damage. While different cancers in different parts of the body behave somewhat differently, almost all cancers share the common features of being abnormal cells that spread throughout the body and lay down roots to penetrate healthy tissue. These common features allow your body to fight cancer with common mechanisms, regardless of where the cancer started in your body.

HOW CANCER SPREADS

Usually, the cancer begins in one spot in the body and spreads via various means. Rarely, several cancers begin in different parts of the body and spread.

Direct extension. Tumors can lay down roots and burrow into the tissue nearby, like carrots growing into the earth.

Travelling through the blood (hematogenous spreading). As a tumor grows beyond 1/4 inch in diameter (about 7 millimeters), it needs a blood supply to bring nutrients and carry away waste products. This form of metastasis involves the tumor sending out "seed" cells into the bloodstream to attach somewhere in the body and begin a new tumor.

Through the lymphatic system. Your body has two separate blood vessel systems. One is the pumping of red blood cells by the heart through 60,000 miles of arteries and veins. The other network involves the much smaller lymphatic vessels, which carry lymph, a milky liquid that is full of immune cells for battle against invaders, as well as toxins and waste products for elimination. The lymphatic system joins the blood circulation of veins at the thoracic duct, in the left side of the neck. Some cancers spread through the lymphatic system, which is why your doctor may choose to remove a lymph node near the cancer to see if it contains malignant tissue. This score card gives your doctor an idea of how far advanced the cancer has spread. Some doctors inject a blue dye into the tumor, then remove the lymph node nearest the tumor, called sentinel node, for the pathologist to look at under the microscope.

DIFFERENT KINDS OF TUMORS

Based on three broad categories (Where is the tumor growing? How fast is it growing? How big has it already grown?), doctors assign a category to the cancer.

Carcinomas. These tumors grow in the tissues that line internal organs (epithelium). Most carcinomas grow in an organ that secretes something. Lung tissue secretes mucus, breast tissue secretes milk, prostate tissue secretes a milky fluid that contributes to sperm semen, and pancreas tissue secretes digestive juices.

Sarcomas. These cancers develop in supporting or connective tissue, such as muscles, tendons, bones, nerves, or blood vessels. A carcinoma may eventually develop a sarcoma, depending on the site of metastasis.

Lymphomas and leukemias. These tumors develop in the lymph glands or bone marrow. Lymphomas (aka lymphosarcomas) develop in the lymph glands, which are small bean-shaped "bus depots" that are spaced regularly throughout the lymphatic vessels. Lymphomas are generally divided into Hodgkin's or non-Hodgkin's lymphomas.

Add the organ name. Body parts are named in Latin and Greek root names. Hence, bone cancer might be osteo (bone) sarcoma. Stomach cancer might be called gastric carcinoma, etc.

MEASURING THE RATE OF GROWTH

Whenever possible, the surgeon removes a section of the tumor and sends it to a doctor who specializes in tissue examinations (pathologist) for assessment on "how fast is this cancer growing?"

Well-differentiated tumors. If the tumor tissue looks similar to the surrounding tissue of healthy cells, then it is called well-differentiated.

Undifferentiated tumors. Other tumor cells look very different and primitive compared to the surrounding healthy tissue and are called poorly differentiated or undifferentiated. In general, undifferentiated tumors grow faster and have a poorer prognosis than well-differentiated tumors.

High grade. A poorly differentiated, fast growing, aggressive tumor is called high grade, while a well-differentiated, slow growing, and less aggressive tumor is called low grade.

DEFINING THE STAGE OF CANCER

By assessing where the cancer is growing, and how fast, and how fast it is spreading, doctors have developed a system of deciding which protocol (precise plan for therapy) to put you on.

The TNM system of defining stage of cancer has been embraced by many oncologists throughout the world. T stands for Tumor size. N stands for Number of lymph nodes found positive with cancer. And M stands for the presence and degree of Metastasis. T0 means that the entire tumor was removed through the biopsy surgical procedure. T1 is a smaller size tumor, with T2, T3, and T4 being larger tumors. N0 means that there were no lymph nodes found with cancer. N1, N2, and N3 indicate increasing involvement of regional lymph nodes with the cancer. M0 means no metastases found. M1 means that metastases were found. So, for example, a breast cancer diagnosis might come back T2 (tumor is 2.5 centimeters=1 inch in diameter), N1 (one lymph node near breast cancer found with malignant cells), and M0 (no evidence of metastasis).

Other oncologists speak of Stage 1 (no metastasis) through stage 2A then B, through stage 3A then B, and culminating in stage 4 (considerable metastasis) cancers.

HOW CANCER IS DIAGNOSED

While early diagnosis of cancer is crucial for improved outcome, most people still do not involve themselves in routine cancer screening techniques. Hence, most cancer patients come to their doctor with a lump, or bump, or soreness, or blood in the stools or urine as the first sign of a health problem.

Physical exam is the starting point for many cancer patients, examining lymph nodes for signs of swelling, Pap smear for cervical cancer, digital rectal exam for prostate cancer, and so on.

Blood tests. There are markers in the blood that can be non-specific indicators of cancer somewhere in the body: alkaline phosphatase (elevated in bone and liver disease), SGOT and SGPT (elevated in liver damage), bilirubin (elevated in liver disease), and LDH (lactate dehydrogenase) elevated in many cancers and indicating how much anaerobic (lacking oxygen) metabolism is going on in the body. Uric acid is elevated in gout and cancers of the blood and lymph nodes. Creatinine and BUN (blood urea nitrogen) are elevated in kidney disease. Calcium is elevated in cancers that have spread to the bone.

Tumor markers. It can be very useful for the doctor to track substances in the blood that relate to the cancer getting better or worse. None of these tumor markers are perfect. All include a certain percentage of false positive (the test came back positive, but you don't have that cancer) and false negative (the test came back negative, but you do have cancer).

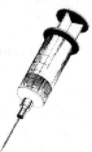

➢ CEA, or carcinoembryonic antigen, may be elevated in cancers of the colon, breast, lung, and pancreas.
➢ CA-125 elevated in cancers of the ovary and uterus.
➢ CA 19-9 elevated in gastrointestinal tract cancers, such as colon, pancreas, stomach, and liver.
➢ CA 15-3 elevated in breast cancer.
➢ AFP, or alpha fetal protein, elevated in liver and testis cancer.
➢ HCG, or human chorionic gonadotropin, elevated in pregnancy and cancers of the testis, ovary, and lung.
➢ PAP, or prostatic acid phosphatase, elevated in prostate cancer.
➢ PSA, or prostate specific antigen, elevated in prostate cancer.
➢ Serum protein electrophoresis, elevated in multiple myeloma.

Testing blood, urine, feces, and spinal fluid may be part of your doctor's exam.

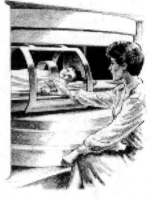

Imaging techniques. Modern medicine has developed some fabulous devices for finding the cancer. What used to require an autopsy can now be done with reasonable accuracy on healthy or sick patients.

X-ray (radiography) can see through tissue and identify differences in the density of tissue, such as a tumor versus healthy tissue. Depending on where your radiologist is examining, the patient may have to consume lightly radioactive material (barium) to add contrast to the diagnosis. X-ray can easily tell the difference between bone and soft flesh. However, in order to determine soft tissue cancers, new techniques, such as nuclear scans, CT (computerized tomography), MRI (magnetic resonance imaging), and ultra sound may be used. PET (positron emission tomography) scans require the doctor to inject radioactively-labeled glucose into the blood stream, then use a "geiger counter"-like device to locate the glucose, because cancer is a sugar feeder, taking up more than its share of sugar in the bloodstream.

The best technique, if possible, is to see the cancer, using a scope. Rigid, thin telescopes can be inserted in various regions of the body to find cancers. A bronchoscope would help examine the lungs. A cytoscope would examine the urethra and bladder. Flexible fiber optic telescopes can not only look inside the body's cavities, but also take out tissue samples for later examination. An endoscope can look into the stomach or colon for signs of cancer.

Biopsy. By taking a sample of the suspect tissue, the doctor can have a pathologist examine the tumor for staging and deciding what protocol to offer the patient. Incisional biopsy involves cutting into the tumor, removing part of it, then stitching the area closed. Excisional biopsy involves removing the entire tumor. It is during the biopsy process that some doctors send the tissue to a lab for determining what forms of chemo might kill this cancer. This process is called "in vitro chemo sensitivity testing" or "ex vivo apoptosis". See RationalTherapeutics.com for more information on this valuable technique for eliminating useless chemo agents and focusing on potentially valuable chemo agents.

YOUR CANCER DOCTOR TEAM

ONCOLOGIST: A Medical Doctor (MD) or Doctor of Osteopathy (DO) who has specialized training in cancer and its treatments with chemotherapy.

RADIOLOGIST: An MD or DO with specialized training in diagnostic use of X-rays and other assessment tools, such as MRI and CT scans.

RADIATION ONCOLOGIST, or radiotherapist: An MD or DO with specialized training in the therapeutic use 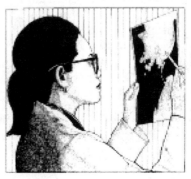 of radiation to treat cancer or palliate cancer symptoms.

SURGICAL ONCOLOGIST: An MD or DO with specialized training in the surgical removal of cancer masses.

PAIN MANAGEMENT SPECIALIST: An MD or DO with specialized training in dealing with the pain that can accompany cancer. It is imperative that patients get adequate pain management. Whether Tylenol or codeine or morphine, whatever it takes to provide reasonable comfort, is crucial for the recovery of the cancer patient.

INTERNIST: An MD or DO trained in internal medicine or the biochemistry of the body and how to adjust problems that arise.

WHAT ABOUT YOUR CANCER?

While there are nearly 200 different cancers, there are only three main categories:

✓ carcinoma, such as breast, lung, colon, and prostate
✓ sarcomas, which are found in the connective tissue
✓ leukemias and lymphomas, which originate in the blood, bone marrow, and lymph nodes

Of the 1.4 million Americans who will be newly diagnosed with cancer this year, and of the 46 main cancers that are tracked, over 50% of these cancer patients will have one of the more common cancers:

➢ Colon/rectum 144,000 per year
➢ Lung 172,000
➢ Breast 212,000
➢ Prostate 232,000

Yet, each of these cancer diagnoses have something in common: the cancer is an abnormal growth that could consume the patient through malnutrition, organ failure, or infection. Nutrition can improve outcome in nearly all cancer patients who are undergoing medical therapies.

PATIENT PROFILE: SURVIVING KIDNEY CANCER

M.M. was diagnosed with renal cell carcinoma stage 4. She took thalidomide and interferon for nearly 2 years, then stopped these medications due to side effects, which included vomiting, headaches, and neuropathy (numb and painful hands and feet). M.M. used the nutrition guidelines in this book along with mistletoe and dendritic cell therapy to shrink her tumor by 30%. She was given 6 months to live, yet has survived 3 years, although she still has tumor burden. Her quality of life is good. M.M. says that "we are all terminal. Just try to make a difference in someone else's life."

CHAPTER 5

CONVENTIONAL CANCER TREATMENTS

※

Courage is being scared to death--but saddling up anyway.
John Wayne (1907-1979)

WHAT'S AHEAD?
In order to know where we are going in cancer
treatment, it helps to know where we have been.
Common treatments for cancer include chemo,
radiation, and surgery. Alternative treatments for
cancer include immune stimulation, herbs, and dietary programs.
Recent innovations filter out an immune inhibitor from the blood of the
cancer patient or use magnetic targeting of cancer cells. None of these
therapies is a universal fix for all cancer patients. Yet, some merit
more attention and availability as an option for all cancer patients.

This chapter looks at both conventional and alternative
cancer treatment methods to give you a better
understanding of our "roots" in cancer treatment options.
For a more thorough discussion of conventional therapies, read:
CANCER THERAPY by Mallin Dollinger, MD
PRACTICAL ONCOLOGY by Robert Cameron, MD

For alternative therapies, read:
CANCER by W.John Diamond, MD and W. Lee Cowden, MD
ALTERNATIVE CANCER THERAPIES by Ron Falcone
ALTERNATIVES IN CANCER THERAPY by Ross Pelton, R Ph, PhD
CANCER AND NATURAL MEDICINE by John Boik
THIRD OPINION by John Fink
THE ALTERNATIVE CANCER THERAPY BOOK by Richard Walters.

CONVENTIONAL THERAPIES

Chemotherapy is a spin-off product from the chemical warfare of World Wars I and II and is now given to 75% of all American cancer patients. Yale University pharmacologists who were working on a government project during World War II to develop an antidote for mustard gas noted that bone marrow and lymphoid tissue were heavily damaged by these poisons. That observation led to experiments in which mustard gas was injected into mice with lymphomas (cancer of the lymph glands) and produced remission. In 1943, researchers found that mustard gas had a similar effect on human Hodgkins disease.[1] Chemo has also become a useful agent against testicular cancer, which is now 92% curable. Most proponents of chemo now recognize the limitations of using chemo as the sole therapy against many types of cancer.

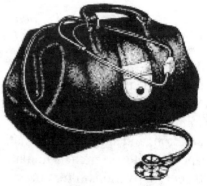

Shortly after these initial exciting discoveries, progress on chemo cures quickly plateaued and forced the innovative thinkers into creative combinations of various chemo drugs, which is now the accepted practice. In the 1980s, oncologists began using chemo by "fractionated drip infusion" in the hospital rather than one large (bolus) injection in the doctor's office. The fractionated method was not only more effective against the cancer, but also less toxic for the patient. Think of the difference in toxicity between taking two glasses of wine with dinner each night, or guzzling all 14 glasses at one time at the end of the week. Also, fractionated drip infusion is more likely to catch the cancer cells in their growth phase, while bolus injections are a random guess to coincide with the growth phase of cancer. In the next evolutionary step, borrowing from technology developed for heart disease, oncologists began using catheters (thin tubes) that could be inserted into an artery (called intra-arterial infusion) to deliver chemo at the site of the tumor, once again improving response and reducing overall toxicity.

Radiation therapy is given to about 60% of all cancer patients. In 1896, a French physicist, Marie Curie discovered radium, a radioactive metal. For her brilliance, Madam Curie was eventually awarded two Nobel prizes and was considered one of the founders of radiation therapy and the nuclear age. For her unprotected use of radioactive materials, she

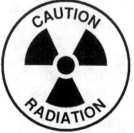

eventually died while still young of leukemia. Cancer patients were soon being treated with a new technique developed by the German physicist, Wilhelm Roentgen, called radiation therapy. This technique relies on regional destruction of unwanted tissue through ionizing radiation that disrupts the DNA of all bombarded cells. Radiation therapy can be externally or internally originated, high or low dose, and delivered with uncanny computer-assisted precision to the site of the tumor. Brachytherapy, or interstitial radiation therapy, places the source of radiation directly into the tumor, as an implanted seed. New techniques use radiation in combination with heat therapy (hyperthermia). Intensity modulated radiation therapy (IMRT) has the potential of being more destructive on the tumor and less harmful to the patient.

Surgery is the first treatment of choice for about 67% of cancer patients. By 1600 B.C., Egyptian physicians were excising tumors using knives or red-hot irons.[2] By physically removing the obvious tumor, physicians feel that they have the best chance for overall success. Unfortunately, many tumors are so entwined with delicate body organs, such as brain and liver, that the tumor cannot be resected (cut out). Another concern is that partial removal of a cancer mass may open the once-encapsulated tumor to spread, like opening a sack of dandelion seeds on your lawn.

Biological therapies, as with most other discoveries, were the product of accidents being observed by a bright mind. William B. Coley, MD, a New York cancer surgeon, scoured the hospital records around 1880 looking for some clue as to why only a minority of patients survived cancer surgery. He found that a high percentage of survivors had developed an infection shortly after the surgery to remove the cancer. This observation led Dr. Coley to inject a wide variety of bacteria, known as Coley's cocktail, into his cancer patients, who then underwent the feverish recovery phase, with noteworthy cancer cures produced. Infections were found to induce the immune system into a higher state of activity, which then helped to destroy tumors. From this crude beginning, molecular biologists have found brilliant ways of producing injectable amounts of the immune factors that can fight cancer.

Biological therapies attempt to fine-tune and focus the immune system into a more vigorous attack on the cancer. Lymphokines are basically "bullets" produced by the immune system to kill invading cells, such as cancer. Lymphokine-activated killer (LAK) cells are incubated in the laboratory in the presence of a stimulator (interleukin-2) and then injected back into the cancer patient's body for an improved immune response.[3]

Interferon, interleukin, monoclonal antibodies, and tumor necrosis factor are among the leading contenders as biological therapies against cancer. The downside of biological therapies is that most forms have extremely toxic side effects.

Heat Therapy (hyperthermia). Cancer cells seem to be more vulnerable to heat than normal healthy cells. Since the time of Hippocrates and the Egyptian Pharoahs, heat therapy has been valued. Experts have shown that applying heat to the patient elevates immune responses. Temperatures of 42 degrees Celsius or 107 degrees Fahrenheit will kill most cancer cells, but can be quite stressful on the patient also. Could it be that exercise induces regular "hyperthermia" to kill off cancer cells before they can become a problem?

Whole body hyperthermia involves a very sophisticated hot tub device, general anesthesia, and medical supervision. Regional hyperthermia can involve either a miniature waterbed-like device applied to the tumor or focused microwaves. Hyperthermia can be useful by itself, or used synergistically to improve the response to chemo and radiation therapy. German oncologist, Friedrich Douwes, MD, has reported superb results using hyperthermia (ph.011-49-8061-398-412, website: klinik-st-georg.de). American hyperthermia units are found throughout the country, including Valley Cancer Institute, Los Angeles, CA ph. 310-398-0013 and Orange County Immune Institute, Huntington Beach, CA, ph. 714-842-1777.

PATIENT PROFILE:BEAT TERMINAL BREAST CANCER
Y.K. was diagnosed with inflammatory stage 4 breast cancer in 2001 and given 6 months to live. Y.K. knew that medical therapy probably couldn't cure her cancer. She asked her oncologist about nutrition as helpful or adjuvant therapy along with the chemo and radiation that had been proposed. Her oncologist said "no nutrients". So Y.K. changed oncologists. Her new oncologist accepted, but did not encourage, the use of nutrients during chemo. Y.K. used an aggressive combination of foods and supplements that she learned about in this book to help put her terminal breast cancer into remission within a year, and she remains disease-free as of 2005. Y.K. told me that she "had to slow down and lose my perfectionism" once she got the cancer diagnosis. Her words of encouragement to you, dear reader, is "Life is worth living. We need to treat our body with respect or we won't have life." As an interesting footnote to Y.K.'s cancer, her dog developed breast cancer. Even after chemo, the dog continued to deteriorate. Y.K. gave her dog nutrition supplements and mistletoe injections subcutaneously, which put her dog into remission. Both Y.K. and all of her dogs are doing well now.

ENDNOTES

[1]. Romm, S, Washington Post, p.Z14, Jan.9, 1990
[2]. Herman, R., Washington Post, p.Z14, Dec.3, 1991
[3]. Boly, W, Hippocrates, p.38, Jan.1989

CHAPTER 6

NOTE TO THE ONCOLOGIST

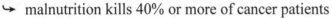

"Cancer metastasis involves a complicated biochemical 'conversation' between the seed and the soil."
                              Stephen Paget, MD, Lancet, 1889
"The time has come to put major emphasis on the soil."
        Isaiah Fidler, MD 2004, MD Anderson Cancer Center

WHAT'S AHEAD?

Nutrition can make medical therapy more of a
selective toxin against the cancer and less damaging to
the patient. Nutrition therapy is an essential part of
comprehensive cancer treatment because:

↪ malnutrition kills 40% or more of cancer patients
↪ nutrition protects the patient against the toxic effects of chemo and
   radiation without reducing their effectiveness in killing cancer
↪ nutrients support the immune system in killing cancer
↪ sugar feeds cancer, which makes diet and supplements crucial
↪ nutrients can become "biological response modifiers" in changing
   the way the body works to re-regulate the cancer cells

Can you imagine any state of being--
heart disease, pregnancy, broken
bone, depression, splinter, flu, or
cancer--in which being malnourished is an
advantage for recovery? This chapter offers some
insights regarding the guided use of nutrition
therapy to help support your cancer patient while
undergoing traditional therapies. You will be spared

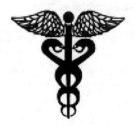

the onslaught of references in this chapter, though ample scientific documentation is found throughout this book to support the use of nutrition as part of comprehensive cancer treatment. No one is saying that nutrition should be the sole therapy in advanced cancer. It is hoped that you will consider using aggressive nutrition to bolster "host defense mechanisms" in your cancer patients.

MISCONCEPTIONS ABOUT NUTRITION & CANCER

The concept of nutrition in cancer treatment comes with a mixed reputation, although its use dates back 2,000 years ago to Chinese medical textbooks.

⇒**FALSE HOPE.** You may have heard the undocumented claims regarding cures from advanced cancer using carrot juice. You have also seen more than a few advanced salvageable cancer patients waste precious time "experimenting" with questionable treatment modalities, only to have the patient succumb to the disease.

⇒**QUESTIONABLE PRACTITIONERS.** To be sure, there are a few unsavory characters in the field of nutritional oncology, just as there are in any profession.

COMMON MISCONCEPTIONS AMONG ONCOLOGISTS

MYTH: Nutrition has nothing to do with cancer.

FACT: The health of all animals and plants is heavily dependent on nutrition. Nutrition improves outcome in cancer treatment.

MYTH: Antioxidants are both expensive urine and will neutralize the benefits of chemo and radiation.

FACT: Then why are the antioxidant drugs Amifostine (cisplatin), Mesna (Ifosphomide), and Dextrazazone (Adria) used with chemo?

MYTH: Sugar has nothing to do with cancer outcome.

FACT: Then why is the $1.5 million PET scan considered such a valuable tool in diagnosing cancer?

⇒**IF YOU FEED THE PATIENT, THEN YOU FEED THE CANCER.** You may have been trained by the founders of chemotherapy, who exploited folic acid antagonists as drugs to slow down neoplasia. It would seem that "if an anti-vitamin (methotrexate) slows down cancer, then a vitamin might accelerate cancer. " In fact, nutrients in general bolster the patient's ability to recover from most diseases. You will see many references throughout this book showing how nutrients improve outcome in cancer treatment. You will also see that some essential nutrients, notably sodium, glucose, iron, copper, and the essential fatty acid of linoleic acid, can accelerate tumor growth when used in excess or in the absence of other controlling nutrients. This book addresses the concepts of nutrient toxicity and provides guidelines for using nutrition as a positive force in the treatment of your cancer patients.

You may have seen the paper from the American College of Physicians (*Annals of Internal Medicine*, vol.110, no.9, p.734, May 1989) claiming that total parenteral nutrition (TPN) may be counterproductive in cancer patients. Paradoxically, malnourished patients were eliminated from this meta-analysis of pooled data. TPN treats malnutrition, not cancer. Also, this collection of studies grouped various TPN protocols together; those that were high in dextrose or low, high in protein or low, with or without fat...all were considered as equal TPN formulas against cancer. Since cancer is an "obligate glucose metabolizer", or sugar-feeder, and since the patient needs adequate amounts of protein to rebuild lost visceral protein stores and replenish the immune system, it is unwise to group all TPN formulas together. Other studies show that the proper formula of TPN along with proper patient-selection criteria can improve the outcome in cancer treatment.

⇒ANTIOXIDANTS WILL REDUCE THE EFFECTIVENESS OF CHEMO AND RADIATION.

In basic theory, this statement makes sense. However, in actual human cancer patients, antioxidants have been shown to dramatically improve the tumor kill from pro-oxidative chemo and radiation, while protecting the host tissue from damage.

CAN VITAMIN E REDUCE NEUROTOXICITY FROM CISPLATIN?

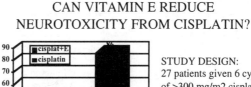

incidence of neurotoxicity

STUDY DESIGN:
27 patients given 6 cycles of >300 mg/m2 cisplatin. 14 received chemo alone. 13 received chemo + E (300 mg/d) during tx + 3 months following tx. $p<0.01$

Pace, A., J.Clin.Oncology, vol.21, no.5, p.927, Mar.2003

Essentially, the proper selection of nutrients taken before and during chemo and radiation can help make the medical therapy more of a selective toxin against the cancer. In one study, cancer patients were given either vitamin E at 300 mg per day or placebo while undergoing cisplatin therapy. Only 31% of the vitamin E group developed neurotoxicity, while 86% of the placebo group developed neurotoxicity. There was no observed difference in tumor kill rate.

Cancer cells are primarily anaerobic, fermenting cells. With the exception of vitamin C, cancer cells do not absorb nor use antioxidants the same way that healthy aerobic cells do. Vitamin C (ascorbic acid) is nearly identical in chemical structure to glucose, which is the favored fuel for cancer cells. With this background, it should not be surprising that researchers at Sloan-Kettering found that radioactively labelled ascorbic acid was preferentially absorbed by implanted tumors in animals. The study admitted that this effect takes place because cancer has many more glucose receptors on the cell surface than healthy normal cells. The researchers then assumed, but never found any evidence, that vitamin C should not be used in conjunction with chemo or radiation because the tumor was absorbing vitamin C to protect itself against the damaging effects of chemo and radiation. Any antioxidant by itself and/or in an anaerobic environment (such as a cancer cell) can become a pro-oxidant. Vitamin C in large doses in cancer patients is both protective of the patient while allowing therapy to be more toxic to the tumor cells.

We can exploit the differences in biochemistry between healthy and malignant cells by combining aggressive nutrition support with restrained cytotoxic therapies.

⇒CANCER MUST BE TREATED WITH CYTOTOXIC THERAPY, NOT NOURISHMENT. That strategy may be changing. An article by an oncologist published in the *Journal of Clinical Oncology* (vol.13, no.4, p.801, Apr.1995) asks the question: "Must we

SHIFTING THE CANCER PARADIGM MUST WE KILL TO CURE?

Journal of Clinical Oncology (ASCO), vol.13, no.4, p.801, Apr.1995
H. Schipper, CR Goh, TL Wang

"the limits of the [cancer killing] model seem to have been reached"
"consider cancer as potentially reversible"
"killing strategies may be counterproductive because they impair host response and drive the already defective regulatory process [of the cancer cell] toward further aberrancy."
"[chemotherapy] treatment strategies have been based on the log-cell-kill hypothesis, derived from leukemia cells in culture...but is rarely seen in nature and only sustained under stringent conditions"
"remission does not predict cure..the failure of adjuvant therapies to flatten disease-free survival curves"
"conventional antineoplastic approaches will play a role as debulkers, ...the strategy will change to one of reregulation."

kill to cure?" Over the past 50 years, we have found that increasing the toxicity and usage of pesticides on insects in the fields has created a net INCREASE in crop loss, with some insects developing near-total immunity to the most potent insecticides. During the same half-century, we have overused antibiotic drugs, with the net effect that infections are now the number three cause of death in America, with some bacteria having become virtually drug-resistant. During that same time frame, we have attempted to use potent systemic chemotherapy to eliminate cancer. Initially, the patient often gets a "response", or a shrinkage of the tumor. In many patients, the tumor soon develops a drug resistance that creates a more virulent tumor, yet at that point the chemotherapy may have compromised the patient's host defense mechanisms and thus, his ability to recover. Attacking cancer with restrained medical intervention COUPLED with aggressive nutrition is the best strategy. These two therapies combine to create a synergistic response that is better than either therapy could achieve on its own.

⇒**WHAT QUALIFIES PATRICK QUILLIN?** You might ask, "With all the conflicting information out there regarding nutrition for cancer patients, why is this guy the one to listen to?" In addition to my three earned degrees in nutrition, and my certified nutrition specialist (CNS) status, I have spent 15 years working with over 3,000 cancer patients and know what works and what doesn't. I organized 3 international continuing medical education scientific symposia on "adjuvant nutrition in cancer treatment" and edited a textbook by the same name. My original release of BEATING CANCER WITH NUTRITION has been translated into Japanese, Korean, and Chinese and was a home-study continuing education course for registered nurses, and was the bestseller in its category on amazon.com for 1999. Please see my complete curriculum vitae at my website: www.NutritionCancer.com.

The bottom line is that a well-nourished cancer patient can better manage the disease, and has fewer infections, fewer side effects from chemo and radiation, a better quality and quantity of life, and improved chances for complete remission. The toxicity of professionally-designed nutrition therapies for the cancer patient is near-zero. The risk-to-benefit-to-cost ratio of nutrition therapy in cancer treatment warrants its inclusion.

I have worked with many cancer patients who came to our centers as the "hospital of last hope" after failing several different chemo and radiation protocols. Many of these patients were in tears as they would tell me about the apathy that their former doctors displayed as the patient asked the doctor: "What about nutrition? Might it help?" As you will see in studies throughout this book, the earlier the cancer patient receives nutrition therapy, the better the outcome. For those patients who are malnourished or who have been through extensive cytotoxic therapies without any nutrition support, the recuperative powers of the human body can be exhausted.

By keeping an open mind and the patient's best interests in the forefront, you will make the right decision in using nutrition for your patients. Thank you in advance for your time and consideration.

CHAPTER 7

NUTRITION CAN IMPROVE OUTCOME IN CANCER TREATMENT

✯

"In the midst of winter, I finally learned that there was in me an invincible summer." Albert Camus

---

WHAT'S AHEAD?
Nutrients can improve cancer outcome by:
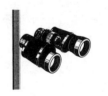
↳ inducing "suicide" (apoptosis) in cancer cells
↳ reverting cancer cells back to healthy cells
↳ improving immune functions to recognize and destroy cancer cells
↳ helping the body to wall off, or encapsulate, the tumor

Nutrition is a low-cost, non-toxic, and scientifically-proven helpful component in the comprehensive treatment of cancer. Adjuvant (helpful) nutrition and traditional oncology are synergistic, not antagonistic. The advantages in using an aggressive nutrition program in comprehensive cancer treatment are, in this critical order of importance:

⇒ 1) avoiding malnutrition
⇒ 2) reducing the toxicity of medical therapy while making chemotherapy and radiation more selectively toxic to the tumor cells
⇒ 3) stimulating immune function
⇒ 4) selectively starving the tumor
⇒ 5) nutrients acting as biological response modifiers assist host defense mechanisms and improve outcome in cancer therapy.

NUTRIENTS AS BIOLOGICAL RESPONSE MODIFIERS

In the early phase of nutrition research, nutrient functions were linked to classical nutrient deficiency syndromes: e.g., vitamin C and scurvy, vitamin D and rickets, niacin and pellagra. Today nutrition researchers find various levels of functions for nutrients. For example, let's look at the "dose-dependent response" from niacin:

⇒20 milligrams daily will prevent pellagra

⇒100 mg becomes a useful vasodilator

⇒2,000 mg is a cholesterol-lowering agent endorsed by the National Institutes of Health. While 10 milligrams of vitamin E is considered the RDA, 800 iu was

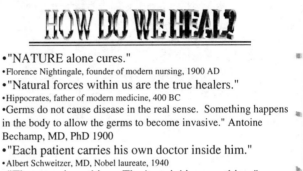

HOW DO WE HEAL?

• "NATURE alone cures."
  • Florence Nightingale, founder of modern nursing, 1900 AD
• "Natural forces within us are the true healers."
  • Hippocrates, father of modern medicine, 400 BC
• Germs do not cause disease in the real sense. Something happens in the body to allow the germs to become invasive." Antoine Bechamp, MD, PhD 1900
• "Each patient carries his own doctor inside him."
  • Albert Schweitzer, MD, Nobel laureate, 1940
• "The germ is nothing. The 'terrain' is everything."
  • Louis Pasteur, founder of microbiology, 1895
• "The doctor of the future will give no medicine, but will involve the patient in the proper use of food, fresh air & exercise."
  • Thomas Edison, inventor with over 1000 patents

shown to improve immune functions in healthy older adults.[1] While 10 mg of vitamin C will prevent scurvy in most adults, the RDA is 60 mg, and 300 mg was shown to extend lifespan in males by an average of 6 years.[2]

The dietary requirement of a nutrient may well depend on the health state of the individual and what you are trying to achieve. In animal studies, 7.5 mg of vitamin E per kilogram of body weight was found to satisfactorily support normal growth and spleen to body weight ratio. Yet, consumption at twice that level of vitamin E was essential to prevent deficiency symptoms of myopathy and testis degeneration. Intake at seven times base level of vitamin E was required to prevent red blood cell hemolysis. Intake of 27 times base level provided optimal T- and B-lymphocyte responses to mitogens.[3]

You can accelerate the rate of a reaction by increasing temperature, surface area, or concentration of substrates or enzymes. Clearly, above-RDA levels of nutrients can offer safe and cost-effective enhancement of metabolic processes, including immune functions. Therapeutic dosages of nutrients may be able to reduce tumor recurrence, selectively slow cancer cells, stimulate the immune system to more actively destroy tumor cells, alter the genetic expression of cancer, and more.

NUTRIENTS ALONE CAN REVERSE EARLY CANCER

Cancer is not an "on or off" switch. No one goes to bed on Sunday night perfectly healthy and then wakes up Monday morning with stage 4 colon cancer metastasis to the liver. Cancer takes months, and probably years to develop. Research has shown that, in the early stages of cancer cell development, nutrients alone can reverse "pre-malignant" cancers[4], which under the microscope are identical to cancer cells, yet have not invaded beyond their own "turf". As the

CAN INDOLE-3-CARBINOL (I3C) REVERSE CERVICAL INTRAEPITHELIAL NEOPLASIA (CIN)?

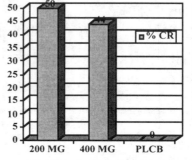

STUDY DESIGN:
30 women biopsy proven CIN stage 2,3 given 200, 400 mg/day I3C or placebo 12 wk. CR in I3C
No toxicity observed.
Dose dependent response
Shifting 16 @hydroxyestrone
To 2 hydroxyestrone
Most HPV positive
P<0.023 for 200 mg/d
P<0.032 for 400 mg/d
50% CIN to neoplasia

Bell, MC, et al., Gynecologic Oncology, vol.78, p.123, 2000

bowling ball of cancer begins its hazardous deterioration downhill, the body has built-in mechanisms to stop this process, including DNA repair, cell-to-cell communication, macrophage engulfment, tumor necrosis factor, collagen encapsulation, and anti-angiogenesis agents to shut down the making of new blood vessels from the tumor.

CAN VITAMINS OR LACTULOSE PREVENT COLON CANCER?

Colon cancer is 3rd most common ca in USA
110,000 cases, 50,000 deaths/yr, liver mets serious complications

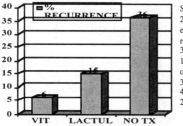

STUDY DESIGN:
209 Patients w. endoscopic polyp removal; given vit. 30,000 iu A, 70 mg E 1 gm C; or lactulose, or no treatment, follow 36 months recurrence 4 of 70 vit., 9 of 61 lact. 28 of 78 no TX recur

Roncucci, L, et al., Dis.Colon Rectum, vol.36, p.227, 1993

This concept is very pivotal to the notion that nutrition can improve outcome in cancer treatment. For decades, researchers have held the notion that "once the cell turns cancerous, only forceful eradication can help the patient." Maybe not. Cancer, in its early stages, can be reversed by nutrients alone. Once cancer has deteriorated to stage 4 malignancy with extensive metastasis, the patient probably needs more than nutrients alone to reverse the disease.

Our 60 trillion cells in the human body are constantly dividing. The DNA, which contains the body's blueprints to make a completely new you, must "unzip" the spiral staircase of chromosomes, then duplicate itself exactly, then "re-zip" the spiral staircase of DNA. This process occurs billions of times daily. The chance for a mistake is quite high, which is why our bodies have many mechanisms in place to correct mistakes in the beginning. Yet, if the mistake cell continues to deteriorate through its many different shades of cancer; including anaplasia, dysplasia, and metaplasia, then the final stage of neoplasia might occur.

Can Nutrients Reverse the Cancer Process?

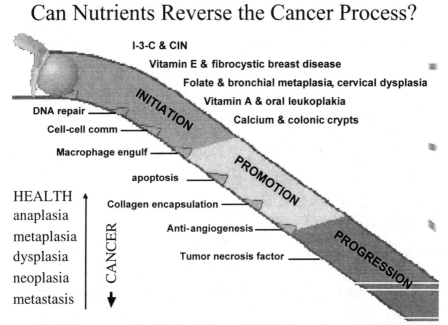

As this process is deteriorating, nutrients have been shown to not only arrest the slippery slide toward cancer, but also to reverse the damage and help the body to generate healthy cells from pre-malignant cancers. In high doses:

- folate and B-12 can reverse bronchial metaplasia[5] or cervical dysplasia
- beta-carotene[6] and vitamin A can reverse oral leukoplakia[7]; so can vitamin E[8]
- selenium can reverse pre-cancerous mouth lesions[9]
- vitamin C[10] and calcium can reverse colon polyps[11]
- vitamins A, C, and E reversed colorectal adenomas[12]
- vitamin E can reverse benign breast disease, such as fibrocystic breast disease, which increases risk for breast cancer by 50-80%[13]
- vitamin E and beta-carotene injected into the tumor reversed mouth cancer in animals[14]

Pre-malignant and malignant cells look almost identical under the microscope. Since nutrients can reverse, or re-regulate, pre-malignant cells, it becomes entirely probably that nutrients can help to re-regulate malignant and metastatic cells. Maybe we don't have to kill all the cancer cells in order to cure the cancer patient.

HOW CAN NUTRIENTS AFFECT THE CANCER PROCESS?

Shklar, G., Alternative & Complementary Therapies, vol.2, no.3, p.156, May 1996
-inhibit angiogenesis
-dysregulate mutant p53 oncogene
-alter immune cytokines
Schwartz, JL, Cancer Prevention Intl., vol.3, p.37, 1997
-upregulate DNA repair
-augment programmed cell death (apoptosis)
Prasad, KN, et al., Arch.Otolaryngol.Head Neck Surg., vol.119, p.1133, Oct.1993
-regulate gene expression
-induce growth inhibition in cancer
-alter cell differentiation
Lupulescu, A., Intl.J.Vit.Nutr.Res., vol.63, p.3, 1993
-A, C, E regulators of cell differentiation, membrane biogenesis, DNA synthesis
-A, C, E may be cytotoxic and cytostatic in certain cell system
-affect oncogenes
Poppel, GV, et al., Cancer Letters, vol.114, p.195, 1997
-immune stimulation
-enhancement of cell to cell communication, defuse carcinogens, etc.

40% OF CANCER PATIENTS DIE FROM MALNUTRITION

A position paper from the American College of Physicians published in 1989 basically stated that total parenteral nutrition (TPN) had no benefit on the outcome of cancer patients.[15] Unfortunately, this article excluded malnourished patients, which is bizarre, since TPN only treats malnutrition, not cancer.[16] Most of the scientific literature shows that weight loss drastically increases the mortality rate for most types of cancer, while also lowering the response to chemotherapy.[17] Chemo and radiation therapy are sufficient biological stressors alone to induce malnutrition.[18]

In the early years of oncology, it was thought that one could starve the tumor out of the host. Pure malnutrition (cachexia) is responsible for somewhere between 22% and 67% of all cancer deaths. Up to 80% of all cancer patients have reduced levels of serum albumin, which is a leading indicator of protein and calorie malnutrition.[19] Dietary protein restriction in the cancer patient does not affect the composition or growth rate of the tumor, but does restrict the patient's well being.[20]

Parenteral feeding improves tolerance to chemotherapeutic agents and immune responses.[21] Malnourished cancer patients who were provided TPN had a mortality rate of 11%, while a comparable group without TPN feeding had a 100% mortality rate.[22] Pre-operative TPN in patients undergoing surgery for gastrointestinal cancer provided general reduction in the incidence of wound infection, pneumonia, major complications, and mortality.[23] Patients who were the most malnourished experienced a 33% mortality and 46% morbidity rate, while those patients who were properly nourished had a 3% mortality rate with an 8% morbidity rate.

In 20 adult hospitalized patients on TPN, the mean daily vitamin C needs were 975 mg, which is over 16 times the RDA, with the range being 350-2,250 mg.[24] Of the 139 lung cancer patients studied, most tested deficient or scorbutic (clinical vitamin C deficiency).[25] Another study of cancer patients found that 46% tested scorbutic, while 76% were below acceptable levels for serum ascorbate.[26] Experts now recommend the value of nutritional supplements, especially in patients who require prolonged TPN support.[27]

WHY USE NUTRITION IN CANCER TREATMENT?

1) Avoiding malnutrition

40% or more of cancer patients actually die from malnutrition, not from the cancer.[28] Nutrition therapy is essential to arrest malnutrition. Among the more effective non-nutritional approaches to reverse cancer cachexia is hydrazine sulfate. Hydrazine sulfate is a relatively non-toxic drug that shuts down energy metabolism in cancer cells. Hydrazine is available through BioTech Labs (800-345-1199) or Great Lakes Metabolics (507-288-2348) or Life Support (209-529-4697) or Life Energy (Vancouver 604-856-0171). Protocol is to take 60 mg capsules: first 3 days 1 cap at brk, day 4-6 take 1 cap at brk and supper, day 7-45 take 3 caps TID (3x/day), off for 1 wk; contraindications are like those of an MAO inhibitor: no aged cheese, yogurt, brewer's yeast, raisins, sausage (tyramine content), excessive B-6, or overripe bananas. See the chapter on malnutrition for more information.

2) Reducing the toxic effects of chemo & radiation

Properly nourished patients experience less nausea, malaise, immune suppression, hair loss, and organ toxicity than patients on routine oncology programs. Antioxidants like beta carotene, vitamin C, vitamin E, and selenium appear to enhance the effectiveness of chemo, radiation, and hyperthermia, while minimizing damage to the patient's normal cells, thus making therapy more of a "selective toxin." An optimally-nourished cancer patient can better tolerate the rigors of cytotoxic therapy. More on this subject is in chapter 9.

3) Bolster immune functions

When the doctor says "We think we got it all", what he or she is really saying is "We have destroyed all DETECTABLE cancer cells, and now it is up to your immune system to find and destroy the cancer cells that inevitably remain in your body." A billion cancer cells are about the size of the page number at the

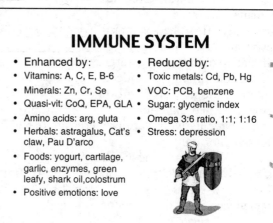

IMMUNE SYSTEM

- Enhanced by:
- Vitamins: A, C, E, B-6
- Minerals: Zn, Cr, Se
- Quasi-vit: CoQ, EPA, GLA
- Amino acids: arg, gluta
- Herbals: astragalus, Cat's claw, Pau D'arco
- Foods: yogurt, cartilage, garlic, enzymes, green leafy, shark oil,colostrum
- Positive emotions: love

- Reduced by:
- Toxic metals: Cd, Pb, Hg
- VOC: PCB, benzene
- Sugar: glycemic index
- Omega 3:6 ratio, 1:1; 1:16
- Stress: depression

top of this page. We must rely on the capabilities of the 20 trillion cells that compose an intact immune system to destroy the undetectable cancer cells that remain after medical therapy. There is an abundance of data linking nutrient intake to the quality and quantity of immune factors that fight cancer.[29] See the chapter on immune functions and nutrition.

4) Sugar feeds cancer

Tumors are primarily obligate glucose metabolizers, meaning "sugar feeders".[30] Americans not only consume about 20% of their calories from refined sucrose, but often manifest poor glucose tolerance curves, due to stress, obesity, low chromium and fiber intake, and sedentary lifestyles. More on this subject is in the chapter on "starving the cancer by controlling blood glucose levels".

5) Anti-proliferative factors

Certain nutrients, like selenium, vitamin K, vitamin E succinate, and the fatty acid EPA, appear to have the ability to slow down the unregulated growth of cancer. Various nutrition factors, including vitamin A, D, folacin, bioflavonoids, and soybeans, have been shown to alter the genetic expression of tumors. More on this subject is in chapter 1 "You have already beaten cancer".

PUTTING IT ALL TOGETHER

Finnish oncologists used high doses of nutrients along with chemo and radiation for lung cancer patients. Normally, lung cancer is a "poor prognostic" malignancy, with a 1% expected survival at 30 months under normal treatment.. In this study, however, 8 of 18 patients (44%) were still alive 6 years after therapy.[31]

In a non-randomized clinical trial, Drs. Hoffer and Pauling instructed patients to follow a reasonable cancer diet (unprocessed food low in fat, dairy, and sugar),
coupled with therapeutic

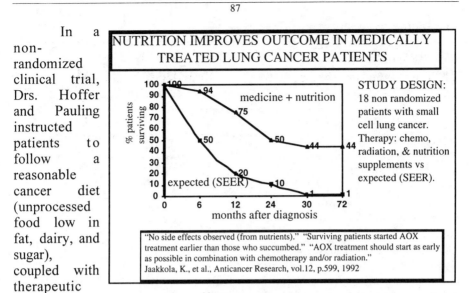

NUTRITION IMPROVES OUTCOME IN MEDICALLY TREATED LUNG CANCER PATIENTS

STUDY DESIGN: 18 non randomized patients with small cell lung cancer. Therapy: chemo, radiation, & nutrition supplements vs expected (SEER).

"No side effects observed (from nutrients)." "Surviving patients started AOX treatment earlier than those who succumbed." "AOX treatment should start as early as possible in combination with chemotherapy and/or radiation." Jaakkola, K., et al., Anticancer Research, vol.12, p.599, 1992

doses of vitamins and minerals.[32] All 129 patients in this study received concomitant oncology care. The control group of 31 patients who did not receive nutrition support lived an average of less than 6 months. The group of 98 cancer patients who did receive the diet and supplement program were categorized into 3 groups:

-Poor responders (n=19) or 20% of treated group. Average lifespan of 10 months, or a 75% improvement over the control group.

-Good responders (n=47), who had various cancers, including leukemia, lung, liver, and pancreas; had an average lifespan of 72 months (6 years) or a 1,200% improvement in lifespan.

-Good female responders (n=32), with involvement of reproductive areas (breast, cervix, ovary, uterus); had

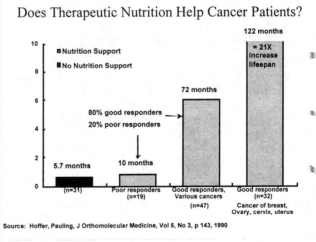

Does Therapeutic Nutrition Help Cancer Patients?

Source: Hoffer, Pauling, J Orthomolecular Medicine, Vol 5, No 3, p 143, 1990

an average lifespan of over 10 years, or a 2,100% improvement in lifespan. Many were still alive at the end of the study.

Oncologists at West Virginia Medical School randomized 65 patients with transitional cell carcinoma of the bladder into either the "one-per-day" vitamin supplement providing the RDA, or into a group which received the RDA supplement plus 40,000 iu of vitamin A, 100 mg of B-6, 2,000 mg of vitamin C, 400 iu of vitamin E, and 90 mg of zinc. At 10 months, tumor recurrence was 80% in the control group (RDA supplement) and

CAN THERAPEUTIC NUTRITION LOWER TUMOR RECURRENCE?

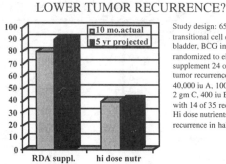

Study design: 65 patients w. transitional cell carcinoma of bladder, BCG immune tx, randomized to either RDA supplement 24 of 30 with tumor recurrence) or RDA + 40,000 iu A, 100 mg B-6, 2 gm C, 400 iu E, 90 mg Zn with 14 of 35 recurrence. Hi dose nutrients cut tumor recurrence in half

% of bladder cancer patients with tumor recurrence
source: Lamm, DL, J.Urol.,151, 21, Jan.1994

40% in the experimental "megavitamin" group. Five year projected tumor recurrence was 91% for controls and 41% for "megavitamin" patients. Essentially, high dose nutrients cut tumor recurrence in half.[33]

Of the 200 cancer patients studied who experienced "spontaneous" regression", 87% made a major change in diet, mostly vegetarian in nature, 55% used some form of detoxification, and 65% used nutritional supplements.[34]

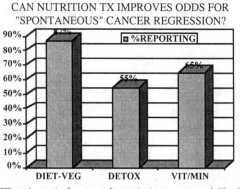

CAN NUTRITION TX IMPROVES ODDS FOR "SPONTANEOUS" CANCER REGRESSION?

Of 200 people reporting "spontaneous" regression in cancer, most made lifestyle changes. Source: Foster,HD, Int.J.Biosocial Res., 10, 1, 17, 1988

Researchers at Tulane University compared survival in patients who used the macrobiotic diet versus patients who continued with their standard Western lifestyle. Of 1,467 pancreatic cancer patients who made no changes in diet, 146 (1%) were alive after one year, while 12 of the 23 matched pancreatic cancer patients (52%) consuming macrobiotic foods were still alive after one year.[35] In examining the diet and lifespan of 675 lung cancer patients over the course of 6 years, researchers found that the more vegetables consumed, the longer the lung cancer patient lived.[36] By adding an aggressive nutrition component to your comprehensive cancer treatment program, you improve the odds for a complete remission/regression and probably add significantly to quality and quantity of life.

NUTRITIONAL ONCOLOGY PROGRAM SHOULD INCLUDE:

1) Food. If the gut works and if the patient can consume enough food through the mouth, then this is the primary route for nourishing the patient. The diet for the cancer patient should be high in plant food (grains, legumes, colorful vegetables, some fruit), unprocessed (shop the perimeter of the grocery store), low in salt, fat, and sugar, with adequate protein (1-2 grams/kilogram body weight).

2) Supplements. Additional vitamins, minerals, amino acids, food extracts (i.e. bovine cartilage), conditionally essential nutrients (i.e. fish, flax, and borage oil; coenzyme Q-10), and botanicals (i.e. echinacea, goldenseal, astragalus) can enhance the patient's recuperative powers.

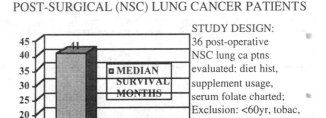

CAN NUTRIENTS EXTEND LIFESPAN IN POST-SURGICAL (NSC) LUNG CANCER PATIENTS

STUDY DESIGN: 36 post-operative NSC lung ca ptns evaluated: diet hist, supplement usage, serum folate charted; Exclusion: <60yr, tobac, alcohol (>2/d),folate antagonists. RESULTS: "Patients (19) took vitamin supplements more likely to be long term survivors." p=.002

Source: Jatoi, A, et al., J.Surg.Oncol., vol.68, no.4, p.231, 1998

3) Total parenteral nutrition (TPN). There are many cancer patients who are so malnourished (weight loss of 10% below usual body weight within a 1 month period and/or serum albumin below 2.5 mg/dl) that we must interrupt this deterioration with TPN. When the patient cannot or will not eat adequately, TPN can be an invaluable life raft during crucial phases of cancer treatment.

4) Assessment. Means of assessment include: health history form to detect lifestyle risk factors; physician's examination; anthropometric measurements of height, weight, and percent body fat; calorimeter measurement of basal metabolic needs; p and various other laboratory tests.

5) Education. A pro-active patient can help reverse the underlying causative factors of cancer.

6) Research. Those who advance the knowledge base have a responsibility to properly gather data and report their findings to the world.

PATIENT PROFILE: SHRINKING LUNG CANCER

C.G. was diagnosed with non-small cell lung cancer stage 3. The tumor was about the size of a tennis ball. C.G. began using the principles in this book along with chemo and radiation. Originally, his doctor gave him 6 months to live. That was 2 years ago. The tumor is now the size of a small marble and shrinking with each chest X ray and CT scan. Doctor said "I don't know what you are doing, but keep doing it." C.G. says "Thank you for writing your book. So far, you have saved my life."

ENDNOTES

[1]. Meydani, SN, et al, Vitamin supplementation enhances cell-mediated immunity in healthy elderly subjects, Am J Clin Nutr, 52,557-63, 1990

[2]. Enstrom, JE, et al., Vitamin C intake and mortality, Epidem, 3, 3:194-6, 1992

[3]. Bendich, A, et al., Dietary vitamin E requirement for optimum immune response in the rat, J Nutr;116:675-681, 1986

[4]. Singh, VN, Am.J.Clin.Nutr., vol.53, p.386S, 1991

[5]. Heimburger, DC, JAMA, vol.259, no.10, p.1525, Mar.11, 1988

[6]. Toma, S., Oncology, vol.49, p.77, 1992

[7]. Stich, HF, Am.J.Clin.Nutr., vol.53, p.298S, 1991

[8]. Benner, SE, J.National Cancer Institute, vol.85, no.1, p.44, Jan.1993

[9]. Toma, S., Cancer Detection & Prevention, vol.15, no.6, p.491, 1991

[10] DeCosse, JJ, Surgery, vol.78, no.5, p.608, Nov.1975

[11]. Wargovich, MJ, et al., Gastroenterology, vol.103, p.92, 1992; see also Steinbach, G., Gastroenterology, vol.106, p.1162, 1994

[12]. Paganelli, GM, J. National Cancer Institute, vol.84,no.1, p.47, Jan.1992

[13]. Krieger, N, American J. Epidemiology, vol.135, no.6, p.619, 1992; see also London, SJ, JAMA, vol.267, no.7, p.941, Feb.1992

[14]. Shklar, G., Nutr Cancer, vol.12, p.321, 1989

[15]. Meta-analysis of survival in cancer patients using TPN, Ann Intern Med, 110, 9, 735-7, May 1989

[16]. Kaminsky, M. (ed.), Hyperalimentation: a Guide , Marcel Dekker, NY, Oct.1985, p.265

[17]. Dewys, WD, et al., Cachexia and cancer treatment, Amer J Med, 69, 491-5, Oct.1980

[18]. Wilmore, DW, Catabolic illness, strategies for recovery, N Engl J Med, 1991, 325:10:695-702

[19]. Dreizen, S., et al., Malnutrition in cancer, Postgrad Med, 87, 1, 163-7, Jan.1990

[20]. Lowry, SF, et al., Nutrient restriction in cancer patients, Surg Forum, 28, 143-9, 1977

[21]. Eys, JV, Total parenteral nutrition and response to cytotoxic therapies, Cancer, 43, 2030-7, 1979

[22]. Harvey, KB, et al., Morbidity in parenterally-nourished cancer patients, Cancer, 43, 2065-9, 1979

[23]. Muller, JM, et al., Nutritional status as a factor in GI cancer morbidity, Lancet, 68-73, Jan.9, 1982

[24]. Abrahamian, V., et al., Ascorbic acid requirements in hospital patients, JPEN, 7, 5, 465-8, 1983

[25]. Anthony, HM, et al., Vitamin C status of lung cancer patients, Brit J Ca, 46, 354-9, 1982

[26]. Cheraskin, E., Scurvy in cancer patients?, J Altern Med, 18-23, Feb.1986

[27]. Hoffman, FA, Micronutrient status of cancer patients, Cancer, 55, 1 sup.1, 295-9, Jan.1, 1985

[28]. Grant, JP, Nutrition, 6, 4, 6S, July 1990 suppl

[29]. Bendich, A, Chandra, RK (eds), Micronutrients and Immune Function, New York Academy of Sciences, 1990, p.587

[30]. Rothkopf, M, Fuel utilization in neoplastic disease: implications for the use of nutritional support in cancer patients, Nutrition, supp, 6:4:14-16S, 1990

[31]. Jaakkola, K., et al., Treatment with antioxidant and other nutrients in combination with chemotherapy and irradiation in patients with lung cancer, Anticancer Res 12,599-606, 1992

[32]. Hoffer, A, Pauling, L, J Orthomolecular Med, 5:3:143-154, 1990

[33]. Lamm, DL, et al., Megadose vitamin in bladder cancer, J Urol, 151:21-26, 1994

[34]. Foster, HD, Lifestyle influences on cancer regression, Int J Biosoc Res, 10:1:17-20, 1988

[35]. Carter, JP, Macrobiotic diet and cancer survival, J Amer Coll Nutr, 12:3:209-215, 1993

[36]. Goodman, MT, Vegetable consumption in lung cancer longevity, Eur J Ca, 28: 2: 495-499, 1992

CHAPTER 8

MALNUTRITION AMONG CANCER PATIENTS

✦

"Each patient carries his own doctor inside him. We are at our best when we give the doctor who resides within a chance to go to work."
Albert Schweitzer, MD, 1940, Nobel Laureate & medical missionary

---

WHAT'S AHEAD?

↪ At least 20% of Americans are clinically malnourished, with 70% being sub-clinically malnourished (less obvious), and the remaining "chosen few" 10% in good to optimal health.

↪ Once these malnourished people get sick, the malnutrition oftentimes gets worse through higher nutrient needs and lower intake

↪ Once at the hospital, malnutrition escalates another notch

↪ Cancer is one of the more serious wasting diseases known

↪ A malnourished cancer patient suffers a reduction in quality and quantity of life, with higher incidences of complications and death

↪ The only solution for malnutrition is optimal nutrition

Howard Hughes, the multi-billionaire, died of malnutrition. It is hard to believe that there can be malnutrition in this agriculturally abundant nation of ours--but there is. At the time of the Revolutionary War, 96% of Americans farmed while only 4% worked at other trades. Tractors and harvesting combines became part of an agricultural revolution that allowed the 2% of Americans who now farm to feed the rest of us. We grow enough food in this country to feed ourselves, to make half of us overweight, to throw away enough food to feed 50 million people daily, to ship food overseas as a major export, and to store enough food in government surplus bins to feed Americans for a year if all farmers quit today. With so much food available, how can Americans be malnourished?

The answer is: poor food choices. Americans choose their food based upon taste, cost, convenience, and psychological gratification--thus ignoring the main reason that we eat, which is to provide our body cells with the raw materials to grow, repair, and fuel our bodies. The most commonly eaten foods in America are white bread, coffee, and hot dogs. Based upon our food abundance, Americans could be the best nourished nation on record. But we are far from it.

MALNUTRITION
in the typical healthy American

average annual consumption of low nutrient foods:

756 doughnuts
60 pound cakes & cookies
23 gallons of ice cream
7 pounds potato chips
22 pounds candy
200 sticks gum
365 cans soft drinks
90 pounds fat
140 pounds sugar

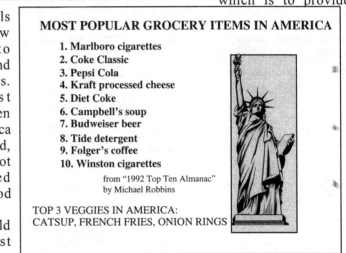

MOST POPULAR GROCERY ITEMS IN AMERICA

1. **Marlboro cigarettes**
2. **Coke Classic**
3. **Pepsi Cola**
4. **Kraft processed cheese**
5. **Diet Coke**
6. **Campbell's soup**
7. **Budweiser beer**
8. **Tide detergent**
9. **Folger's coffee**
10. **Winston cigarettes**

from "1992 Top Ten Almanac"
by Michael Robbins

TOP 3 VEGGIES IN AMERICA:
CATSUP, FRENCH FRIES, ONION RINGS

CAUSES OF NUTRIENT DEFICIENCIES:

There are many reasons for developing malnutrition:

⇒ We don't eat well due to poor food choices, loss of appetite, discomfort in the gastrointestinal region, or consuming nutritionally bankrupt "junk food"; many people just don't get enough nutrients into their stomachs.

⇒ We don't absorb nutrients due to loss of digestive functions (including low hydrochloric acid or enzyme output), allergy, "leaky gut", or intestinal infections, like yeast overgrowth.

⇒ We don't keep enough nutrients due to increased excretion or loss of nutrients because of diarrhea, vomiting, or drug interactions.

⇒ We don't get enough nutrients due to increased requirements caused by fever, disease, alcohol, or drug interactions.

Anyone who is confused about why we spend so much on medical care with such poor results in cancer treatment might glean some wisdom by reading what sells best in American grocery stores. Overwhelming evidence from both government and independent scientific surveys shows that many Americans are low in their intake of:[1]

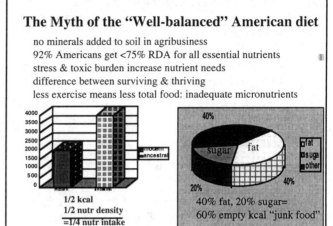

The Myth of the "Well-balanced" American diet

no minerals added to soil in agribusiness
92% Americans get <75% RDA for all essential nutrients
stress & toxic burden increase nutrient needs
difference between surviving & thriving
less exercise means less total food: inadequate micronutrients

1/2 kcal
1/2 nutr density
=1/4 nutr intake

40% fat, 20% sugar=
60% empty kcal "junk food"

-VITAMINS: A, D, E, C, B-6, riboflavin, folacin, pantothenic acid

-MINERALS: calcium, potassium, magnesium, zinc, iron, chromium, selenium; and possibly molybdenum and vanadium. With many common micronutrient deficiencies in the Western diet, it makes sense that a major study in Australia found that regular use of vitamin supplements was a protective factor against colon cancer.[2]

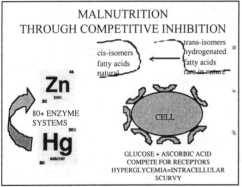

MALNUTRITION
THROUGH COMPETITIVE INHIBITION

trans-isomers
hydrogenated
fatty acids
rare in nature

cis-isomers
fatty acids
natural

Zn

80+ ENZYME
SYSTEMS

CELL

Hg

GLUCOSE + ASCORBIC ACID
COMPETE FOR RECEPTORS
HYPERGLYCEMIA=INTRACELLULAR
SCURVY

-MACRONUTRIENTS: fiber, complex carbohydrates, plant protein, special fatty acids (EPA, GLA, ALA), clean water

Meanwhile, we also eat alarmingly high amounts of: fat, salt, sugar, cholesterol, alcohol, caffeine, food additives, and toxins.

This combination of too much of the wrong things along with not enough of the right things has created epidemic proportions of degenerative diseases in this country. The Surgeon General, Department of Health and Human Services, Center for Disease Control, National Academy of Sciences, American Medical Association, American Dietetic Assocation, and most other major public health agencies agree that diet is a major contributor to our most common health problems, including cancer.

The typical diet of the cancer patient is high in fat, while being low in fiber and vegetables--"meat, potatoes, and gravy" is what many of my patients lived on. Data collected by the United States Department of Agriculture from over 11,000 Americans showed that on any given day:

-41% did not eat any fruit
-82% did not eat cruciferous vegetables
-72% did not eat vitamin C-rich fruits or vegetables
-80% did not eat vitamin A-rich fruits or vegetables

% OF AMERICANS NOT EATING THE RDA
Recommended Dietary Allowance=92%

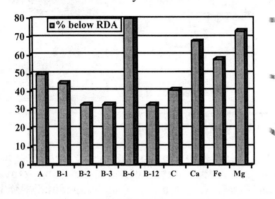

-84% did not eat high fiber grain food, like bread or cereal[3]

The human body is incredibly resilient, which sometimes works to our disadvantage. No one dies on the first cigarette inhaled, or the first drunken evening, or the first decade of unhealthy eating. We misconstrue the fact that we survived this ordeal to mean we can do it forever. Not so. Malnutrition can be as blatant as the starving babies in third world countries, but malnutrition can also be much more subtle.

SEQUENCE IN DEVELOPING NUTRIENT DEFICIENCY

⇒ 1) *Preliminary.* Reduction of tissue stores and depression of urinary excretion.

⇒ 2) *Biochemical.* Reduction of enzyme activity due to insufficient coenzymes (vitamins). Urinary excretion at minimum levels.

⇒ 3) *Physiological.* Behavioral effects, such as insomnia or somnolence. Irritability accompanied by loss of appetite and reduced body weight. Modified drug metabolism and reduced immune capabilities.

⇒ 4) *Clinical.* Classical deficiency syndromes as recognized by the scientific pioneers in the developmental phases of nutrition science.

⇒ 5) *Terminal.* Severe tissue pathology resulting in imminent death.

It was the Framingham study done by Harvard University that proclaimed: "Our way of life is related to our way of death." Typical hospital food continues or even worsens malnutrition. While many Americans are overfed, the majority are also poorly nourished. If proper nutrition could prevent from 30 to 90% of all cancer, then doesn't it seem foolish to continue feeding the cancer patient the same diet that helped to induce cancer in the first place?

MALNUTRITION AMONG CANCER PATIENTS

From 25-50% of hospital patients suffer from protein calorie malnutrition. Protein calorie malnutrition leads to increases in mortality and surgical failure, with a reduction in immunity, wound healing, cardiac output, response to chemo and radiation therapy, and plasma protein synthesis, and generally induces weakness and apathy. Many patients are malnourished before entering the hospital, and another 10% become malnourished once in the hospital. Nutrition support, as peripheral parenteral nutrition, has been shown to reduce the length of hospital stay by 30%. Weight loss leads to a decrease in patient survival. Common nutrient deficiencies, as determined by experts at M.D. Anderson Hospital in Houston, include protein calorie, thiamin, riboflavin, niacin, folate, and K.

So nutrition therapy has two distinct phases

1) Take the clinically malnourished patient and bring him/her up to "normal" status.

2) Take the "normal" sub-clinically malnourished person and bring him/her up to "optimal" functioning. For at least the few nutrients tested thus far, there appears to be a "dose-dependent" response--more than RDA levels of intake provide for more than "normal" immune functions.

Not only is malnutrition common in the "normal" American, but malnutrition is extremely common in the cancer patient. A theory has persisted for decades that one could starve the tumor out of the host. That just ain't so. The tumor is quite resistant to starvation, and most studies find

MALNUTRITION KILLS >40% OF CANCER PATIENTS
REDUCED NUTRIENT INTAKE:
loss of appetite (anorexia), chemo, disease, stress
maldigestion, chemo, disease, stress
ELEVATED NUTRIENT NEEDS
hypermetabolic state
squandering calories via anaerobic glycolysis
needs in fighting disease; host defense mechanisms
AS DETECTED BY
Subjective Global Assessment score "C"
rapid weight loss, >10% loss in 6 mo, 5% 1 mo.
bio-impedance (BCA), lean body mass< ideal
TREATMENT
dietary intervention; foods, Dragonslayer shake
metabolic support: TPN/TNA, enteral, G-tube
enzymes, anabolic hormones, hydrazine sulfate

more harm to the host than to the tumor in either selective or blanket nutrient deficiencies.[4] Pure malnutrition (cachexia) is responsible for at least 22%

and up to 67% of all cancer deaths. Up to 80% of all cancer patients have reduced levels of serum albumin, which is a leading indicator of protein and calorie malnutrition.[5] Dietary protein restriction in the cancer patient does not affect the composition or growth rate of the tumor, but does restrict the patient's well being.[6]

A commonly used anti-cancer drug is methotrexate, which interferes with folate (a B vitamin) metabolism. Many scientists guessed that folate in the diet might accelerate cancer growth. Not so. Depriving animals of folate in the diet allowed their tumors to grow anyway.[7] Actually, in starved animals, the tumors grew more rapidly than in fed animals, indicating the parasitic tenacity of cancer in the host.[8] Other studies have found that a low folate environment can trigger "brittle" DNA to fuel cancer metastasis.

There is some evidence that tumors are not as flexible as healthy host tissue in using fuel. A low carbohydrate parenteral formula may have the ability to slow down tumor growth by selectively starving the cancer cells.[9] Overall, the research shows that starvation provokes host wasting while tumor growth continues unabated.[10] Weight loss drastically increases the mortality rate for most types of cancer, while also lowering the response to chemotherapy.[11]

Parenteral feeding improves tolerance to chemotherapeutic agents and immune responses.[12] Of 28 children with advanced malignant disease, 18 received parenteral feeding for 28 days with resultant improvements in weight gain, increased serum albumin and transferrin, and major benefits in immune functions. In comparing cancer patients on TPN versus those trying to nourish themselves by oral intake of food, TPN provided major improvements in calorie, protein, and nutrient intake, but did not encourage tumor growth. Malnourished cancer patients who were provided TPN had a mortality rate of 11%, while the group without TPN feeding had a 100% mortality rate.[13] Pre-operative TPN in patients undergoing surgery for GI cancer provided general reduction in the incidence of wound infection, pneumonia, major complications, and mortality.[14] Patients who were the most malnourished experienced a 33% mortality and 46% morbidity (problems and illness) rate, while those patients who were properly nourished had a 3% mortality rate with an 8% morbidity rate. In 49 patients with lung cancer receiving chemotherapy with or without TPN, complete remission was achieved in 85% of the TPN group versus 59% of the non-TPN group.[15] A TPN formula that was higher in protein, especially branched chain amino acids, was able to provide better nitrogen balance in the 21 adults tested than the conventional 8.5% amino acid TPN formula.[16]

A finely-tuned nutrition formula can also nourish the patient while starving tumor cells. Enteral (oral) formulas fortified with arginine, fish oil, and RNA have been shown to stimulate the immune system, accelerate wound repair, and reduce tumor burden in both animals and humans.

In 20 adult hospitalized patients on TPN, the mean daily vitamin C needs were 975 mg, which is over 16 times the RDA, with the range being

350-2250 mg.[17] Of the 139 lung cancer patients studied, most tested deficient or scorbutic (clinical vitamin C deficiency).[18] Another study of cancer patients found that 46% tested scorbutic, while 76% were below acceptable levels for serum ascorbate.[19] Experts now recommend the value of nutritional supplements, especially in patients who require prolonged TPN support.[20] The Recommended Dietary Allowance (RDA) is inadequate for many healthy people and nearly all sick people.

PATIENT PROFILE: J.H. was a wasting 38 year old male with advanced lymphoma when he was admitted to our hospital as a medical emergency, having failed prior therapies. He was dying more from malnutrition than the cancer. We put him on total parenteral nutrition, with a disease-specific formula that is higher in protein and fats and lower in glucose than standard TPN formulas. Within a month, he was able to eat solid foods. He rebounded from his malnutrition so that he could resume chemo. Within 6 months he was disease-free. Eight years later, still in remission, he attended our Celebrate Life festival and planted a tree.

ENDNOTES

[1]. Quillin, P., HEALING NUTRIENTS, p.43, Vintage Books, NY, 1989
[2]. Kune, GA, and Kune, S., Nutrition and Cancer, vol.9, p.1, 1987
[3]. Patterson, BH, and Block, G., American Journal of Public Health, vol.78, p.282, Mar.1988
[4]. Axelrod, AE, and Traketelis, AC, Vitamins and Hormones, vol.22, p.591, 1964
[5]. Dreizen, S., et al., Postgraduate Medicine, vol.87, no.1, p.163, Jan.1990
[6]. Lowry, SF, et al., Surgical Forum, vol.28, p.143, 1977
[7]. Nichol, CA, Cancer Research, vol.29, p.2422, 1969
[8]. Norton, JA, et al., Cancer, vol.45, p.2934, 1980
[9]. Dematrakopoulos, GE, and Brennan, MF, Cancer Research, (sup.),vol.42, p.756, Feb.1982
[10]. Goodgame, JT, et al., American Journal of Clinical Nutrition, vol.32, p.2277, 1979
[11]. Dewys, WD, et al., American Journal of Medicine, vol.69, p.491, Oct.1980
[12]. Eys, JV, Cancer, vol.43, p.2030, 1979
[13]. Harvey, KB, et al., Cancer, vol.43, p.2065, 1979
[14]. Muller, JM, et al., Lancet, p.68, Jan.9, 1982
[15]. Valdivieso, M., et al., Cancer Treatment Reports, vol.65, sup.5, p.145, 1981
[16]. Gazzaniga, AB, et al., Archives of Surgery, vol. 123, p.1275, 1988
[17]. Abrahamian, V., et al., Journal of Parenteral and Enteral Nutrition, vol.7, no.5, p.465, 1983
[18]. Anthony, HM, et al., British Journal of Cancer, vol.46, p.354, 1982
[19]. Cheraskin, E., Journal of Alternative Medicine, p.18, Feb.1986
[20]. Hoffman, FA, Cancer, vol.55, 1 sup.1, p.295, Jan.1, 1985

CHAPTER 9

MAKING CHEMO AND RADIATION MORE EFFECTIVE

✶

"God heals and the doctor takes the fee."   Benjamin Franklin

WHAT'S AHEAD?
Nutrients can improve cancer treatment by:
↪ protecting the patient from the damaging effects
  of chemotherapy and radiation while allowing
  these therapies to kill the tumor
↪ nutrition makes chemo and radiation therapy more of a selective
  toxin against cancer and not a general toxin upon the patient

Cancer patients often feel like a child in a wicked divorce custody battle. The oncologist tells the patient "Don't take that nutrition therapy. It is nothing more than expensive urine. And it will reduce the effectiveness of my chemo and radiation therapies." The nutritionist tells the same patient "Don't take that poisonous chemo or radiation therapy. It will do you no good." In fact, when the oncologist and nutritionist work together, both are more successful at

---

DOES NUTRITION THERAPY REDUCE THE
EFFECTIVENESS OF CHEMO OR RAD TX?
i.e. antioxidant + prooxidant = 0?

LITERATURE REVIEWS SHOWING NUTRITION MAY
HELP, BUT NEVER HINDERS CHEMO & RAD TX
Alternative Medicine Review, vol.5, no.2, p.152, 2000
J.American College of Nutrition, vol.18, no.1, p.13, 1999
J.American Nutraceutical Association, vol.4, no.1, p.11, 2001

EXPLANATION: Antioxidant nutrients are best absorbed
by aerobic (healthy) cells and poorly absorbed by anaerobic
(sick/cancerous) cells. AOX protect healthy cells, but not
cancerous cells from prooxidative therapies. Vitamin C
becomes selective anti-cancer agent as "sugar feeding" cancer
cells absorb excessive vit.C (similar to glucose in structure)
which becomes prooxidant in anaerobic environment.

helping the cancer patient. Nutrients make medical therapy more toxic to the tumor and less toxic to the patient.

Linus Pauling, PhD, earned one of his Nobel prizes in chemistry in the 1950s by discovering how atoms bond together to become molecules. Picture the sun with Earth, Saturn, and Mars among other planets orbiting around the sun. Atoms and molecules are a tiny rendition of our solar system. Electrons orbit the nucleus of an atom just like planets orbit around the sun in our solar system. Atoms

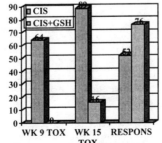

FREE RADICALS & ANTIOXIDANTS

TYPE OF RADICAL "electron thief"	ANTIOXIDANT "electron donor"
Superoxide O2	SOD, lipoic acid
Hydrogen peroxide H2O2	Catalase, glutathione peroxidase
Hydroxyl radical OH-	Vit.C, lipoic acid, melatonin
Peroxyl radical (PUFA+O2)	Vit. E, CoQ, beta carot, lycopene
Singlet oxygen O2	Lycopene, carotenes, lutein, Canthaxanthin, lipoic acid, Glutathione, vit.E
Hypochlorous radical OCl	Lipoic acid
Peroxynitrite radical ON	Lipoic acid
Ozone O3	Vit.C

Cadenas, E. et al., HANDBOOK OF ANTIOXIDANTS, Marcel Dekker, NY. 1996
Levine, SA, et al., ANTIOXIDANT ADAPTATION, Biocurrents, SF, 1985

"The amount of antioxidants that you maintain in your body is directly Proportional to how long you will live." Richard Cutler, MD, Director Anti-aging Research, National Institutes of Health

bond together, such as hydrogen with oxygen to yield water, by sharing electrons, as if two suns came close together and shared planets or moons to keep in balance and to be complete. Now imagine if a planet was missing from a solar system. There is an imbalance in forces that makes this solar system unstable. Free radicals, or pro-oxidants, are like unstable solar systems, because they lack a planet in their outer orbit. Free radicals will grab a planet from a nearby solar system to make that solar system now unstable. And on its goes in domino fashion, disrupting solar systems (or atoms and molecules) until tissue damage occurs and cancer or premature aging sets in. Though there are many variations of pro-oxidants and antioxidants (see table below), the theme is always the same: pro-oxidants can destroy tissue, while antioxidants can protect tissue.

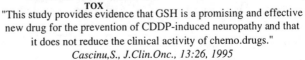

CAN GLUTATHIONE REDUCE CISPLATIN-INDUCED NEUROTOXICITY IN PATIENTS WITH GASTRIC CANCER?

STUDY DESIGN:
50 patients w. advanced gastric cancer weekly tx (CDDP) cisplatin w.glutathione (GSH) IV prior to cisplatin then IM on days 2-5 or placebo. Patients assessed at wk 9&15. GSH reduced hemotransfusion 32 vs 64 (by 50%) & TX delay 55 vs 94 weeks due to toxicity.

WK 9 TOX   WK 15   RESPONS
TOX

"This study provides evidence that GSH is a promising and effective new drug for the prevention of CDDP-induced neuropathy and that it does not reduce the clinical activity of chemo.drugs."
Cascinu,S., J.Clin.Onc., 13:26, 1995

Oxygen, hydrogen peroxide (which

we constantly create inside of our bodies as part of living), air pollution (ozone), tobacco smoke, most chemotherapy drugs, radiation therapy, and alcohol are among the more common and noteworthy free radicals in life. Chemo and radiation are free radicals that work by, hopefully, killing more cancer cells than healthy cells. We are constantly "rusting" from within, just like a nail rusts outside. We can slow down this rusting with antioxidants, such as vitamin C and lipoic acid, but we cannot stop it. Basically, free

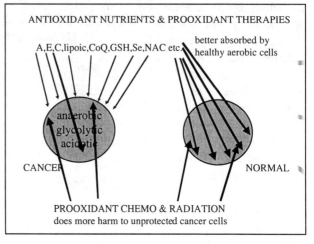

radicals are electron (planet) thieves, and antioxidants, such as vitamin C, are electron donors. Antioxidants perform like a sacrificial warrior, giving up their life so that your tissue is not harmed. However, in an anaerobic environment, such as cancer, antioxidants can become pro-oxidants. Vitamin C can become a targeted anti-cancer agent because it resembles the preferred fuel of cancer, glucose, and is absorbed in abundance. The ascorbic acid by itself in an anaerobic environment then becomes a powerful pro-oxidant and destroys the cancer cell--but only the cancer cells, since healthy cells have built-in mechanisms for absorbing the right amount of vitamin C along with the entire "symphony" of other antioxidants.

Researchers "assume" that antioxidant nutrients (such as coenzyme Q, glutathione, and vitamin E) will reduce the tumor kill rate from chemo and radiation. In simplistic chemistry, one might think this

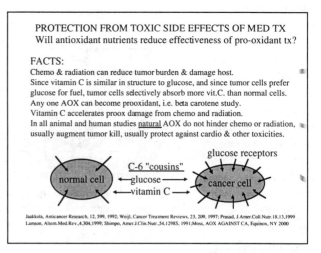

to be true. However, in test tubes (in vitro), in animals, and in human cancer patients, such is not the case. Since cancer is usually an oxygen-deprived tissue, or anaerobic cell, the cancer cell has very poor mechanisms for absorbing proper amounts of antioxidants. A cancer cell has no more use for antioxidants than a gopher needs sunglasses. The exception is vitamin C, which is remarkably similar in chemical structure to glucose, the favorite fuel for cancer cells.

Antioxidants have been shown to dramatically improve the tumor kill from pro-oxidative chemo and radiation, while protecting the host tissue from damage. Cancer cells are primarily anaerobic (meaning "without oxygen") cells. With the exception of vitamin C, cancer cells do not absorb nor use antioxidants the same way that healthy aerobic cells do. Vitamin C (ascorbic acid) is nearly identical in chemical structure to glucose, which is the favored fuel for cancer cells. When researchers found that radioactively labeled ascorbic acid was preferentially absorbed by implanted tumors in animals, they admitted that this effect takes place because cancer has many more glucose receptors

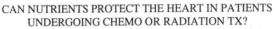

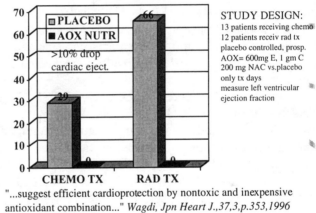

CAN NUTRIENTS PROTECT THE HEART IN PATIENTS UNDERGOING CHEMO OR RADIATION TX?

STUDY DESIGN: 13 patients receiving chemo 12 patients receiv rad tx placebo controlled, prosp. AOX= 600mg E, 1 gm C 200 mg NAC vs.placebo only tx days measure left ventricular ejection fraction

">10% drop cardiac eject."

"...suggest efficient cardioprotection by nontoxic and inexpensive antioxidant combination..." *Wagdi, Jpn Heart J.,37,3,p.353,1996*

on the cell surface than healthy normal cells. Antioxidants protect healthy tissue, but leave the cancer cells more vulnerable to the damage from chemo or radiation.

VITAMIN K. While in simplistic theory, vitamin K might inhibit the effectiveness of anticoagulant therapy (coumadin), actually vitamin K seems to augment the anti-neoplastic activity of coumadin. In a study with human rheumatoid arthritis patients being given methotrexate, folic acid supplements did not reduce the antiproliferative therapeutic value of methotrexate.[1] In one study, patients with mouth cancer who were pre-treated with injections of K-3 prior to radiation therapy doubled their odds (20% vs. 39%) for 5-year survival and disease-free status.[2] Animals with implanted tumors had greatly improved anti-cancer effects from all chemotherapy drugs tested when vitamins K and C were given in combination.[3] In cultured leukemia cells, vitamins K and E added to the chemotherapy drugs of 5FU (fluorouracil) and leucovorin provided a 300% improvement in growth inhibition when compared to 5FU by itself.[4] Animals given methotrexate and K-3 had improvements in cancer reversal, with no increase in toxicity to the host tissue.[5]

VITAMIN C. Tumor-bearing mice fed high doses of vitamin C (antioxidant) along with adriamycin (pro-oxidant) had a prolonged life and no reduction in the tumor-killing capacity of adriamycin.[6] Lung cancer patients who were provided antioxidant nutrients prior to, during, and after radiation and chemotherapy had enhanced tumor destruction and significantly longer life span.[7] Tumor-bearing mice fed high doses of vitamin C experienced an increased tolerance to radiation therapy without reduction in the tumor-killing capacity of the radiation.[8]

FISH OIL. A special fat in fish (eicosapentaenoic acid, EPA) improves tumor kill in hyperthermia and chemotherapy by altering cancer cell membranes for increased vulnerability.[9] EPA increases the ability of adriamycin to kill cultured leukemia cells.[10] Tumors in EPA-fed animals are more responsive to Mitomycin C and doxorubicin (chemo drugs).[11] EPA and another special fat from plants (gamma linolenic acid, GLA) were selectively toxic to human tumor cell lines while also enhancing the cytotoxic effects of chemotherapy.[12]

VITAMIN A & BETA-CAROTENE. There is a synergistic benefit of using vitamin A with carotenoids in patients who are being treated with chemo, radiation, and surgery for common malignancies.[13] Beta-carotene and vitamin A together provided a significant improvement in outcome in animals treated with radiation for induced cancers.[14]

VITAMIN E. Vitamin E protects the body against the potentially damaging effects of iron (pro-oxidant) and fish oil. Vitamin E deficiency, which is common in cancer patients, will accentuate the cardiotoxic effects of adriamycin.[15] The worse the vitamin E deficiency in animals, the greater the heart damage from adriamycin.[16] Patients undergoing chemo, radiation, and bone marrow transplant for cancer treatment had markedly depressed levels of serum antioxidants, including vitamin E.[17] Vitamin E protects animals against a potent carcinogen, DMBA.[18] Vitamin E supplements prevented the glucose-raising effects of a chemo drug, doxorubicin,[19] while improving the tumor-kill rate of doxorubicin.[20] Vitamin E modifies the carcinogenic effect of daunomycin (chemo drug) in animals.[21] One study found that vitamin E supplements (300 mg/day) could reduce the neurotoxicity commonly caused by cisplatin (a chemo drug) from 86% of patients getting the placebo and cisplatin down to 31% of the patients getting vitamin E and cisplatin, which is a 55% reduction in tingling and painful nerves. There was no loss in tumor kill rate from the cisplatin.

CAN VITAMIN E REDUCE NEUROTOXICITY FROM CISPLATIN?

STUDY DESIGN:
27 patients given 6 cycles
of >300 mg/m2 cisplatin.
14 received chemo alone.
13 received chemo + E
(300 mg/d) during tx +
3 months following tx.

incidence of neurotoxicity

Pace, A., J.Clin.Oncology, vol.21, no.5, p.927, Mar.2003

NIACIN. Niacin supplements in animals were able to reduce the cardiotoxicity of adriamycin while not interfering with its tumor-killing capacity.[22] Niacin combined with aspirin in 106 bladder cancer patients receiving surgery and radiation therapy provided for a substantial improvement in 5-year survival (72% vs. 27%) over the control group.[23] Niacin seems to make radiation therapy more effective at killing hypoxic cancer cells.[24] Loading radiation patients with 500 mg to 6,000 mg of niacin has been shown to be safe and is one of the most effective agents known to eliminate acute hypoxia in solid malignancies.[25]

SELENIUM. Selenium-deficient animals have more heart damage from the chemo drug, adriamycin.[26] Supplements of selenium and vitamin E in humans did not reduce the efficacy of the chemo drugs against ovarian and cervical cancer.[27]   Animals with implanted tumors who were then treated with selenium and cisplatin (chemo drug) had reduced toxicity to the drug with no change in anti-cancer activity.[28] Selenium supplements helped repair DNA damage from a carcinogen in animals.[29] Selenium was selectively toxic to human leukemia cells in culture.[30]

CARNITINE. Carnitine may help the cancer patient by protecting the heart against the damaging effects of adriamycin.[31]

QUERCETIN.   Quercetin reduces the toxicity and carcinogenic capacity of substances in the body[32], yet at the same time may enhance the tumor-killing capacity of cisplatin.[33] Quercetin significantly increased the tumor-kill rate of hyperthermia (heat therapy) in cultured cancer cells.[34]

GINSENG. Panax ginseng was able to enhance the uptake of mitomycin (an antibiotic and anti-cancer drug) into the cancer cells for increased tumor kill.[35]

PATIENT PROFILE: REVERSING PRE-CANCER OF CERVIX
M.M. was a 46 year old female with excessive pain and discharge in the vaginal region. Metrogel and Diflucan were prescribed with no improvement. Gynecologist scheduled cryosurgery (removal) of entire cervix due to benign tumor (leiomyoma). M.M. followed principles in this book along with colloidal silver-soaked tampon inserted twice daily. All inflammation and discharge cleared up within one week. Ultrasound showed decrease in leiomyoma. Doctor states "no surgery warranted at present."

ENDNOTES

[1]. Leeb, BF, Clin.Exper.Rheum, 13,459,1995
[2]. Krishanamurthi, S., et al., Radiology, vol.99, p.409, 1971
[3]. Taper, HS, et al., Int.J.Cancer, vol.40, p.575, 1987
[4]. Waxman, S., et al., Eur.J.Cancer Clin.Oncol., vol.18, p.685, 1982
[5]. Gold, J., Cancer Treatment Reports, vol.70, p.1433, Dec.1986
[6]. Shimpo,K, Am.J.Clin.Nutr.54,1298S,1991
[7]. Jaakkola, K. Anticancer Res., 12, 599, 1992
[8]. Okunieff, P, Am.J.Clin.Nutr.54, 1281S, 1991
[9]. Burns, CP, et al., Nutrition Reviews, vol.48, p.233, June 1990
[10]. Guffy, MM, et al., Cancer Research, vol.44, p.1863, 1984
[11]. Cannizzo, F., et al., Cancer Research, vol.49, p.3961, 1981
[12]. Begin, ME, et al., J.Nat.Cancer Inst., vol.77, p.1053, 1986
[13]. Santamaria, L., et al., Nutrients and Cancer Prevention, p.299, Prasad, Humana Press, 1990
[14]. Seifter, E., et al., J.Nat.Cancer Inst., vol.71, p.409, 1983
[15]. Singal, PK, et al., Mol.Cell.Biochem., vol.84, p.163, 1988
[16]. Singal, PK, et al., Molecular Cellular Biochem., vol.84, p.163, 1988
[17]. Clemens, MR, et al., Am.J.Clin.Nutr., vol.51, p.216, 1990
[18]. Shklar, G., et al., J.Oral Pathol.Med., vol.19, p.60, 1990
[19]. Geetha, A., et al., J.Biosci., vol.14, p.243, 1989
[20]. Geetha, A., et al., Current Science, vol.64, p.318, Mar.1993
[21]. Wang, YM, Molecular Inter Nutr.Cancer, p.369, , Arnott, MS, (eds), Raven Press, NY, 1982
[22]. Schmitt-Graff, A., et al, Pathol.Res.Pract., vol.181, p.168, 1986
[23]. Popov, AI, Med.Radiol. Mosk., vol.32, p.42, 1987
[24]. Kjellen, E., et al., Radiother.Oncol., vol.22, p.81, 1991
[25]. Horsman, MR, Radiotherapy Oncology, vol.22, p.79, 1991
[26]. Coudray, C., et al., Basic Res.Cardiol., vol.87, p.173, 1992
[27]. Sundstrom, H., et al., Carcinogenesis, vol.10, p.273, 1989
[28]. Ohkawa, K., et al., Br.J.Cancer, vol.58, p.38, 1988
[29]. Lawson, T., et al.,Chem.Biol.Interactions, vol.45, p.95, 1983
[30]. Milner, JA, et al., Cancer Research, vol.41, p.1652, 1981
[31]. Furitano, G, et al., Drugs Exp.Clin.Res., vol.10, p.107, 1984
[32]. Wood, AW, in PLANT FLAVONOIDS IN BIOLOGY, p.197, Cody, V. (eds), Liss, NY, 1986
[33]. Scambia, G., et al., Anticancer Drugs, vol.1, p.45, 1990
[34]. Kim, JH, et al., Cancer Research, vol.44, p.102, Jan.1984
[35]. Kubo, M., et al., Planta Med, vol.58, p.424, 1992

CHAPTER 10

NUTRITION THERAPY IMPROVES IMMUNE FUNCTIONS

✷

"Every cell in your body is eavesdropping on your thoughts."
Deepak Chopra, MD

WHAT'S AHEAD?
Your immune system consists of 20 trillion specialized "warrior" cells in your body that are responsible for killing lethal invaders, such as cancer, yeast, bacteria, and virus. Breakdown in the immune system is at least partly responsible for cancer taking over a human body. There are many ways to get your immune system working:

→ protein, calories, vitamins, minerals, amino acids, food extracts, fatty acids, and other nutrition components feed the immune system
→ certain nutrition factors, such as enzymes, colostrum, cartilage, and medicinal mushrooms can help your immune system better recognize the cancer
→ toxins and stress shut down the immune system
→ sugar slows the immune system to a crawl

Imagine being a special forces cop in downtown New York City. There are millions of people of all different sizes, shapes, colors, languages, manner of dress, and movement. Most are good people. Some are bad people. Some are terrorists with very evil intentions. Your job is to find the bad guys and get rid of them. No easy chore. That is what your immune system is trying to do in your body: recognize self from non-self. Good guys from bad guys. Workers from traitors. You have trillions of cells in your body of many different sizes, shapes, and various functions. Most are cooperative cells. Some are defective cells. A few are cancerous and could take over the body. Your immune system's job is to eliminate cancer.

IMMUNOLOGY 101A

function: recognize self from non-self
major histocompatibility complex (MHC) or
human leukocyte antigen (HLA in humans)
IMMUNE SURVEILLANCE IS CRITICAL

destruction via: phagocytosis
oxidative burst, membrane pen
enzymatic breakdown

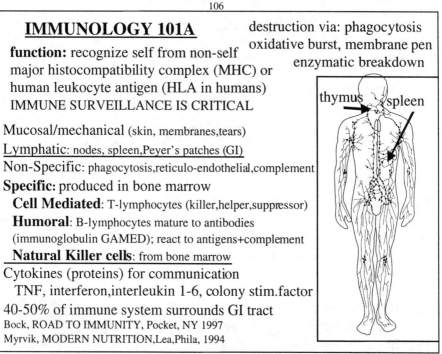

thymus   spleen

Mucosal/mechanical (skin, membranes,tears)
Lymphatic: nodes, spleen,Peyer's patches (GI)
Non-Specific: phagocytosis,reticulo-endothelial,complement
Specific: produced in bone marrow
  Cell Mediated: T-lymphocytes (killer,helper,suppressor)
  Humoral: B-lymphocytes mature to antibodies
  (immunoglobulin GAMED); react to antigens+complement
  Natural Killer cells: from bone marrow
Cytokines (proteins) for communication
  TNF, interferon,interleukin 1-6, colony stim.factor
40-50% of immune system surrounds GI tract
Bock, ROAD TO IMMUNITY, Pocket, NY 1997
Myrvik, MODERN NUTRITION,Lea,Phila, 1994

When the doctor says "We think we got it all," what he or she is really saying is "We have destroyed all DETECTABLE cancer cells, and now it is up to your immune system to find and destroy the cancer cells that inevitably remain in your body." A billion cancer cells are about the size of the page number at the top of this page. We must rely on the capabilities of the 20 trillion cells that compose an intact immune system to destroy the undetectable cancer cells that remain after medical therapy. There is an abundance of data linking nutrient intake to the quality and quantity of immune factors that fight cancer.[1]

The immune system of Americans is under serious attack by the forces of malnutrition, toxins, and stress. Cancer, drug-resistant infections, and auto-immune diseases (like arthritis and lupus) all conspire to make us sicker.

We have an extensive network of protective factors that circulate throughout our bodies to kill any bacteria, virus, yeast, or cancer cells. Think of these 20 trillion immune cells as both your Department of Defense and your waste disposal company. The immune system of the average American is "running on empty". Causes for this problem include toxic burden, stress, no exercise, poor diet, unbridled use of antibiotics and vaccinations, innoculations from world travelers, and less breast feeding.

Most experts now agree to the "surveillance" theory of cancer. Cells in your body are duplicating all day every day at a blinding pace. This process of growth is fraught with peril. When cells are not copied exactly as they should be, then an emergency call goes out to the immune system to find and destroy this abnormal saboteur cell. This process occurs frequently in most people throughout their lives. Fortunately, only 42% of Americans will actually develop detectable cancer, yet most experts agree that everyone gets cancer about six times per lifetime with one cancer cell sprouting up in everyone each day. It is the surveillance of an alert and capable immune system that defends most of us from cancer.

A healthy adult body includes around 60 trillion cells, of which nearly a third, or 20 trillion cells, are immune factors. Among the primary aspects of the immune system are:

⇒ **Birth place.** The bone marrow generates most immune cells, primarily in the long bones, especially the ribs.

⇒ **Maturation.** Bone immune cells (B-cells) move into the thymus gland for maturation and activation, and are then called "T" cells.

⇒ **Gastrointestinal (GI) tract.** 40% of the immune system surrounds the GI tract as lymph nodes, not only to absorb fat soluble nutrients (like essential fatty acids) and to protect against bacterial translocation (crossing of the intestinal barrier into the bloodstream by disease-causing bacteria), but also to stimulate the production of various immunoglobulins (IgA etc.) A healthy gut is a critical aspect of a healthy immune system.

⇒ **Filtering.** The immune cells move through the lymphatic ducts, not unlike the blood moving through the arteries and veins. Dead immune cells and invaders are filtered out of this "freeway" system in the spleen and lymph nodes.

⇒ **Quantity.** There are many factors that can influence the sheer numbers of immune warriors.

⇒ **Quality.** Not all immune cells have the same level of ferocity against an invading tumor cell. Some immune cells become confused about "who to shoot at" and end up creating an autoimmune response (often called an allergic response), which imbalances the immune system and detracts from the critical task of killing cancer cells. Some nutrients provide the immune warriors with a protective coating, like an asbestos suit, so that the immune cell is not destroyed in the process of killing a cancer cell with some "napalm". Some nutrients provide the immune cells with more "napalm" or "bullets" in the form of granulocytes and nitric oxide.

Many nutrition factors affect the ability of the immune system to recognize and destroy cancer cells and invading bacteria. In the cancer patient, for a variety of reasons, the immune system has not done its work.

We are going to bolster your immune army with improved:

-quantity by producing more natural killer cells, tumor necrosis factor, lymphocytes, interleukin, and interferon.

-quality by:

1) reducing the ability of cancer cells to hide from the immune system. A healthy immune system will attack and destroy any cells that do not have the "secret pass code" of host DNA. Both the fetus and cancer are able to survive by creating a hormone, HCG, which allows the fetus to hide from the immune system. Tumor necrosis factor (TNF), which is specifically made by the immune system to kill cancer cells, is like a sword. TNF-inhibitor is produced in the presence of HCG and is like putting a sheath on the sword. Digestive enzymes and vitamins E and A help to clear away the deceiving "stealth" coating on the tumor and improve tumor recognition by the immune system.

2) providing antioxidants. We can put special shielding on the immune soldiers so that when they douse a cancer cell with deadly chemicals, the immune soldier is protected and can go on to kill other cancer cells. Otherwise, you seriously restrict the "bag limit" of any given immune soldier.

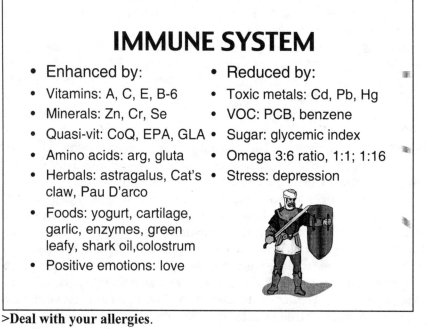

IMMUNE SYSTEM

- Enhanced by:
  - Vitamins: A, C, E, B-6
  - Minerals: Zn, Cr, Se
  - Quasi-vit: CoQ, EPA, GLA
  - Amino acids: arg, gluta
  - Herbals: astragalus, Cat's claw, Pau D'arco
  - Foods: yogurt, cartilage, garlic, enzymes, green leafy, shark oil,colostrum
  - Positive emotions: love

- Reduced by:
  - Toxic metals: Cd, Pb, Hg
  - VOC: PCB, benzene
  - Sugar: glycemic index
  - Omega 3:6 ratio, 1:1; 1:16
  - Stress: depression

>Deal with your allergies.

Your immune system cannot fully direct its energies toward destroying cancer cells if it spends too much time mistakingly destroying your dinner. Food allergies are caused by food proteins being absorbed into the bloodstream, then your immune system attacking the food as if it were an invading bacteria. Many food allergies can be caused by a leaky gut, which may be caused by yeast overgrowth. See the section on purging yeast or fungus from the body.

If nutrition itself is a controversial subject, then allergies represent controversy to the cubed power. From 25% to 50% of the population suffer from allergies, which can come from foods that we eat (ingestant), air particles that we breath (inhalant), or substances on our skin (contact). Allergies can cause an amazing array of diseases, including immune problems, arthritis, diabetes, heart disease, mental illness, and more. The reason allergies are so complicated to detect and treat is the limitless combinations of chemicals in the human body. You might react to wheat products only if you consume citrus at the same meal and are under stress. Otherwise, wheat may not create any problems. Some people have transient food allergies, that come and go along with the pollen seasons. Because of this trend, some allergists subscribe to the "rain barrel" theory, in which you only have allergic reactions when the rain barrel is overflowing, such as combined allergies with stress.

Allergies are generated by an over-reactive immune system or a porous digestive tract. What happens is that small undigested particles (polypeptides and peptides) of food pass through the intestinal wall into the blood stream and are recognized by the immune system as an invading bacteria (since its DNA is not yours). Now, you may be thinking that an over-reactive immune system should help to fight cancer, yet the immunoglobulins that instigate allergies will depress the production of cancer-killing immune factors, like natural killer cells and tumor necrosis factor. Allergies create an imbalanced immune system. Correct the allergies and you can re-establish a vigorous immune attack on the cancer.

Allergic reactions can be:

-Type I. Immediate reaction of less than 2 hours. It is estimated that less than 15% of all food allergies are of this easily-detected type.

-Type 2. Delayed cytotoxic reaction which may require days to develop into subtle and internal symptoms. It is estimated that 75% of food allergies involve this category of cell destruction. The ELISA/ACT test detects type 2 delayed reactions.

-Type 3. Immune complex mediated reactions. In this reaction, a "wrestling match" goes on between the antigen (offending factor) and antibody (immune factor trying to protect the body), which can easily slip through the permeable blood vessels due to large amounts of histamine release.

-Type 4. T cell dependent reactions. Within 36-72 hours after exposure to the offending substance, inflammation is produced by stimulating T-cells.

Allergies are common, complex to diagnose, difficult to treat, and closely related to a variety of diseases, including cancer. A primitive and not terribly accurate way to find allergies involves the hypoallergenic diet. For 4 days, eat nothing but rice, apples, carrots, pears, lamb, turkey, olive, and black tea. If you find relief from any particular symptoms, then add back a new food every four days and record the results. The most common allergenic foods are milk, wheat, beef, eggs, corn, peanut, soybeans, chicken, fish, nuts, mollusks, and shellfish. Outside of humans, no other creature on earth consumes milk after weaning. Only 11-20% of Americans breast feed, which helps explain why the most allergenic food in the world is cow's milk.

Detecting and treating food allergies is a real challenge. The food rotation program basically states that you can only have a food once within a 4-day period, hoping that the body has time to reset the switch on your immune system and not create an allergic reaction. To resolve food allergies, work with your nutritionally oriented doctor listed in the appendix.

NUTRIENTS AFFECT THE IMMUNE SYSTEM

There is an abundance of scientific documentation linking nutrient intake with immune quality and quantity. This is a very crucial issue for the cancer patient.

Many nutrients taken orally can provide pharmacological changes in immune function in humans. Protein, arginine, glutamine, omega-6 and omega-3 fats, iron, zinc, vitamins E, C, and A have all been proven to modulate immune functions.[2]

Vitamin A deficiency causes reduced lymphocyte response to antigens and mitogens, while beta-carotene supplements stimulate immune responses.[3]

There is extensive literature supporting the importance of vitamin B-6 on the immune system. In one study, B-6 supplements (50 mg/day) provided a measurable improvement in immune functions (T3 and T4 lymphocytes) for 11 healthy, well-fed older adults.[4]

Various B vitamins have been linked to the proper functioning of antibody response and cellular immunity.

Folate deficiency decreases mitogenesis.

Deficiency of vitamin C impairs phagocyte functions and cellular immunity.

Vitamin E deficiency decreases antibody response to T-dependent antigens, all of which gets worse with the addition of a selenium deficiency. In test animals, normal vitamin E intake was not adequate to optimize immune functions.[5] Modest supplements of vitamin E have been shown to enhance the immune response.

While iron deficiency can blunt immune functions, iron excess can increase the risk for cancer.[6] Iron presents an interesting case: 1) because it is the most common nutritional problem worldwide, 2) because low levels of iron will depress the immune system, and 3) because high levels of iron will stimulate both bacterial and tumor growth. Iron intake needs to be well regulated...not too much, and not too little.

Zinc exerts a major influence on the immune system. Lymphocyte function is seriously depressed, and lymphoid tissues undergo general atrophy in zinc-deficient individuals. The lymphocytes in zinc-deficient animals quickly lose their killing abilities (cytotoxicity) and engulfing talents (phagocytosis) for tumor cells and bacteria. Natural killer cell and neutrophil activity is also reduced. All of these compromised immune activities elevate the risk for cancer.

Copper plays a key role in the production of superoxide dismutase and cytochrome systems in the mitochondria. Hence, a deficiency of copper is manifested in a depressed immune system, specifically reduced microbicidal activity of granulocytes.

Selenium works in conjunction with vitamin E to shield host cells from lipid peroxidation. Humoral immune response is depressed in selenium deficient animals. Selenium and vitamin E deficiencies lead to increased incidence of enteric lesions. Lymphocyte proliferation is reduced in selenium deficiency. The theory is that selenium and vitamin E help to provide the host immune cells with some type of "bullet-proof plating" against the toxins used on foreign cells. Hence, one immune body can live on to destroy many invaders if enough vitamin E and selenium allow for these critical chemical shields.

In magnesium deficiency, all immunoglobulins (except IgE) are reduced, along with the number of antibody forming cells. Magnesium is crucial for lymphocyte growth (involvement in protein metabolism) and transformation in response to mitogens. Prolonged magnesium deficiency in animals leads to the development of lymphomas and leukemia.

Iodine plays an important role in the microbicidal activity of polymorphonuclear leukocytes. Activated neutrophils may use the conversion of iodide to iodine to generate free radicals for killing foreign invaders.

Boron is an interesting trace mineral, since it is now recognized for its role in preventing osteoporosis, yet is still not considered an essential mineral. Boron deficiency in chicks creates immune abnormalities like arthritis.

Toxic trace minerals, like cadmium, arsenic, and lead all blunt the immune system.

The quality and quantity of fat in the diet play a major role in dictating the health of the immune system. A deficiency of the essential fatty acid (linoleic acid) will lead to atrophy of lymphoid tissue and a depressed antibody response. And yet, excess intake of polyunsaturated fatty acids will also diminish T-cell immune responsiveness. Since fat directly affects prostaglandin pathways, and prostaglandins (depending on the pathway) can either depress or enhance immune function, fat intake is crucial in encouraging a healthy immune system. Oxidized cholesterol is highly immuno-suppressive. Cholesterol is less likely to oxidize while in the presence of antioxidants, like vitamin E, C, and beta-carotene.

PATIENT PROFILE: REVERSING KIDNEY CANCER: C.H. was diagnosed with renal cell carcinoma stage 4 that had spread to his liver and spleen. All 3 oncologists said that C.H. had less than 6 months to live with no chance of recovery. C.H.'s daughters gathered the information in this book to create a diet, supplement, and detoxification program. Within a few weeks, his pain was significantly less and his pain medications could be reduced. "The doctor was amazed and said the patient's tumors are shrinking and there has been no new tumor growth in 2 months." Six months after his initial diagnosis C.H. is in good spirits, out of pain, and has much less tumor burden than the beginning. "Thank you for writing your wonderful book." states the daughters who provided their father with his nutrition program.

ENDNOTES

[1]. Bendich, A, Chandra, RK (eds), Micronutrients and Immune Function, New York Academy of Sciences, 1990, p.587

[2]. Alexander, JW, et al., Critical Care Medicine, vol.18, p.S159, 1990

[3]. Rhodes, J., and Oliver, S., Immunology, vol.40, p.467, 1980

[4]. Talbott, MC, et al., American Journal of Clinical Nutrition, vol.46, p.659, 1987

[5]. Bendich, A., et al., Journal of Nutrition, vol.116, p.675, 1986

[6]. Cerutti, PA, Science, vol.227, p.375, 1985

CHAPTER 11

SUGAR FEEDS CANCER

✷

SLOW CANCER GROWTH BY LOWERING BLOOD AND GUT GLUCOSE

✷

"Cancer cells demonstrate a 3 to 5 fold increase in glucose uptake compared to healthy cells."
Demetrakopoulos, GE, Cancer Research, vol.42, p.756S, Feb.1982

"Sugar is the most hazardous foodstuff in the American diet."
Linus Pauling, PhD, twice Nobel laureate

WHAT'S AHEAD?
Cancer cells feed almost exclusively on sugar.
You can slow tumor growth by:
↪ eating a diet that lowers blood and gut sugar
↪ exercise to burn up any extra glucose in the blood
↪ taking supplements such as chromium, CLA, and gymnema
↪ using medications, if necessary, for better control of diabetes

---

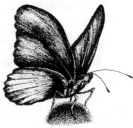

A moth is attracted to bright light, which can be its own demise if the bright light is a flame. Americans consume 140 pounds of refined sugar per year, mostly in the form of sucrose (white sugar) and corn syrup. Our incidence of obesity, diabetes, and many cancers has escalated parallel to our rise in sugar intake. We consume 15 billion gallons of soft drinks, 2.7 billion Krispy Cremes, and 500 million Twinkies per year. Our appetite for sugar is like a hummingbird sucking on sweet food all day long.

Problem is, we are not exercising like a hummingbird. A special region of our tongue is exclusively reserved for finding and appreciating sweet foods. This makes good sense. Sweet foods are more likely to have carbohydrates for nourishment and

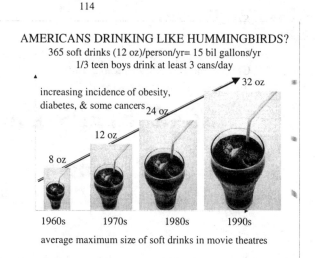

AMERICANS DRINKING LIKE HUMMINGBIRDS?
365 soft drinks (12 oz)/person/yr= 15 bil gallons/yr
1/3 teen boys drink at least 3 cans/day

increasing incidence of obesity, diabetes, & some cancers

32 oz
24 oz
12 oz
8 oz

1960s   1970s   1980s   1990s

average maximum size of soft drinks in movie theatres

less likely to be poisonous, such as some bitter plants. Our hunter-gatherer ancestors were hard pressed to find sweet foods, and thus their bodies were

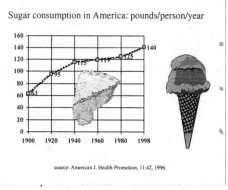

Sugar consumption in America: pounds/person/year

160
140   140
120   115   115   125
100   95
80
60   63
40
20
0
1900 1920 1940 1960 1980 1998

source: American J. Health Promotion, 11:42, 1996

forced to make glucose out of proteins in the body. However, once mankind developed the technology for growing and concentrating refined sugars in unimaginable levels, that sweet tooth of ours has become our enemy within. That sweet tooth leads us on to greater and greater heights of sugar intake like a moth drawn to a flame.

Cut back dramatically on total sweetener intake: either caloric or non-caloric. By doing so, you will begin to taste the flavors of the food and begin to lose that sweetness craving. Once you have cut back your intake of caloric sugars from the current average of 140 pounds per year per person to a more reasonable 20 pounds per year and have removed all aspartame (NutraSweet) from your diet, then choose from the preferred sweeteners listed below.

The alphabet of sugars:
Disaccharide means 2 sugar molecules together, like table sugar, or sucrose.
Monosaccharide means 1 sugar molecule, like fructose in honey or fruits.
glucose + fructose=sucrose (table sugar)
glucose + glucose=maltose
glucose + galactose=lactose (milk sugar)

CALORIC SWEETENERS
contain 4 kcal per gram & can cause cavities

SUGAR: Based upon federal laws passed after World War II to protect the California and Hawaii sugar industry, a "sugar" must have at least 96% of all other plant matter stripped from it in order to be called sugar. 90% of the bulk of cane sugar is fiber, protein, and other matter. All of this is lost in the sugar refining process. Therefore, turbinado sugar, brown sugar, and other health food store sugars are virtually identical to white sugar in nutrient density and glycemic index.

Barley malt is a mild natural sweetener made from barley sprouts that is less sweet and less hazardous on blood glucose levels than other sweeteners listed here, yet very expensive.

Blackstrap molasses: what's left over at the bottom of the barrel from the sugar refining industry. Molasses contains the concentrated vitamins and minerals that were once in the cane sugar, though it still can create havoc with blood glucose levels and has an unusual wild taste. It has more calcium than milk, more iron than eggs, and is a rich source of potassium.

Brown sugar: can be made by blending white sugar with molasses. Little advantage over white sugar.

Corn syrup is commercial glucose from cornstarch with some sucrose syrup added. Very refined food, with a very high glycemic index.

Date sugar is ground and dried dates from desert climates. Tasty whole food, but high glycemic index.

Fructose is found in many fruits, honey, and as pure crystalline fructose. It is slowly absorbed in the intestinal tract, and requires the liver to convert fructose to glucose for body use. Glycemic index of 20. Very useful for diabetics.

Fruit juice concentrate is usually made from grape juice and, due to a high fructose concentration, has a favorable glycemic index.

Glucose/dextrose: Here is the gold currency of sugar in the blood. Glucose is usually extracted from corn syrup and is rapidly absorbed from the intestines into the bloodstream. Foods high in glucose (watermelon, parsnips) or starches easily digested into glucose (like rice cakes or white bread) can create rapid and dangerous rises in blood glucose.

Gymnema sylvestre is a valuable herb that can block the taste of sugar in the mouth. Using gymnema tea with those occasional sweet snacks can help to reduce the amount of sugar that you crave.

Honey is formed when bees partially digest nectar from flowers. Honey has well documented value as an antiseptic, antibiotic, and stomach calming food. Honey from your nearby vicinity can help with allergies and is a real food vs. the "cadaver" state of most other highly refined caloric sweeteners. Honey varies in taste and content based on the hives and flowers in your region. Honey is usually about 31% glucose, 38% fructose, 18% water, 9% other sugars, and 2% sucrose. Yet, honey, in excess, can create problems with glycemic index and weight. Once honey has been heated, which neutralizes many of its benefits, the honey will become more water-like. Rich honey (Y.S. Farms 800-654-4593) is thick and organically-raised.

Lactose (milk sugar). About 50-90% of adults are lactose intolerant and therefore do not digest this sugar well, which then generates intestinal cramps, constipation, gas, or diarrhea. In yogurt, the lactose has been fermented by healthy bacteria into lactic acid, hence the slightly tart taste. People who are lactose intolerant can usually consume yogurt with no problem.

Maltitol is a relatively new sugar found in health food stores. Made from corn, maltitol has a better glycemic index than sucrose and 25% fewer calories per gram. However, it is expensive and not as sweet as table sugar.

Maple syrup is concentrated sweetener from the sap of sugar maple trees. It requires 30-40 gallons of sap to make 1 gallon of maple syrup. Unless the product is labelled "pure" maple syrup, then it is probably diluted with corn syrup to cut the cost. Though the flavor is unique, the glycemic index is little better than white sugar.

Rice syrup is made by culturing rice with digestive enzymes to break down the starch into glucose. Tasty whole food, but high glycemic index.

Sorghum molasses is the concentrated juice from the sorghum plant, a cereal grain. Has a lighter flavor than blackstrap molasses.

Sucanat: trade name that means "SUgar CAne NATural" and comes from ground up organically grown sugar cane. 85% is sugar, with the balance of 15% being fiber, vitamins, minerals, amino acids, and molasses. Though Sucanat is a whole food, it is more expensive and provides a minor advantage in nutrient density and glycemic index vs white table sugar.

Sucrose is basic table sugar and merits a special discussion here. It was around 600 AD that Persians began growing and refining sugar cane into something similar to our white table sugar. Since then, sugar has been a pivotal point in history, wars, taxes, and even the Declaration of Independence of the United States of America. The immoral trade route that connected the continents of Europe, Africa, and North America for centuries involved buying slaves from Africa with rum in order to sell the slaves to sugar cane plantations in the Caribbean, then bring the sugar, molasses, and rum to Europe and back to Africa for more trade.

Long before the Boston Tea Party, the Molasses Act of 1733 put British rule in the crosshairs of American colonists. At the time of the Revolutionary War, the average annual consumption of molasses rum was 4 gallons per man, woman, and child. One could argue that the enthusiastic consumption of sugar and its by-products have been instrumental in bringing us the "diseases of civilization", including tuberculosis, diabetes, heart disease, many forms of cancer (which is a sugar-feeder), various mental disorders (including hyperactivity), and more. Suffice it to say that sucrose is more of a drug than a food. Consume it with all due caution.

Turbinado sugar is raw sugar that has been washed of its molasses content in a centrifuge. Basically, it is over-priced white sugar.

CALORIC BUT NON-CARIOGENIC
contain 4 kcal per gram and cannot cause cavities

Sorbitol is derived from corn, absorbed slowly, requires little insulin, and is used in many foods for diabetics. Probably safe, but may cause diarrhea in some sensitive individuals. Use in moderation.

Xylitol (Xylitol.com) is extracted from birchwood chips and used in chewing gum. May reduce cavities by neutralizing the acids in the mouth. Use in moderation.

Tagatose (Naturlose.com) is the new kid on the block among sugar substitutes. Tagatose is nearly identical (C-4 epimer) to D-fructose, the common simple sugar found in many fruits. Tagatose has full GRAS (generally regarded as safe) approval from the FDA. Tagatose provides only 37% of the calories found in an equal amount of sucrose, has a mild laxative effect and seems to have no toxicity. Currently, tagatose can only be found in mixed products, but may soon be available by itself as a sugar substitute.

NON-CALORIC SWEETENERS
no calories & no cavities

Stevia, or stevioside, is extracted from a sweetening herb, stevia rebaudiana, and does not have either calories or a long and checkered past like many of the other artificial sweeteners listed here. Stevia was commercialized in the 1970s by a Japanese firm and still enjoys over 40% of the food sweetener market in both South America and Asia. Stevia has been used as a natural sweetener for over 1,500 years in South America. The herb is actually beneficial for people with poorly regulated blood glucose, though the concentrated extract, stevioside, sold in health food stores, does not retain these healing properties. The FDA created a bizarre and suspicious import ban on stevia for years, which was recently lifted. Stevioside and stevia are the safest and most recommended of the artificial sweeteners available today.

Splenda, or sucralose, is a relatively new artificial sweetener invented in 1976, patented by a subsidiary of Johnson & Johnson, and approved by the Food and Drug Administration in 1998. Splenda is made from sugar, is stable in cooking, tastes like sugar, but cannot cause dental caries and does not raise blood sugar. Splenda has a molecule that is slightly different in shape from normal table sugar and has a chlorine atom added.

Preliminary evidence indicates that Splenda is relatively safe, especially compared to aspartame.

✖ Aspartame provides us with a classical example of how the FDA is not protecting the American consumer, but rather creating extremely profitable monopolies for those who can afford the $150-800 million investment required to pass the "safety tests". Aspartame, Equal, or NutraSweet (trademark of the NutraSweet Company) is consumed by over 100 million people in the US alone. It is 180 times sweeter than table sugar, is included in over 1,200 products in America, and was approved by the FDA in 1981. Over a billion pounds of aspartame are used annually in the US. I will spare you the detailed accounts of how aspartame has been linked to our 250% rise in brain cancer since its approval[1], or the double blind study by psychiatrists that was halted because aspartame created such blatant depression in the test subjects[2], or the study showing that aspartame caused headaches in a double blind trial[3], or the fact that of the 2800 FDA approved food additives, 80% of all complaints are regarding aspartame.[4] Aspartame breaks down after long term storage, heating, and in the body into wood alcohol (methyl alcohol) and dangerous isomers of the amino acid phenylalanine. Researcher Richard Wurtman, MD of MIT cautioned the FDA on the approval of aspartame, noting the rise in brain tumors among animals fed aspartame. Along with the meteoric rise in the consumption of aspartame has come a parallel rise in the incidence of both obesity and morbid obesity (people who are dangerously overweight). I strongly discourage the use of aspartame. I would rather have the judicious use of white table sugar than aspartame.

Saccharin is a chemical derivative of petroleum and toluene, a solvent used to reduce the knocking in automobile engines.[5] Saccharin was found to increase the incidence of bladder cancer in animals, but under pressure from lobbyists, the FDA allowed saccharin to remain on the market with a warning label. I discourage the use of saccharin.

Acesulfame K, sold as Sunette or Sweet One, was approved by the FDA in 1988 as a sugar substitute. Early studies show that Acesulfame may cause cancer: "Acesulfame K...might be carcinogenic." David Rall, MD, PhD, Assistant Surgeon General of America. Don't use it.

THE SUGAR-CANCER LINK

At the world-famous Sloan-Kettering Cancer hospital in New York City, researchers found that tumors sucked up radioactively-labeled vitamin C like thirsty sponges because cancer cells thought they were getting their favorite fuel, glucose, which is nearly identical in chemical structure to vitamin C. Meanwhile, across the globe in a modern clinic in Germany, oncologists were injecting glucose into cancer patients to activate the cancer growth, then whack the cancer with intensive chemo, radiation, or hyperthermia. Their results have doubled 5-year survival for these patients undergoing Systemic Cancer Multistep Therapy. Researchers at Harvard University have developed a special Total Parenteral Nutrition formula for cancer patients that uses much less sugar (glucose) and more protein and fats. The net result of this "disease-specific" formula for starving cancer patients is to feed the immune system and not the cancer. In most major cancer hospitals around the world, oncologists use a $2 million device, called a PET scan (positron emission tomography), which detects cancer by finding hot spots of sugar feeding cells in the body. All of these world-class scientists are using the same principle: sugar feeds cancer. When we can lower blood glucose, we can slow cancer growth.

Tumors are primarily obligate glucose metabolizers, meaning "sugar feeders".[6] The average American consumes 20% of calories from refined white sugar, which is more of a drug than a food. We also manifest poor glucose tolerance due to stress, obesity, low chromium and fiber

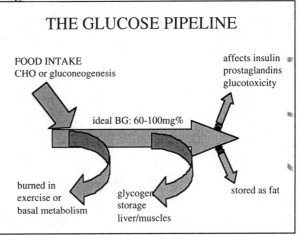

THE GLUCOSE PIPELINE

FOOD INTAKE
CHO or gluconeogenesis

affects insulin
prostaglandins
glucotoxicity

ideal BG: 60-100mg%

burned in exercise or basal metabolism

glycogen storage liver/muscles

stored as fat

intake, and sedentary lifestyles. Blood glucose is basically there to feed the brain and other glucose-dependent organs, while also supplying fuel for muscle movement. When we sit all day, the sugar in our blood is like a teenager with nothing to do--trouble is bound to happen. Elevated sugar levels in the blood will "tan" proteins (glycosylation), which makes immune cells and red blood cells less capable of doing their jobs. Elevated sugar in the blood has a number of ways in which it promotes cancer:

✓ Rises in blood glucose generate corresponding rises of insulin, which then pushes prostaglandin production toward the immune-suppressing and stickiness-enhancing PGE-2. While fish oil (EPA) and borage oil (GLA) have a favorable impact on cancer, these potent fatty acids are neutralized when the blood glucose levels are kept high.

✓ Cancer cells feed directly on blood glucose, like a fermenting yeast organism. Elevating blood glucose in a cancer patient is like throwing gasoline on a smoldering fire.

✓ Elevating blood glucose levels suppresses the immune system

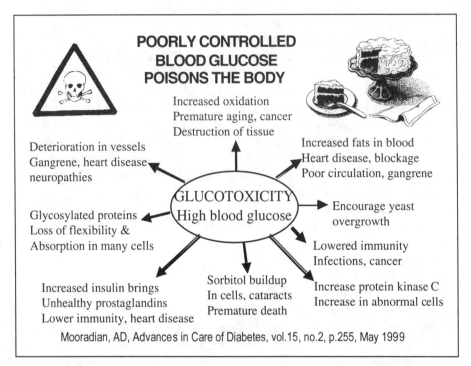

POORLY CONTROLLED BLOOD GLUCOSE POISONS THE BODY

Increased oxidation
Premature aging, cancer
Destruction of tissue

Deterioration in vessels
Gangrene, heart disease
neuropathies

Increased fats in blood
Heart disease, blockage
Poor circulation, gangrene

Glycosylated proteins
Loss of flexibility &
Absorption in many cells

GLUCOTOXICITY High blood glucose

Encourage yeast
overgrowth

Lowered immunity
Infections, cancer

Increased insulin brings
Unhealthy prostaglandins
Lower immunity, heart disease

Sorbitol buildup
In cells, cataracts
Premature death

Increase protein kinase C
Increase in abnormal cells

Mooradian, AD, Advances in Care of Diabetes, vol.15, no.2, p.255, May 1999

Cancer cells primarily use glucose for fuel, with lactic acid as an anaerobic by-product, thus generating a lower pH, fatigue (lactic acid buildup), and enlarged liver (where lactic acid is converted back to pyruvate in the Cori cycle). This inefficient pathway for energy metabolism yields only 5% of the ATP energy available in food, which is one of the reasons why 40% of cancer patients die from malnutrition or cachexia. Cancer therapies need to regulate blood glucose levels via diet, supplements, enteral and parenteral solutions for cachectic patients, medication, exercise, gradual weight loss, stress reduction, etc. The role of glucose in the growth and metastasis of cancer cells can be utilized to help the

HYPERGLYCEMIA CREATES VITAMIN C DEFICIENCY SCORBUTIC IMMUNE CELLS

15% rise in blood glucose creates 50% drop in intracellular vit.C

FACTS:
√ Vitamin C is similar in structure to glucose
√ Vitamin C and glucose share receptors for cellular absorption
√ Leukocytes and macrophages have 50x more vitamin C than plasma
√ Phagocytic index of granulocytes falls 50% when BG at 120 mg%, healthy
√ Requires 5 hours for phagocytic index to return to normal
√ Pharmacological ascorbate supplementation will not enhance cell-mediated
√ immunity unless hyperglycemia is corrected.
√ When blood glucose is lowered, vitamin C therapy more effective in
√ cancer patients. Cheraskin, E, Acta.Cytologica, vol.12, p.433, 1968

vitamin C & glucose
receptors

macrophage

Santisteban, GA, Biochem. Biophysical Res.Comm., vol.132, no.3, p.1174, Nov.1985 cancer patient with such therapies as:

-diets designed with glycemic index in mind to regulate rises in blood glucose, hence selectively starving the cancer cells

-low glucose total parenteral nutrition (TPN) solution

-positron emission tomography (PET) assays of tumor progress

-hydrazine sulfate to inhibit gluconeogenesis in cancer cells

-avocado extract (mannoheptulose), which inhibits glucose uptake in cancer cells

-Systemic Cancer Multistep Therapy, which injects glucose into the cancer patient to initiate malignancy growth, then uses hyperthermia to selectively destroy tumor tissue.

DOES SUGAR (GLUCOSE) FEED CANCER CELLS?

Nobel laureate (1931 Medicine) Otto Warburg, PhD, first discovered that cancer cells have a fundamental difference in energy metabolism compared to healthy undifferentiated cells. Cancer cells ferment glucose anaerobically.[7] Since Warburg's pivotal study published in *Science* in 1956, many other researchers have corroborated his conclusions.

"A frequent characteristic of many malignant tumors is an increase in anaerobic glycolysis, that is the conversion of glucose to lactate, when compared to normal tissues."

"The high rate of glucose consumption by malignant cells, their heavy dependence on the inefficient glycolytic mode for energy production, their increased energy expenditures, and the susceptibility to carbohydrate deprivation prompted several attempts to exploit the tumoricidal potential of manipulations interfering with carbohydrate and/or energy metabolism, hoping that such interventions could preferentially impair the malignant cells."[8]

"In normoglycemic hosts the in vivo consumption of glucose by neoplastic tissues was found to be very high. Cerebral tissue is reported to use from 0.23 to 0.57 gm of glucose per hour per 100 gm wet brain and rates as one of the highest consumers among the normal tissues. However, hepatomas and fibrosarcomas consumed roughly as much glucose as the brain does and carcinomas about twice as much."[9]

"The glucose utilization rate in neoplastic tissues, unlike in host tissues, is high. Glucose, in fact, is the preferred energy substrate, utilized mainly via the anaerobic glycolytic pathway. The large amount of lactate produced by this process is then transported to the liver where it is converted to glucose, thus contributing to further increase host's energy wasting."[10]

ELEVATED LACTATE LEVELS. "Our laboratory has been interested in the metabolic derangements of cancer, particularly lactate overproduction, in view of our work linking lactate overproduction in obesity to insulin resistance…Thus, in all four studies listed above, lactate levels were 27-83% higher in cancer patients than in related controls."[11]

LOWER PH THROUGH LACTIC ACID ACCUMULATION.

If cancer cells use glucose through anaerobic fermentation, then lactic acid must accumulate as the inefficient by-product of energy metabolism. Human tumors were implanted in rats, which were then given IV solutions of glucose. pH in the tumor tissue was reduced to an average of 6.43, given the logarithmic scale of hydrogen ions in pH measurement, "This pH value corresponds to a ten-fold increase in H+ ion activity in tumor tissue as compared to arterial blood."[12]

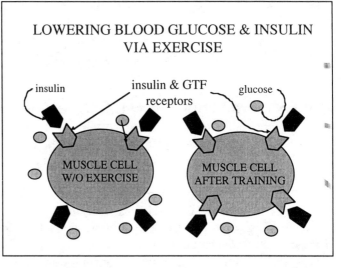

By lowering pH in tumor cells, we can effectively create a selective systemic therapy which will kill cancer cells and not healthy tissue. "After IV glucose, tumor acidification occurred in 9 out of 10 patients…Larger tumors tended to exhibit a greater decrease in pH…We conclude that IV and IV + oral glucose administration are equally effective inducing tumor acute acidification."[13]

ELEVATED BLOOD GLUCOSE MAY SUPPRESS IMMUNE FUNCTIONS. Ten healthy human volunteers were assessed for fasting blood glucose levels and phagocytic index of neutrophils. "Oral 100 gm portions of carbohydrates from glucose, fructose, sucrose, honey, or orange juice all significantly decreased the capacity of neutrophils to engulf bacteria as measured by the slide technique. Starch ingestion did not have this effect."[14]

INSULIN-CANCER RELATIONSHIP. "Insulin is a major anabolic hormone in mammals and its involvement in malignancies is well documented."[15]

EPIDEMIOLOGICAL EVIDENCE. "Risk associated with the intake of sugars, independent of other energy sources, is more than doubled [for biliary tract cancer]".[16] "In older women, a strong correlation was found between breast cancer mortality and sugar consumption…"[17]

ACTION PLAN: STARVE CANCER CELLS

HYDRAZINE SULFATE. Since cancer cells derive most of their energy from anaerobic glycolysis, Joseph Gold, MD, developed hydrazine sulfate to inhibit the excessive gluconeogenesis that occurs in cancer patients. Hydrazine inhibits the enzyme phosphoenol pyruvate carboxykinase (PEP-CK), and in placebo-controlled clinical trials at UCLA, hydrazine was proven to slow and reverse cachexia in advanced cancer patients.[18] Unfortunately, this non-toxic and inexpensive substance has been banished by the FDA. Hydrazine for cancer cachexia is a troubling story of stupidity and greed preventing the American public from having easy access to a useful anti-cancer substance. Hydrazine sulfate may be available from: Life Support 209-529-4697, Life Energy 604-856-0171, Nutrilogics 800-618-1881, Biotech 800-345-1199.

IV GLUCOSE WITH HYPERTHERMIA. Since cancer growth can be accelerated with intravenous glucose solutions, researchers in Germany have developed a technique, Systemic Cancer Multistep Therapy (SCMT), in which the cancer patient is given injections of glucose to elevate blood glucose to around 400 mg%, which generates a substantial reduction in pH in all malignant tissues due to lactic acid formation, then the patient is given whole body hyperthermia (42°C core temp.). Patients may then be treated with chemotherapy and radiation, which are optional. Five year survival in these SCMT treated patients increased by 25-50%, and complete regression of tumor increased by 30-50%.[19]

LOW GLUCOSE TOTAL PARENTERAL NUTRITION (TPN) SOLUTION. When a cancer patient cannot eat enough food to prevent lean tissue wasting, nutrients may be injected into a port implanted in the sub-clavian artery. Since "tumors appear to be obligate glucose utilizers..."[20], we can capitalize on

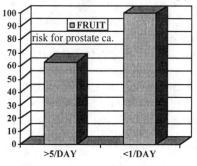

DOES FRUIT (SUGAR?) CAUSE CANCER?

whole fruit is rich in phytochemicals, antioxidants (ORAC), apoptosis agents, enzymes, low glycemic index

STUDY DESIGN: Prospective study of 47,781 men 1986-1994; 1369 cases prostate cancer. "Fruit intake inversely associated with risk of advanced prostate cancer." 47% lower risk in higher fruit intake (>5 servings/day) vs. lower intake <1 serving.

Giovannucci, E., et al., Cancer Res., vol.58, no.3, p.442, Feb.1998

the differences in energy metabolism between healthy and differentiated malignant cells by providing starving cancer patients with TPN solutions that are relatively low in glucose and higher in amino acids and lipids.[21] Many starving cancer patients are offered either no nutrition support or the standard TPN solution developed for intensive care units with 70% of kcal from glucose (dextrose). Disappointing results have been found when using standard high glucose TPN solutions for cachectic cancer patients.[22]

PET SCANS MAP TUMOR PROGRESS AND AGGRESSIVENESS. PET (positron emission tomography) scans use radioactively-labeled glucose (fluoro-2-deoxy-D-glucose, FDG) to tag areas of the body with unusually high levels of glycolysis. "Enhanced glucose utilization by tumor cells via

ORAL GLUCOSE TOLERANCE CURVES

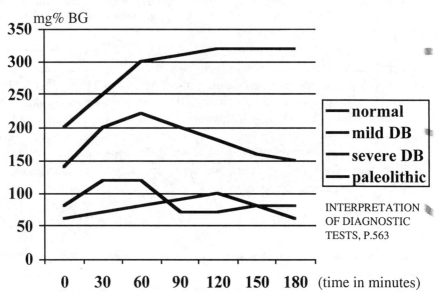

INTERPRETATION OF DIAGNOSTIC TESTS, P.563

glycolysis, identified by Warburg, is a characteristic exploited in cancer imaging using FDG-PET."[23] "Specific parameters of the glucose consumption curves are predicted to be markedly different in normal and neoplastic tissues and critical to the tumor-host interaction. Tumor invasability and patient prognosis can be linked to these parameters." PET scans can be used to plot the progress of cancer patients and decide if current protocols are effective, or if different protocols need to be employed.[24]

TUMOR HYPOXIA AND TREATMENT RESISTANCE. "...tumor hypoxia is present in at least one third of cancers in the clinical setting."[25] "Tumors differ from normal tissues because there is not enough oxygen to meet demand, even under baseline conditions."[26] Since solid tumors can develop pockets of hypoxic tissue that are particularly resistant to radiotherapy, a unique protocol using niacin (to improve aerobic energy metabolism) has been used by Jae Ho Kim, MD, PhD, at Ford Hospital in Detroit with noteworthy successes.

DOES BLOOD SUGAR IMPACT BREAST CA SURVIVAL?

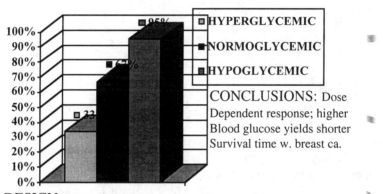

CONCLUSIONS: Dose Dependent response; higher Blood glucose yields shorter Survival time w. breast ca.

STUDY DESIGN: Mice (BALB/C) injected with aggressive mammary tumor and then placed on 3 different diets to alter blood glucose. Survival after 70 days was 8 of 24 (hyper), 16 of 24 (normo) & 19 of 20 (hypo). Santisteban, GA, Biochem.& Biophys Res. Comm., vol.132, no.3, p.1174, Nov.1985

GLYCEMIC CONTROL OF CANCER PATIENT'S DIET.

Humans are not built to withstand the rigors of many aspects of modern life. We are going deaf at an alarming rate due to noise pollution. The same thing is happening with respect to sugar. Our bodies are not built to withstand the constant flood of simple sugars entering our bloodstream. If we were active and burning up the sugar in exercise, then the sugar would be of less consequence. But we sip and munch on sweet foods all day long while sitting at our desks or in front of the TV, then wonder why morbid obesity has increased by 300% since 1982.

Animals were injected with an aggressive strain of breast cancer, then fed diets that would provide either 1) hypoglycemia, 2) normoglycemia, or 3) hyperglycemia. There was a dose-dependent response in which the lower the blood glucose, the greater the survival percentage at 70 days.[27] In rats exposed to a carcinogen, then fed isocaloric intake levels of 49% of kcal as either sucrose or wheat starch, there was a doubling of the tumor incidence in the sugar-fed group (14 of 20 animals with tumors vs 7 out of 20).[28] Educating the cancer patient on the importance of regulating glycemic index can become a key strategy in slowing tumor growth.

IMPROVING INSULIN SENSITIVITY IN CELLS

Magnesium supplementation improved insulin response in aging non-obese human subjects. Paolisso, G., Am.J.Clin.Nutr., vol.55, p.1161, 1992

Vitamin E (900 mg/d) improves insulin action in healthy subjects & type 2 diabetics. Paolisso, G., Am.J.Clin.Nutr., vol.57, p.650, 1993

CLA normalizes impaired glucose tolerance and reduces insulin in pre-diabetic rat. Housekneckt, Biochem.Biophys.Res.Comm.,244,678,1998

Vanadium (100 mg/d vanadyl sulfate) improves insulin sensitivity in type 2 diabetics. Halberstam, M., Diabetes, 45, 659, 1996

Chromium decreases insulin resistance at a fraction of drug cost. Linday,LA, Med.Hypotheses, vol.49, p.47, 1997

Chromium suppl (1000 mcg/d) improved glucose and insulin variables in type 2 diabetics. Anderson, RA, Diabetes, vol.46, p.1786, 1997

Biotin improves hyperglycemia in animals. J.Nutr.Sci.Vitam.42,517,1996

Fish oil reversed hyperinsulinemia in animals. J.Nutr.126,1951, 1996

Lipoic acid supplementation improves insulin sensitivity in type 2 diabetics. Jacob,S., Free Rad.Biol.Med., 27, 3, 309, 1999

Glycemic index is a scientific approach to measuring the role of dietary carbohydrates in blood glucose levels and was developed in 1981 by Dr. David Jenkins. Though glycemic index does not take into consideration "nutrient density", it is a useful means of helping people to select foods that will create a more favorable blood glucose level.

With that caveat in mind, let's explain how the GI was developed and what it means to you. Human subjects, both healthy and diabetic, are fed 50 grams of carbohydrates from various foods. For instance, people are fed 200 grams of spaghetti in order to get 50 grams of carbohydrates, because spaghetti also contains some protein, fat, water, and fiber. Researchers then compare the size of the Oral Glucose Tolerance Test curve. If a food creates only half the rise in blood glucose compared to consuming a

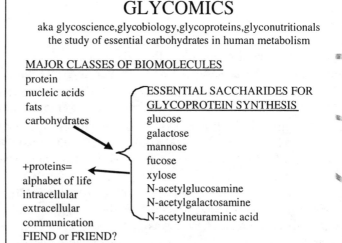

GLYCOMICS
aka glycoscience,glycobiology,glycoproteins,glyconutritionals
the study of essential carbohydrates in human metabolism

MAJOR CLASSES OF BIOMOLECULES
protein
nucleic acids
fats
carbohydrates

ESSENTIAL SACCHARIDES FOR GLYCOPROTEIN SYNTHESIS
glucose
galactose
mannose
fucose
xylose
N-acetylglucosamine
N-acetylgalactosamine
N-acetylneuraminic acid

+proteins=
alphabet of life
intracellular
extracellular
communication
FIEND or FRIEND?

pure glucose drink, then the food gets a GI rating of 50, and so on.

The more that you process a food, the higher the GI becomes. Cooked whole wheat berries have a GI of 41, white bread has a GI of 70. The more the food is stripped of its fiber and ground into smaller particles, the higher the GI and the worse that food becomes for the diabetic.

You might say that ice cream has a better GI than whole wheat bread, so eat more ice cream? Actually, the sugar in ice cream may create havoc for the cancer patient. Use this glycemic index table[29] as it was meant to be used: as a guideline to help people make the right food choices, not as the only nutrition tool for good judgment at the dinner table.

RECOMMENDATIONS FOR IMPROVING
CANCER OUTCOME VIA DIETARY CARBOHYDRATES

EAT LESS/NO SUGAR
USE MICRONUTRIENTS TO AUGMENT GLUCOSE TOLER.
chrom (400 mcg), Mag 400 mg, van sulfate (1 mg), lipoic 100 mg,
niacin (500 mg), zinc (15-50 mg), B-6 (50-100 mg), E (400 mg)
HERBS: bitter melon, gymnema sylv., fenugreek, salt bush,
gingko, glucosol, ginseng
USE FATTY ACIDS TO AUGMENT INSULIN SENSITIVITY
Conjugated Linoleic Acid, fish oil, Gamma Linolenic Acid
FOODS WITH HEALTHY INSULIN & GLUCOSE SCORE
ADD vinegar, onions, & cinnamon to foods to slow gastric
emptying & reduce blood glucose
MONITOR BLOOD GLUCOSE: home diabetes kits <110 mg%
Glycated (glycosylated or glyco) hemoglobin HbA1C < 7%

PATIENT PROFILE: S.D. was diagnosed with stage 4 lung cancer in January of 2004. Surgery was unsuccessful since the tumor had spread to the lining of her lungs. She was put in a clinical trial using 3 chemo drugs that caused a brain hemorrhage (burst blood vessel). In February 2004, S.D. began an aggressive nutrition program along with the drug Arissa. Her doctors told her not to take any nutrients on her days of chemotherapy. Patient ignored this advice. Her doctor has evolved from a skeptic of the value of nutrition to actually writing a prescription for S.D.'s nutrition supplements, after observing the incredible progress patient showed and lack of toxic side effects from chemo. S.D. followed the inspirational message found in Vicki Girard's NO PLACE LIKE HOPE. S.D.'s disease is stable. Her quality of life is excellent as of January 2005. S.D. believes that nutrition helped her to beat the odds on her poor prognostic cancer.

ENDNOTES

[1] . Olney, JW, et al., J.Neuropathol.Exp.Neurol., vol.55, p.1115, 1996

[2] . Walton, RG, et al., Biol.Psychiatry, vol.34, p.13, 1993

[3] . VanDen Eeden, SK, et al., Neurology, vol.44, p.1787, Oct.1994

[4] . Roberts, HJ, ASPARTAME: IS IT SAFE?, p.12, Charles Press, Philadelphia, 1990

[5] . Page, LR, HEALTHY HEALING, p.199, Healthy Healing Publ, 1996

[6]. Rothkopf, M, Fuel utilization in neoplastic disease: implications for the use of nutritional support in cancer patients, Nutrition, supp, 6:4:14-16S, 1990

[7] . Warburg, O., Science, vol.123, no.3191, p.309, Feb.1956

[8] . Demetrakopoulos, GE, Cancer Research, vol.42, p.756S, Feb.1982

[9] . Gullino, PM, Cancer Research, vol.27,p.1031, June 1967

[10] . Rossi-Fanelli, F., J.Parenteral Enteral Nutr., vol.15, p.680, 1991

[11] .Digirolamo, M., in DIET AND CANCER: MARKERS, PREVENTION, AND TREATMENT, p.203, Plenum Press, NY, 1994

[12] . Volk, T., Br.J.Cancer, vol.68, p.492, 1993

[13] . Leeper, DB, Int.J.Hyperthermia, vol.14, no.3, p.257, 1998

[14] . Sanchez, A., Amer.J.Clin.Nutr., vol.26, p.1180, Nov.1973

[15] . Yam, D., Medical Hypotheses, vol.38, p.111, 1992

[16] . Moerman, CJ, Int.J.Epidemiology, vol.22, no.2, p.207, 1993

[17] . Seeley,S.,, Med.Hypotheses, vol.11, p.319, 1983

[18] . Chlebowski, RT, J.Clin.Oncology, vol.8, no.1, p.9, Jan.1990; see also Chlebowski, RT, Cancer, vol.59, p.406, 1987; see also Gold, J., Nutrition & Cancer, vol.9, p.59, 1987

[19] . von Ardenne, M., Strahlentherapie und Onkologie, vol.170, p.581, 1994

[20] . Rothkopf, M, Nutrition, vol.6, no.4, p.14S, July 1990 supp

[21] . Tuttle-Newhall, JE, Cancer & Nutrition, in ADJUVANT NUTRITION IN CANCER TREATMENT, Quillin, P (ed), p.145, Cancer Treatment Research Foundation, Arlington Heights, IL 1994

[22] . Sakurai, Y, Japanese J. Surgery, vol.28, p.247, 1998

[23] . Smith, TAD, Nuclear Med.Comm., vol.19, p.97, 1998

[24] . Gatenby, RA, J.Nuclear Medicine, vol.36, p.893, 1995

[25] . Vaupel, P., Int.J.Rad.OncologyBiol.Phys., vol.42, no.4, p.843, 1998

[26] . Gulledge, CJ, Anticancer Research, vol.16, p.741, 1996

[27] . Santisteban, GA, Biochem. & Biophys.Res.Comm., vol.132, no.3, p.1174, Nov.1985

[28] . Hoehn, SK, Nutrition & Cancer, vol.1, no.3, p.27, 1982

[29] . Brand-Miller, J., et al., THE GLUCOSE REVOLUTION, Marlowe, NYC, 1999

GLYCEMIC INDEX (Brand-Miller, J. et al., Glucose Revolution, Marlow, NY 1999:

how fast does the carbohydrate food get into the blood compared to glucose (=100)

	bread/grain	vegetables	fruit	legumes	dairy	beverages	snack food
90-100		parsnip, baked white potato	dried dates (103)				glucose, maltose (105)
80-89	corn flakes, crispbread	red skinned potato					
70-79	raisin bran, vanilla wafers, graham crackers, waffles, white & wheat bread, bagel, cocoa krispies	french fries, pumpkin	watermelon	broad beans		Gatorade	corn chips, Life Savers, Skittles Fruit Chews
60-69	taco shells, shredded wheat, arrowroot cookies, shortbread	beets, new potatoes	cantaloupe, pineapple, raisins		ice cream	soft drink syrup, Fanta	sucrose (white sugar), Mars almond bar
50-59	all bran, whole wheat, buckwheat, brown & white rice, blueberry muffin, pita & sourdough bread	sweet corn, sweet potato, yam	banana, kiwi, mango, papaya				Power bar, potato chips, honey, popcorn
40-49	noodles, sponge cake, spaghetti, oatmeal, banana bread	carrots, green peas	grapes, orange	baked beans		orange juice, apple juice	chocolate, Twix Cookie, Snickers, lactose
30-39	pasta fettuccine, ravioli		apple, apricot, pear, plum	butter beans, chick peas (garbanzo), lentils, navy beans	low fat yogurt, skim milk, chocolate milk		
20-29			cherries, grapefruit	kidney beans	whole milk		fructose
10-19				soybeans			peanuts

CHAPTER 12

THE POWER OF NUTRITIONAL SYNERGISM

✳

"The deeper that sorrow carves into your being, the more joy you can contain."　　　　　　*Kahlil Gibran in THE PROPHET, p.29*

Synergism: the action of two or more substances to achieve an effect of which each is individually incapable

---

WHAT'S AHEAD?
Synergism means that 1 + 1 = 3 or 500, greater than what would be expected. Nutrients work together in an elegant symphony to heal the body from cancer. There is no one "magic bullet" nutrient against cancer, since we need 50 essential nutrients and probably hundreds of other nutrition factors for optimal health.
↪ take nutrition supplements in the proper ratio, i.e. zinc to selenium
↪ take an assortment of antioxidants together, since they work in the body to play "hot potato" in defusing the damage from free radicals
↪ eat a wide variety of food in its natural state to include valuable nutrients for healing that are not yet accepted as essential

---

There are two primary lessons to be learned in nutritional synergism:
1) Enhanced effects.
⇒ **Nutrient & nutrient combinations** augment each other to achieve greater healing capacity. Either vitamin C or essential fatty acids were able to inhibit the growth of melanoma in culture, yet when combined, their anti-cancer activity was much stronger.[1]
⇒ **Nutrient & medicine combinations** help to protect the patient while selectively destroying the cancer cells. Maitake D-fraction inhibited tumor growth by 80%, while the drug Mitomycin C inhibited tumor

growth by 45%. Yet when both were given together, but at half the dosage for each, tumor inhibition was 98%.

2) Lower doses are required when nutrients are used synergistically. In animals with implanted tumors, vitamin C and B-12 together provided for significant tumor regression and 50% survival of the treated group, while all of the animals not receiving C and B-12 died by the 19th day.[2] C and B-12 seemed to form a cobalt-ascorbate compound that selectively shut down tumor growth. When vitamin C and K were added to cancer cells in culture, the dosage required to kill cancer cells dropped by 98% compared to the dosage required by either of these vitamins alone.[3] Combining vitamins C and K-3 against cultured human breast cancer cells allowed for inhibition of the cancer growth at doses 90-98% less than what was required if only one of these vitamins was used against the cancer.[4]

Listening to the rapture of a symphonic orchestra, I was impressed with the complex synergistic nature of most aspects of our lives. No one and nothing operates in isolation. Both 20th century research and our multi-billion dollar pharmaceutical-based medical system are rooted in the concept of using a single agent to treat a single symptom. Unfortunately, life is much more complicated than that.

NEGATIVE SYNERGISM OF TOXINS

We know that barbiturates have a certain toxicity on the liver, which is synergistically enhanced when alcohol is consumed at the same time. We know that tobacco brings a major risk for lung cancer, as does asbestos exposure, yet when a person is exposed to both, there is a 500% greater risk for lung cancer than would have been expected by adding the two risks (1+1=2). Scientists recently found that pesticides amplify one another's toxicity by 500-1,000 fold.[5] Thus, 1+1=500. This discovery of synergistic toxicity presents the chilling possibility that the 1.2 billion pounds of pesticides sprayed on our domestic food supply may not be as safe as we once thought.

In 1976, a study examined animals that were fed 2% of their diet as either red dye, sodium cyclamate, or an emulsifier--all approved at the time by the Food and Drug Administration. Animals fed one food additive showed no harmful effects. Animals fed two of the food additives exhibited balding scruffy fur, diarrhea, and retarded weight gain. Animals fed all three additives all died within 2 weeks.[6] The take-home lesson is that poisons probably amplify another's toxicity in logarithmic fashion. Given the cavalier spirit with which Americans have nonchalantly discarded and intentionally added toxins to our air, food, and water supply, synergistic toxicity gives me an uneasy feeling about the future health of our nation.

POSITIVE SYNERGISM OF NUTRIENTS

While the prospects of synergistic toxicity are daunting, the prospects of synergistic nutritional healing may be the key to solving many of our health problems. Perusing any biochemistry textbook, we find an abundance of synergistic nutritional relationships: calcium with magnesium with potassium with sodium, vitamin E with selenium, polyunsaturated fats with vitamin E, protein with B-6, and so on.

Antioxidants have surfaced as the "fire extinguishers" that minimize the cellular damage from reactive oxygen species, or free radicals. Yet, these antioxidants work in a hierarchy, not unlike a game of "hot potato", trying to pass along the unpaired electron until the energy dissipates. In this hierarchy, vitamin C recharges vitamin E. Biologists find this complex hierarchy of antioxidants consists of 20,000 bioflavonoids; 800 carotenoids; known essential vitamins, such as C and E; conditionally essential vitamins, such as lipoic acid and coenzyme Q; and endogenously-synthesized antioxidants like superoxide dismutase (SOD) and glutathione peroxidase (GSH-Px). The possible combinations and permutations of antioxidants in the human body make the combinations in the Rubik's cube look like mere child's play. When these antioxidants are all in their proper place in optimal amounts, we have a relatively impenetrable barrier against oxidative damage. Researching any one of these nutrients in isolation is overly simplistic and doomed to misleading results.

The National Cancer Institute reported in 1994 that beta-carotene supplements provided a slightly elevated risk for lung cancer in heavy smokers.[7] Yet other prominent researchers in nutrition and cancer have published papers showing that antioxidants such as beta-carotene can become pro-oxidants in the wrong

BETA-CAROTENE CAUSES LUNG CANCER?	
YES	**NO**
1994 Finnish study	Over 200 epidemiology studies show
29,000 smokers	fruits & veg lower risk
beta 5-8 yrs	11 studies show beta protective
1996 CARET study	against lung ca
18,000 smoker/asbestos	8+ studies show beta reverses
30 mg beta 25,000 A	premalignant lesions
NO BENEFIT	3 studies show beta improves
1995 Phys Health Study	human cancer outcome
22,000 MDs	4 animal studies show beta cures ca
50 mg beta 12 yr	As sole nutrient, AOX can be PROX

RECOMMENDATIONS: Eat a diet rich in green & orange fruits & veg. Take beta, mixed carot, other AOX. Don't smoke.

biochemical environment, such as the combat zone of free radicals generated by heavy tobacco use.[8] At the International Conference on Nutrition and Cancer, sponsored by the University of California at Irvine, held in July

1997, there were several watershed presentations showing that one nutrient alone may be ineffective or counterproductive, while a host of compatible nutrients in the proper ratio can be extremely effective at slowing or reversing cancer.

NUTRITIONAL SYNERGISM AGAINST CANCER

While vitamin C or K alone had mild anti-neoplastic activity against cancer cells in culture, when combined together, these nutrients showed improved tumor cell destruction at 10 to 50 times lower dosages.[9] Other scientists found that vitamins C and B-12 have a synergistic action at slowing cancer growth in animal studies.[10] Apparently, the cobalt from the B-12 attaches to the ascorbic acid to form cobalt ascorbate, a selective toxin against cancer cells.

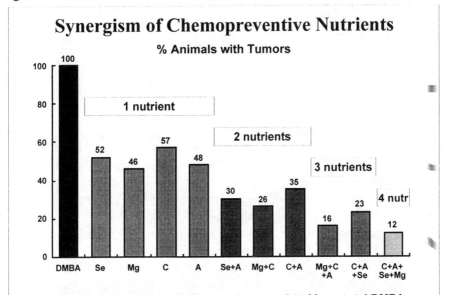

Synergism of Chemopreventive Nutrients

% Animals with Tumors

Study design: female rats (15-30/group) exposed to 30 mg total DMBA begin at day 50 after birth, provided nutrient supplements from d 40-240;
Rao, AR, et al, Jpn J Ca Res, vol 81, p 1239, Dec 1990

In another animal study, researchers found that all DMBA-exposed animals died. When provided a single chemopreventive nutrient (either selenium, magnesium, vitamin C, or vitamin A), cancer incidence after DMBA exposure was cut in half. When two nutrients were combined, the cancer incidence was cut by 70%; with 3 chemopreventive nutrients the cancer incidence was cut by 80%; and with 4 nutrients the cancer incidence was cut by 88%.[11]

Lamm and colleagues found that a multi-nutrient packet of vitamins A, E, C, B-6, and the mineral zinc cut cancer recurrence more than half in

CAN THERAPEUTIC NUTRITION LOWER TUMOR RECURRENCE?

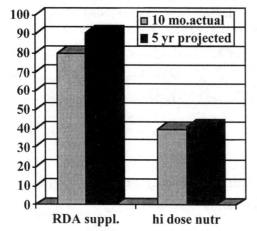

Study design: 65 patients w. transitional cell carcinoma of bladder, BCG immune tx, randomized to either RDA supplement 24 of 30 with tumor recurrence) or RDA + 40,000 iu A, 100 mg B-6, 2 gm C, 400 iu E, 90 mg Zn with 14 of 35 recurrence. Hi dose nutrients cut tumor recurrence in half.

% of bladder cancer patients with tumor recurrence
source: Lamm, DL, J.Urol.,151, 21, Jan.1994

bladder cancer patients treated with BCG.[12] A group of Finnish oncologists treated 18 non-randomized lung cancer patients with chemotherapy, radiation, and a collection of nutrition factors. The anticipated outcome in this group of poor prognostic patients is 1% survival at 30 months after diagnosis. In these nutritionally-supported lung cancer patients, 44% were still alive 6 years (72 months) after diagnosis, with half of these surviving patients in remission.[13] Something in multi-nutrient synergism had provided a major boost over the anticipated outcome in these patients.

One of the brightest nutritional physicians of the 20th century, Abram Hoffer, MD, PhD, and his colleague, twice Nobel laureate, Linus Pauling, PhD, tracked 129 human cancer patients for over 11 years. Of the 31 patients who received only medical intervention for their cancer, the average lifespan was about 6 months. Of the remaining 98 patients who received a combination of medical and nutritional therapies, the average lifespan was about 6 years, a 1,200% increase in lifespan, with poor responders (20%) somewhat offsetting exceptional responders (33%).[14]

EASY SCIENCE OR REALISTIC SCIENCE?

Our bodies are composed of around 60 trillion cells, working in synergistic unison. While our textbooks speak of around 50 essential nutrients for the human body, the number is probably much higher if the endpoint were "thriving" versus the Recommended Dietary Allowance goal of "surviving". Those nutrients work in synergism, not isolation. While mono-nutrient studies are easier to get funded, easier to statistically interpret, and more likely to lead to some drug patent application, these projects fail miserably at appreciating the grandiose complexities of the human body. Nutritional synergism is a biological law that we can either ignore or capitalize on, in order to improve outcome in a variety of disease states.

PATIENT PROFILE: REVERSING COLON CANCER
G.K. was diagnosed with stage 4 colon cancer that had spread to the liver and multiple lymph nodes. His doctor gave him surgery then chemo and told the patient to "get his affairs in order." G.K. began using the principles in this book along with quitting his high stress job. Since no one seemed to hold any hope for chemo helping him, G.K. quit the chemo regimen and began travelling and enjoying himself. G.K. still has the disease 2 years later, but it is a minor inconvenience and is not stopping him from savoring life. "I really owe what is left of my life to your book." states G.K.

ENDNOTES

[1] . Gardiner, N, et al., Pros.Leuk., vol.34, p.119, 1988
[2] . Poydock, ME, Am.J.Clin.Nutr., vol.54, p.1261S, 1991
[3] . Noto, V., et al., Cancer, vol.63, p.901, 1989
[4] . Noto, V., et al., Cancer, vol.63, p.901, 1989
[5] . Arnold. SF, et al., Science, vol.272, p.1489, 1996
[6] . Ershoff, BH, Journal of Food Science, vol.41, p.949, 1976
[7] . Alpha tocopherol beta-carotene cancer prevention study group, New England Journal of Medicine, vol.330, p.1029, 1994
[8] . Schwartz, JL, Journal of Nutrition, vol.126, 4 suppl, p.1221S, 1996
[9] . Noto, V., et al., Cancer, vol.63, p.901, 1989
[10] . Poydock, ME, American Journal of Clinical Nutrition, vol.54, p.12661S, 1991
[11] . Rao, AR, et al., Japanese Journal Cancer Research, vol.81, p.1239, Dec.1990
[12] . Lamm, DL, et al., Journal of Urology, vol.151, p.21, Jan.1994
[13] . Jaakkola, K., et al., Anticancer Research, vol.12, p.599, 1992
[14] . Hoffer, A., et al., Journal Orthomolecular Medicine, vol.5, no.3, p.143, 1990

CHAPTER 13

HEALING POWER OF WHOLE FOODS

✴

"Humor is the balancing stick that allows us to walk the tightrope of life." John F. Kennedy, 35th president of the United States

---

WHAT'S AHEAD?
Whole food contains more than just essential nutrients. There are minor dietary constituents, conditionally essential nutrients, phytochemicals, enzymes, pH stabilizing factors, substances required for a healthy colony of bacteria in the gut, and much more. Whole foods are irreplaceable in your quest for healing from cancer. No vitamin pill can substitute for the thousands of useful anti-cancer agents in Nature's treasure trove of delicious, fresh, unprocessed foods. This chapter will teach you good judgment and how to navigate through the confusing waters of nutrition information.
↪ if a food will not rot or sprout, then throw it out
↪ shop the perimeter of the grocery store for more of Nature's finest and less of mankind's nutrient-depleted junk food
↪ human-altered food is almost always an inferior substitute for Nature's original creation
↪ eat foods in as close to their natural state as is possible

---

Nutrition and health. It makes so much sense: "you are what you eat." Veterinarians know the irreplacable link between nutrient intake and health. Actually, most pets and all zoo creatures eat better than most Americans. Your dog or cat probably gets a balanced formula of protein, carbohydrate, fat, fiber, vitamins, and minerals. Yet, most of us eat

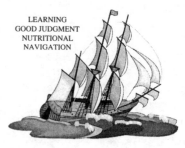

LEARNING GOOD JUDGMENT NUTRITIONAL NAVIGATION

for taste, cost, and convenience. The most commonly eaten food in America is heavily refined and nutritionally bankrupt white flour. Meanwhile, our livestock eat the more nutritious wheat germ and bran that we discard. When our crops are not doing well, we examine the soil for nutrients, fluid, and pH content. Our gardens prosper when we water, fertilize, and add a little broad-spectrum mineral supplement, such as Miracle Gro.

A sign posted near the junk food vending machines in a major city zoo warns: "Do not feed this food to the animals or they may get sick and die." Think about it. The food that might kill a 400 pound ape is okay for a 40 pound child who is biologically very similar? If our gardens, field crops, pets, exotic zoo creatures, and every other form of life on earth are all heavily dependent on their diet for health, then what makes us think that humans have transcended this dependence?

Like all forms of life, humans adapt to our environment. After 40,000 years, Eskimos have adapted to their unique diet and harsh cold environment. After thousands of years, humans adapted to a diet of small amounts of lean and clean meat (wild game, fish) along with fresh vegetables, fruit, whole grains, legumes, nuts, seeds, and kelp (seaweed). In the past 50 years, we have substantially deviated from this "factory specification" diet and have suffered the consequences with unprecedented levels of new diseases that were relatively rare or unknown prior to the later 20th century: obesity, diabetes, auto immune disease, Alzheimer's, Parkinson's, cancer, and depression.

ADAPTIVE FORCES OF NATURE. The first and worst pollutant on the planet earth was oxygen. Blue green algae soaked up the sun's energy in photosynthesis and produced sugar in the process, with oxygen as the waste by product. The oxygen killed everything around it. Eventually life adapted to tolerating oxygen. Eventually higher forms of life adapted to needing oxygen. The same goes for sunshine producing vitamin D in our skin and the need for iron and other nutrients. Over time, our bodies adapt to,

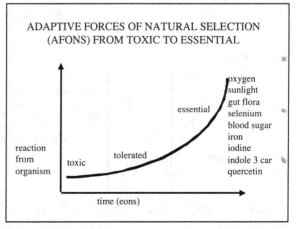

then tolerate and eventually need these substances. Xenobiotics are substances that are not commonly found in the body. Most drugs are

xenobiotics and have enormous potential for harm, unless used in the proper dosage and for limited time. This is why nutrients, in general, are safer than drugs, in general, because our body has had millennia to adapt and tolerate whatever is in our food supply.

MAKING SENSE OUT OF NUTRITION

One of our quests in this chapter is to help you better understand the concepts of nutrition. It never ceases to amaze me how people graduate from high school or college in America with no clue as to how to feed their body, or take care of the body, or how to best choose a mate, if and when to have a family, how to apply for work, and so on. Basic survival skills seem to be deleted from the academic curriculum in favor of less relevant topics.

Nutrition is logical. You cannot make a silk purse out of a sow's ear. You cannot squeeze blood from a rock. And you cannot fuel the processes of life from dead food. Much of what America eats is low in essential nutrients and high in harmful additives. While 2/3 of America is overweight, most Americans are suffering from malnutrition from excesses (calories, sugar, hydrogenated fat, additives), deficiencies (vitamins, minerals, fiber, essential fats, water), and imbalances between nutrients (sodium to potassium, omega 3 to omega 6, protein to B-6).

Some nutrients we need entirely from our diet, such as all minerals. Some nutrients we can make inside of us (endogenous), such as vitamin D from sunshine on the skin. Some nutrients we both eat and make, such as niacin can be made from the essential amino acid tryptophan. Some nutrients become

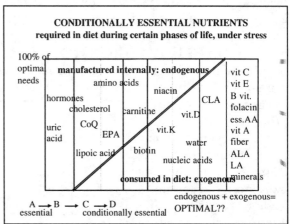

essential as we age or get sick, because the body can no longer make enough of it for good health, such as lipoic acid or coenzyme Q. Note the chart nearby for the complexities of this issue.

TIME REQUIRED TO DEVELOP MALNUTRITION. In 5
minutes without oxygen, a human can die. As little as 1 day without water might cause a lethal nutritional deficiency of water. It takes weeks or months for most nutrient deficiencies to surface. It might take years before a

chronic sub-clinical nutrient deficiency becomes a serious health challenge. New evidence shows us that heart disease is sometimes due to a 20 year deficiency of chromium, or folate, or vitamin E. In some cases, cancer is a long term deficiency of various nutrients, which is why it is so crucial

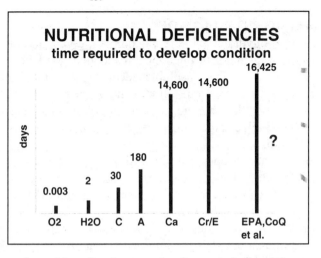

NUTRITIONAL DEFICIENCIES
time required to develop condition

to properly nourish the patient. Note the chart nearby for more information.

MALNUTRITION

Though America is the most agriculturally productive nation in the history of the world, there is indeed malnutrition among us. There are a set of nutritional guidelines that will allow you to survive long enough to reproduce, found in the Recommended Dietary Allowances, or Dietary Reference Intakes. There is a separate set of more complex nutritional requirements that will allow you to thrive beyond the normal 72 years and perhaps recover from cancer.

For instance, while the RDA for vitamin B-3 (niacin) is 20 milligrams daily, studies show that 100 mg of niacin becomes a potent vasodilator, while 2,000 mg of niacin can therapeutically lower serum cholesterol. Nutrients develop additional valuable duties in the body when taken in higher than survival doses. There is a limit to this, of course. More is not always better. See

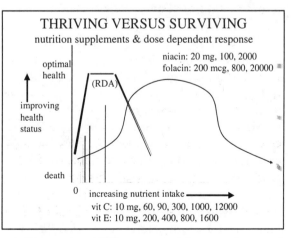

THRIVING VERSUS SURVIVING
nutrition supplements & dose dependent response

niacin: 20 mg, 100, 2000
folacin: 200 mcg, 800, 20000

vit C: 10 mg, 60, 90, 300, 1000, 12000
vit E: 10 mg, 200, 400, 800, 1600

the chapters on micronutrients for more guidelines on making supplemental nutrition safe and valuable.

MACRONUTRIENTS OF:
⇒ Carbohydrates (simple vs complex, glycemic index of foods, regulating prostaglandins through insulin and glucagon levels)
⇒ Fiber (soluble vs insoluble, adequate for regular bowel movements)
⇒ Fat: Useful include olive, canola, medium chain triglycerides, lecithin, fish oil, flax, borage, evening primrose, black current, hemp. Unhealthy fats include: too much fat (40% kcal vs 20%), hydrogenated, saturated, oxidized.
⇒ Protein: Proper quantity and quality necessary. Lean and clean protein found in chicken, fish, turkey, and beans. Vegetarians must match grains with legumes for complementary amino acids to create a high quality (biological value) protein.
⇒ Water. 2/3 of our body is water. Must consume high quality clean water throughout the day to improve hydration.

MICRONUTRIENTS OF:
⇒ Vitamins, such as C, E, A, D, B-6, B-12, B-1, B-2, biotin, etc.
⇒ Minerals, such as calcium, magnesium, potassium, iron, chromium, etc.
⇒ Ultra trace minerals, such as cesium, rubidium, lithium, etc.
⇒ Minor dietary constituents (i.e., lycopenes from tomato, allicin from garlic, sulforaphane from cabbage)
⇒ Conditionally essential nutrients (i.e., coenzyme Q-10; taurine; arginine; the fats of EPA, CLA, GLA; trimethylglycine; lipoic acid, etc.).

Too much, too little, or an imbalance of any nutrient leads to malnutrition. Most malnutrition in the US is via the cumulative effects of long term, sub-clinical deficiencies.

JUICING VERSUS PUREEING. Some of the earlier efforts at treating cancer with nutrition involved diets high in vegetables with regular fruit and vegetable juices offered throughout the day. Juicing has its advantages, because one glass of carrot juice is equal to about a pound of carrots, which few of us could eat. Unfortunately, much of the valuable anti-cancer nutrients in the

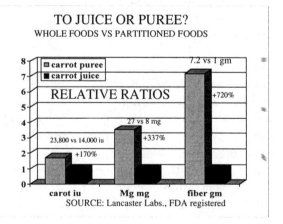

TO JUICE OR PUREE?
WHOLE FOODS VS PARTITIONED FOODS

RELATIVE RATIOS

□ carrot puree
■ carrot juice

7.2 vs 1 gm
+720%

27 vs 8 mg
+337%

23,800 vs 14,000 iu
+170%

carot iu   Mg mg   fiber gm
SOURCE: Lancaster Labs., FDA registered

vegetables get tossed out with the pulp that is discarded. That is why I recommend complete liquification of the vegetable or fruit rather than just extracting juice from it. High speed blenders, such as Vitamix (800-848-2649), will keep all the valuable nutrients in while allowing you to consume more vegetables in a liquid form. There are 10 times more cancer-fighting agents in pureed whole vegetables than in juice extracted from vegetable pulp.

>The KISS (keep it simple, student) method of optimal nutrition.

-Go natural. Eat foods in as close to their natural state as possible. Refining food often adds questionable agents (like food additives, salt, sugar, and fat), removes valuable nutrients (like vitamins, minerals, and fiber) and always raises the cost of the food.

-Expand your horizons. Eat a wide variety of foods. By not focusing on any particular food, you can obtain nutrients that may be essential, but are poorly understood, while also avoiding a buildup of any substance that could create food allergies or toxicities.

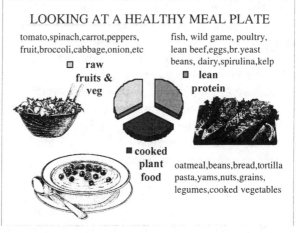

LOOKING AT A HEALTHY MEAL PLATE

tomato,spinach,carrot,peppers, fruit,broccoli,cabbage,onion,etc

☐ raw fruits & veg

fish, wild game, poultry, lean beef,eggs,br.yeast beans, dairy,spirulina,kelp

▣ lean protein

■ cooked plant food

oatmeal,beans,bread,tortilla pasta,yams,nuts,grains, legumes,cooked vegetables

-Nibbling is better. Eat small frequent meals. Nibbling is better than gorging. Our ancestors "grazed" throughout the day. Only with the advent of the industrial age did we begin the punctual eating of large meals. Nibbling helps to stabilize blood sugar levels and minimize insulin rushes, therefore it has been linked to a lowered risk for heart disease, diabetes, obesity, and mood swings.

-Avoid problem foods. Minimize your intake of unhealthy

FOOD PYRAMID FOR CANCER PATIENTS

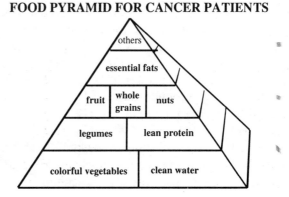

others

essential fats

fruit | whole grains | nuts

legumes | lean protein

colorful vegetables | clean water

foods that are high in fat, salt, sugar, cholesterol, caffeine, alcohol, processed lunch meats, and most additives.

-Seek out nutrient-dense foods. Maximize your intake of life-giving foods, including fresh vegetables, whole grains, legumes, fruit, low fat meat (turkey, fish, chicken), and clean water. Low-fat dairy products, especially yogurt, can be valuable if you do not have milk allergies or lactose intolerance.

-Monitor your quality of weight, rather than quantity of weight. Balance your calorie intake with expenditure so that your percentage of body fat is reasonable. Pinch the skinfold just above the hipbone. If this skin is more than an inch in thickness, then you may need to begin rational efforts to lose weight. Obesity is a major factor in cancer. For a more exact way to track your percent body fat, use the Tanita scale for bio-impedence (800-826-4828).

-Eat enough protein. Cancer is a serious wasting disease. I have counseled far too many cancer patients who looked like war camp victims, having lost 25% or more of their body weight due to insufficient protein intake. Take in 1 to 2 grams of protein for each kilogram of body weight. Example: 150 pound patient. Divide 150 pounds by 2.2 to find 68 kilograms, multiply times 1 to 2, yields 68 to 136 grams of protein daily that are needed to generate a healthy immune system. While a protein excess can have some harmful side effects, a protein deficiency is disastrous for the cancer patient.

-Use supplements in addition to, rather than instead of, good food. Get your nutrients with a fork and spoon. Do not place undue reliance on pills and powders to provide optimal nourishment. Supplements providing micronutrients (vitamins and minerals) cannot reverse the major influence of foods providing macronutrients (carbohydrate, fat, protein, fiber, water). Foods are top priority in your battle plan against cancer.

-Shop the perimeter of the grocery store. On outside aisles of your grocery store, you will find fresh fruits, vegetables, bread, fish, chicken, and dairy. When you venture into the deep dark interior of the grocery store, nutritional quality of the foods goes way down and prices go way up. Organic produce is raised without pesticides and may be valuable in helping cancer patients. However, organic produce is unavailable or unaffordable for many people. Don't get terribly concerned about having to consume organic produce. Any produce that cannot be peeled (like oranges or bananas) should be soaked for 5 minutes in a solution of one gallon lukewarm clean water with 2 tablespoons of vinegar

-If a food will not rot or sprout, then don't buy it, or throw it out. Your body cells have similar biochemical needs to a bacteria or yeast cell. Foods that have a shelf life of a millenium are not going to nourish the body.

Think about it: if bacteria is not interested in your food, then what makes you think that your body cells are interested? Foods that cannot begin (sprouting) or sustain (bacterial growth) life elsewhere will have a similar effect in your body.

-Dishes should be easy to clean. Foods that are hard to digest or unhealthy will probably leave a mess on plates and pots. Dairy curd, such as fondue, is both difficult to clean and very difficult for your stomach to process--same thing with fried, greasy, or burned foods.

>Essential nutrient pyramid.

We need to recognize the priority placed on essential nutrients. We can live weeks without food, a few days without water, and only a few minutes without oxygen. Keep in mind the relative importance of these essential nutrients.

Oxygen and water form the basis of human life. Make sure that your quality and quantity of intake pay homage to this fact. Protein, carbohydrate, fiber, and fat form the next level of importance. Vitamins and minerals are the essential micronutrients required for health.

Above these essential substances are two levels of quasi (meaning "as if it were") nutrients. Conditionally essential nutrients include coenzyme-Q10, carnitine, EPA and GLA (fatty acids), and much more. Some people may require these nutrients in the diet during certain stressful phases of their lives. Minor dietary constituents (MDC) include a wide variety of plant compounds that have shown remarkable anti-cancer abilities. Indoles in the cabbage family, lycopenes in tomatoes, allicin in garlic, immune stimulants in sea vegetables, and others make up this new and exciting category. Eating a wide variety of unprocessed plant foods will help to ensure adequate intake of these quasi-nutrients.

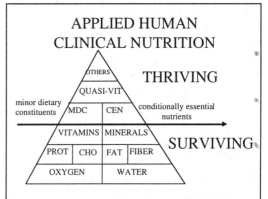

FOOD

Food is a rich tapestry of various chemicals. For some advanced cancer patients, TPN is often the only route that can provide adequate nutrient intake.

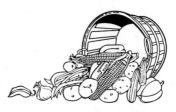

However, for most cancer patients, food is an integral part of their recovery. Food contains anti-cancer agents that we are only beginning to understand. One third of all prescription drugs in America originated as plant products. It is food that provides macronutrients, like carbohydrate, fat, and protein, which drive extremely influential hormones and prostaglandins in your body. It is food that establishes your pH balance and the electrolyte "soup" that bathes every cell in your body. While supplements are valuable, they cannot replace the fundamental importance of a wholesome diet.

Our eating habits are all acquired. We base our current diet on what mother cooked when we were younger; what our society, ethnic, and religious groups prefer; what is advertised in print and electronic media; and what is available in the local grocery store. People in the Phillipines or the Amazon are born with structurally-identical taste buds to Americans, yet they eat entirely different foods.

It takes about 3 weeks to acquire new eating habits. Try this program for 3 weeks, at which time it will become easier to stay with, and you may just find that the nutrient-depleted junk food of yesterday really doesn't satisfy your taste buds like the following whole foods outlined by Noreen Quillin.

GET ALL VECTORS WORKING IN THE RIGHT DIRECTION

Health is generated by many forces, or vectors, working in the right direction. Nutrition, stress, exercise, toxin avoidance, and energy alignment constitute the main vectors that allow our bodies to stay well or recover from any illness.

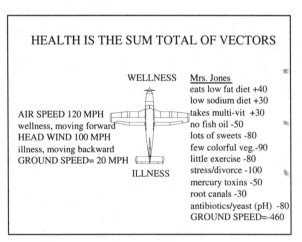

HEALTH IS THE SUM TOTAL OF VECTORS

WELLNESS

AIR SPEED 120 MPH
wellness, moving forward
HEAD WIND 100 MPH
illness, moving backward
GROUND SPEED= 20 MPH

ILLNESS

Mrs. Jones
eats low fat diet +40
low sodium diet +30
takes multi-vit +30
no fish oil -50
lots of sweets -80
few colorful veg.-90
little exercise -80
stress/divorce -100
mercury toxins -50
root canals -30
antibiotics/yeast (pH) -80
GROUND SPEED=-460

I have worked with patients who were doing a few minor things right and a lot of major things wrong. The net effect is little or no healing.

TRUE CONFESSIONS

Patrick Quillin has not always eaten as he does now. I now talk the talk and walk the walk. But I was raised in middle America, with roast beef, potatoes, and gravy every Sunday afternoon; Captain Crunch for breakfast; and a soda pop if you were good. White bread and bologna were the standard fare at home. My parents provided what they felt were lavish and well-balanced meals to the best of their knowledge, as do millions of other American families.

I remember one semester of my undergraduate degree when studying nutrition at San Diego State University. I was taking 19 units, 3 labs, and working part time. I had no spare time to cook or even eat, so I kept a large box of Twinkies in the back of my van to provide "sustenance" when needed. Right now, it seems humorous to have a nutrition student buying Twinkies in bulk. For many months, those Twinkies baked in the hot southern California sun and were always as fresh as the day they were bought. I began to question the shelf life of this food: "If bacteria is not interested in this food, then what makes me think that my body cells are interested in it!!" I no longer eat dead foods. If a food will not rot or sprout, then throw it out.

At that turning point in my life, my lovely and talented wife Noreen began exploring alternative cooking styles. For the 10 years that I worked with patients in cancer hospitals, Noreen taught cooking classes. What you have in the next chapter is a condensed and extremely practical approach to making your anti-cancer diet practical and tasty. Bon appetit!

SYNERGISTIC FORCES IN FOODS

Although 1,000 mg daily of vitamin C has been shown to reduce the risk for stomach cancer, a small glass of orange juice containing only 37 mg of vitamin C is twice as likely to lower the chances for stomach cancer. Something in oranges is even more chemo-protective than vitamin C. Although most people only absorb 20-50% of their ingested calcium, the remaining calcium binds up potentially damaging fats in the intestines to provide protection against colon cancer.

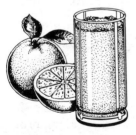

In 1963, a major "player" in the American drug business, Merck, tried to patent a single antibiotic substance that was originally isolated from yogurt. But this substance did not work alone. Since then, researchers have found no less than seven natural antibiotics that all contribute to yogurt's unique ability to protect the body from infections. There are many anti-cancer agents in plant food, including beta-carotene, chlorophyll, over 800 mixed carotenoids, over 20,000 various bioflavonoids, lutein, lycopenes, and canthaxanthin. The point is: we can isolate and concentrate certain factors in foods for use as therapeutic supplements in cancer therapy, but we must always rely heavily on the mysterious and elegant symphony of ingredients found in wholesome food.

USING GUIDELINES THAT ARE UNIVERSAL

There have been a number of diets developed for the cancer patient: Drs. Moerman[1], Livingston[2], Gerson[3], and the macrobiotic[4] diets to mention a few. Each of these visionaries was a physician who spent at least several decades ministering to cancer patients. While there are some differences in these diets, there is also some common ground. Peculariarities about each program include:

-Dr. Moerman recommends supplements of iron for cancer patients, yet other data show that elemental iron may accelerate cancer growth. He allows the yolk of the egg, but not the white part.

-Macrobiotics allow liberal amounts of soy sauce and pickles, yet restrict intake of fruit and fish.

-Dr. Gerson used to encourage raw pureed calf's liver, which can contain a number of dangerous bacteria.

-Dr. Livingston prohibits any chicken intake, since they think that a cancer-causing organism thrives in chicken.

The points just mentioned are the oddities about each program that lack a good explanation. Yet, we don't want to "throw out the baby with the bath water". Each of these programs embraces a common thread, which includes a number of explanable nutrition principles. They all provide a diet that:

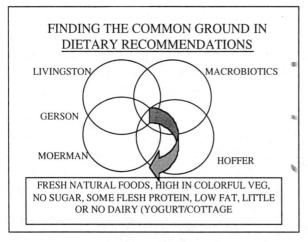

FINDING THE COMMON GROUND IN
DIETARY RECOMMENDATIONS

LIVINGSTON   MACROBIOTICS

GERSON

MOERMAN   HOFFER

FRESH NATURAL FOODS, HIGH IN COLORFUL VEG,
NO SUGAR, SOME FLESH PROTEIN, LOW FAT, LITTLE
OR NO DAIRY (YOGURT/COTTAGE

-uses only unprocessed foods, nothing in a package with a label

-uses high amounts of fresh vegetables

-employs a low fat diet

-emphasizes the importance of regularity

-uses little or no dairy products, with yogurt as the preferred dairy selection

-stabilizes blood sugar levels, with no sweets and never eat something sweet by itself

-increases potassium and reduces sodium intake

TOP TEN ANTI-CANCER FOOD CATEGORIES

There are many very nourishing foods. Creating a short list of superfoods is challenging and open to debate. Many of these foods are rich in antioxidants. Antioxidants are "electron donors", and free radicals are "electron thieves" that take away electrons in a cell membrane or DNA to destabilize that tissue. That could be the beginning of cancer. Scientists have developed a new technique for measuring the antioxidant capacity of foods, called ORAC, or oxygen radical antioxidant capacity. Basically, foods that are rich in color are usually rich in antioxidants.

How narrow do we limit the diet of the cancer patient? Some nutritionists will only encourage raw vegetables, which may induce malnutrition, weight loss, cachexia, and diarrhea. Some nutritionists insist on all food being organically raised. While organic food is cleaner, it is also much more expensive and difficult if not impossible for some

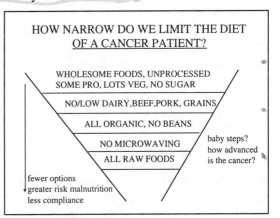

HOW NARROW DO WE LIMIT THE DIET OF A CANCER PATIENT?

WHOLESOME FOODS, UNPROCESSED SOME PRO, LOTS VEG, NO SUGAR

NO/LOW DAIRY, BEEF, PORK, GRAINS

ALL ORGANIC, NO BEANS

NO MICROWAVING

ALL RAW FOODS

baby steps? how advanced is the cancer?

fewer options
greater risk malnutrition
less compliance

people to obtain. Hence, I try to make the diet for the cancer patient realistic, yet nourishing. No unnecessary restrictions will be found. The more you restrict the diet, the more likely that malnutrition will set in, and the lower the chances for compliance.

1) **VEGETABLES.** Vegetables are rich in antioxidants and anti-cancer nutrients, have a preferred lower glycemic index, and are rich in cleansing fiber. Best categories of vegetables include:

COLORFUL: Beets, spinach, carrots, tomatoes, squash, and more. The deeper the color, the more "phytochemicals". In these pigments lay 20,000 bioflavonoids and 800 carotenoids, which provide extraordinary antioxidant protection for the human body, plus immune stimulation to destroy cancer cells.

CABBAGE FAMILY. Cabbage, broccoli, brussel sprouts, cauliflower. In these unique cruciferous vegetables lay a series of anti-cancer, detoxifying substances, including indole-3-carbinol and sulforafane.

ALLIUM FAMILY. Onions and garlic contain bioflavonoids, like quercetin, that can actually revert a cancer cell back to a healthy cell. Other components of this special anti-cancer vegetable family include allicin, S-allyl cysteine, selenium, and probably unknown components that contribute to the powerful cancer-protective effects of having garlic and onions regularly.

2) COLD WATER FISH. Salmon, haddock, halibut, bass, cod, mackerel, sardine, and tuna are loaded with anti-cancer fats, which slow down the spreading of cancer, stimulate immune functions, and contain trace minerals from the sea that are not commonly found in foods from our mineral-depleted soil. Due to mercury content, avoid tilefish, swordfish, king mackerel, shark, red snapper, and orange roughy.

3) LEGUMES. Soybeans, garbanzo, kidney beans, pinto beans, and many others constitute this group of plant food, which is rich in protease inhibitors for cancer fighting, inositol hexaphosphate (phytic acid, also sold as IP-6), and genistein for shutting down the making of blood vessels from tumors (anti-angiogenesis). Legumes have the cleansing activity of soluble fibers.

4) WHOLE GRAINS. Oats, rice, millet, amaranth, buckwheat, barley, corn, rye, and the American standard wheat all contain components that can help stem the cancer deterioration, like fiber that gets broken down in the gut to butyric acid, which is a powerful anti-cancer agent. Modern wheat has been hybridized many times to achieve a much higher, but not necessarily healthier, gluten content. Sprout and/or puree barley, oats, rice, quinoa, rye, and flax in your blender in place of wheat flour.

5) KELP. Sea vegetables have been a staple in the diet of people who lived near the ocean for many centuries. Only recently have we turned away from kelp for a food. Kelp, including dulse, nori, wakame, and other varieties, is rich in anti-microbial agents that keep pathogens from invading our guts. Kelp has a special soluble fiber that carries harmful fats, pro-oxidants, hormone residues, and other toxins out of the gut. Kelp is also the best source of the many trace minerals that are in the ocean, and need to be in the human diet, yet are not added to the soil to grow our food crops.

6) COLORFUL BERRIES. In raspberries, boysenberries, strawberries, dark cherries, blueberries, and blackberries lay a powerful anti-cancer agent, ellagic acid, which causes cancer cells to self destruct (apoptosis).

7) YOGURT. When the bacteria, Lactobacillus,

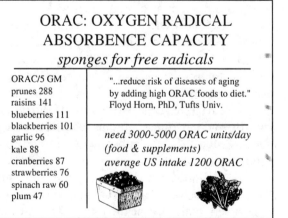

ORAC: OXYGEN RADICAL ABSORBENCE CAPACITY
sponges for free radicals

ORAC/5 GM	
prunes 288	"...reduce risk of diseases of aging by adding high ORAC foods to diet." Floyd Horn, PhD, Tufts Univ.
raisins 141	
blueberries 111	
blackberries 101	
garlic 96	*need 3000-5000 ORAC units/day*
kale 88	*(food & supplements)*
cranberries 87	*average US intake 1200 ORAC*
strawberries 76	
spinach raw 60	
plum 47	

ferments milk sugar, a variety of healthy by-products are created that nourish the gut and immune system. Since 80% of the immune system lines the gastrointestinal tract, yogurt can fortify the body's defenses against infections and cancer.

8) GREEN TEA. Containing catechins and other microscopic phytochemicals, green tea is a treasure trove of cancer-fighting agents. Researchers at the National Cancer Institute in Japan and China have found numerous mechanisms explaining why green tea can prevent and even reverse some forms of cancer.

9) HEALTHY SEASONINGS. Mustard, curry, hot peppers, salsa, cinnamon, garlic, onions, ginger, sage, rosemary, thyme, and other seasonings replace the typical unhealthy American "fat, salt, and sugar" approach to flavoring foods. These seasonings add flavor and therapeutic anti-cancer and immune-stimulating ingredients.

10) CLEAN WATER. Two thirds of the earth's surface is covered with water. And two thirds of the human body is filled with water. Water is the medium of life on the planet earth. Water in the human body helps to cleanse and dilute impurities, stabilize acid/base balance, and provide a healthy flow of nutrients into the cells and toxins out of the cells through a newly discovered "cell membrane dynamics".

SUPERFOODS

Though there are many nourishing foods, there are only a few superfoods that contain such a potent collection of protective factors that they deserve regular inclusion in most diets.

-Garlic. This stinky little vegetable has been used for 5,000 years in various healing formulas. Pasteur noted that garlic killed all of the bacteria in his petri dishes. More importantly, garlic has been found to stimulate natural protection against tumor cells. Tarig Abdullah, MD, of Florida found that white blood cells from garlic-fed people were able to kill 139% more tumor cells than white cells from non-garlic eaters.[5] Garlic and onions fed to lab animals helped to decrease the number of skin tumors.[6] Researchers found that onions provided major protection against expected tumors from DMBA in test animals.[7] Mice with a genetic weakness toward cancer were fed raw garlic with a lower-than-expected tumor incidence.[8]

The most common form of cancer worldwide is stomach cancer. Chinese researchers find that a high intake of garlic and onions cuts the risk for stomach cancer in half.[9] Garlic provides the liver with a certain amount of protection against carcinogenic chemicals. Scientists find that garlic is deadly to invading pathogens or tumor cells, but is harmless to normal healthy body cells, thus offering the hope of the truly selective toxin against cancer that is being sought worldwide.

-Carotenoids. Green plants create sugars by capturing the sun's energy in a process called photosynthesis. The electrons that must be corralled in this process can be highly destructive. Hence, nature has evolved an impressive system of free radical protectors, including carotenoids and bioflavonoids, that act like the lead lining in a nuclear reactor to absorb dangerous unpaired electrons. Both of these substances have potential in stimulating the immune system, while there is preliminary evidence that carotenoids may be directly toxic to tumor cells.

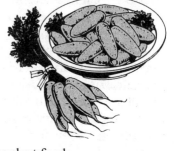

Carotenoids are found in green and orange fruits and vegetables. Bioflavonoids are found in citrus, whole grains, honey, and other plant foods.

-Cruciferous vegetables. Broccoli, brussel sprouts, cabbage, and cauliflower were involved in the "ground floor" discovery that nutrition is linked to cancer. Lee Wattenberg, PhD, of the University of Minnesota found in the 1970s that animals fed cruciferous vegetables had markedly lower cancer rates than matched controls. Since then, the active ingredient "indoles" have been isolated from cruciferous vegetables and found to be very protective against cancer. Scientists at Johns Hopkins University found that lab animals fed cruciferous vegetables and then exposed to the deadly carcinogen aflatoxin had a 90% reduction in their cancer rate.[10]

Cruciferous vegetables are able to increase the body's production of glutathione peroxidase, which is one of the more important protective enzyme systems in the body.

-Mushrooms. Gourmet chefs have long prized various mushrooms for their subtle and exotic flavors. Now there is an abundance of scientific evidence showing that Rei-shi, Shiitake, and Maitake mushrooms are potent anti-cancer foods.[11] Actually, Maitake literally means "dancing mushroom" since people would dance with joy when finding these delicate mushrooms on a country hillside. Oral extract of Maitake provided complete elimination of tumors in 40% of animals tested, while the remaining 60% of animals had a 90% elimination of tumors. Maitake contains a polysaccharide, called beta-glucan, which stimulates the immune system and even lowers blood pressure.

-Legumes. Seed foods (like soybeans) have a substance that can partially protect the seed from digestion, called protease inhibitors (PI). For

many years, these substances were thought to be harmful. New evidence finds that PIs may squelch tumor growth.[12] Researchers at the National Cancer Institute find a collection of substances in soybeans, including isoflavones and phytoestrogens, that appear to have potent anti-cancer properties.[13] Dr. Ann Kennedy has spent 20 years researching a compound in soybeans that:

-prevents cancer in most animals exposed to a variety of carcinogens

-retards cancer in some studies

-lowers the toxic side effects of chemo and radiation therapy

-reverts a cancer cell back to a normal healthy cell.[14]

-Others. There are numerous foods that show an ability to slow tumor growth in some way. Apples, apricots, barley, citrus fruit, cranberries, fiber, figs, fish oil, fish, ginger, green tea, spinach, seaweed, and other foods are among the reasons that I heavily favor the use of a mixed highly nutritious diet as the foundation for nutrition in cancer therapy.

Food treats malnutrition. Food contains known essential nutrients that stimulate the immune system and provide valuable protection against carcinogens. Foods also contain poorly understood factors that may add measurably to the recovery of the cancer patient. Many foods have tremendous therapeutic value in helping the patient to internally fight cancer.

DRAGON-SLAYER SHAKE

I hate taking pills, even when I know the value of using supplements to improve my health. That's why I developed this "shake". While most of us are familiar with milkshakes, there are many variations on that theme that can provide nutrient-dense foods in a convenient format. I have found that many cancer patients would avoid taking their supplements of vitamins, minerals, and botanicals because they didn't like swallowing pills. To solve that problem, I have developed this shake, which can incorporate many nutrients in powder form, thus eliminating taking pills at all, and the remaining pills are easier to swallow with the lubricating ability of this smooth shake.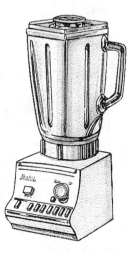

Shakes can be a quick and easy breakfast. Depending on your calorie requirements, use this shake in addition to or instead of the breakfast suggestions listed later. My typical breakfast consists of this Dragon-Slayer shake, whole grain tortillas, 2 eggs, salsa, and avocado.

Take up to half of your pills with the "Dragon-Slayer shake" and save the remaining pills for later in the day. Taking supplements in small divided dosages helps to maintain sustained levels of nutrients in the bloodstream.

DRAGONSLAYER SHAKE: general combination of ingredients				
liquid 4-8 oz	protein1-4 T	vegetables	thicken 2T	other 1-3 T.
water	egg,soy, rice	raw or cook	froze banana	MCT
fruit juice	powder beef	carrots, beets	apple sauce	lecithin
vegetable j.	whey	broccoli	agar	powdr greens
V8	bee pollen	cauliflower	carragenan	aloe
ice cubes	dry milk	cabbage	guar gum	Perfect 7
milk	wheat germ	tomato,onion	gelatin	vit/min powd
soy milk	flax meal	asparagus	ice cubes	ImmunoPwr
rice milk	spirulina	spinach, kale		flax oil
	brewer yeast	collards		

Ingredients:
➤ 4-8 ounces of liquid
➤ 10-15 grams (1-4 tablespoons) of powdered protein
➤ 1/4 to 1/2 cup vegetables, cooked or raw
➤ 1-3 tablespoons thickening agent
➤ 1-3 tablespoons of other ingredients, including ImmunoPower (888-741-LIFE), Perfect 7 (Agape 800-767-4776), or flax oil.

Banana adds texture via pectin to make this shake have true milk shake viscosity. If the banana is frozen, it will give a thick "milkshake-like" texture to your drink.

For those who need to gain weight, add 2 tablespoons of MCT (medium chain triglyceride) oil from your health food store.

Directions:
Using a powerful blender, such as a Vitamix (800-VITAMIX), puree all ingredients.

EAT YOUR ANCESTRAL DIET

There has been an endless parade of diets that were hailed as "the perfect diet". But there is no one perfect diet. Behold the fascinating spectrum of 6 billion people on the planet earth. We are all different. While macrobiotics may be helpful for some, it is counterproductive for a few. In order to have a decent grasp on the core diet for humans, we need to take a ride in our time machine back to our hunter and gatherer ancestors, who roamed the earth before the dawn of agriculture. By examining the diet of primitive hunter gatherer societies plus archeological findings, a trio of modern day "Indiana Jones" researchers turned up some of the most important nutrition data of the 20th century.[15]

Paleolithic vs. Modern Diet

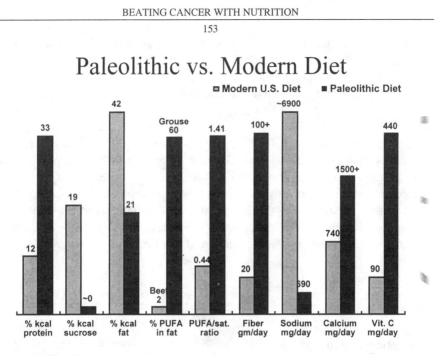

Source: Paleolithic Prescription by Eaton, Shostak, Konner, Harper & Row, 1988

Most of our hunter-gatherer ancestors ate a diet consisting of about 1/3 lean animal tissue with the remaining 2/3 of the diet unprocessed plant food; mostly vegetables, some grains, some fruit, nuts, seeds, and legumes. If the creature runs, flies, or swims, then it may be about 4% body fat, with obvious exceptions including duck and salmon. Cows, the staple meat of America, do none of the above and are about 30-40% body fat. While there are certainly variations on this theme, this is the basic diet of our ancestors and a good starting point for our cancer-fighting diet. Both studies and my clinical experience

REASONS FOR OMNIVOROUS DIET

CARNIVORE NUTRIENTS	HERBIVORE nutrients
conjugated linoleic acid (CLA)	carotenoids
eicosapentaenoic acid (EPA)	bioflavonoids
cartilage (glycosaminoglycans)	sterolins (beta sitosterol)
carnitine	fiber (butyrate)
CoQ	potassium
B-12	anti-fungals (veg., mushr.,kelp)
zinc	chlorophyll
quarternary amino acid sequence	
biological value of protein	

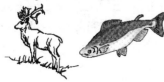

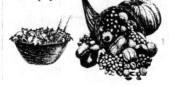

show that a low fat diet with lots of fresh vegetables will improve cancer outcome. Take a look at the graphic illustration of the contrast between the modern American diet and our "factory specification" ancestral diet. Notice how far we have strayed from our ancestral diet.

Keep in mind that you may have to "fine tune" this diet to suit your ethnic background. The macrobiotic diet was developed by a Japanese physician who cured himself of cancer in the 19th century. The macrobiotic diet tends to encourage anything Oriental (even soy sauce and pickles) and discourage anything Western, including chicken, turkey, fish, and fruit. Macrobiotics may be ideally suited for many Orientals and has helped some Caucasians, because it is such a vast improvement over the nutritional quality of the typical American diet. I encourage people to determine the diet of their ancestors 5,000 years ago and use that food pattern as a starting point.

Imagine the following experiment. Dr. Rabbit, Dr. Cat, and Dr. Squirrel are conducting a study of the nutrient needs of their patients, consisting of 100 subjects of 33 cats, 33 rabbits, and 34 squirrels. Dr. Rabbit puts everyone on a vegetarian diet, because Dr. Rabbit is

MERITS OF FOLLOWING YOUR ETHNIC DIET

- Nutrition & Physical Degeneration, Price, 1945
- Pottenger's Cats, Pottenger, 1983
- Paleolithic Prescription, Eaton, 1988
- Native Nutrition, Schmid, 1994
- Coronary Heart Disease, Mann, 199
- The Zone, Sears, 1995
- 10 adult male aborigine diabetics, return to wild, diet high in meat, 7 wk: 18 lb loss, TG 75% drop, BG 50% drop, "cured", *O'Dea, Diabetes, vol.33, p.596, 1984*

a vegan. Some of the 100 "patients" get much better, some get worse, and some stay the same. Dr. Cat steps up to the plate and takes the same "mono-mania" approach of putting everyone on a carnivorous diet, just like Dr. Cat. Same results: 1/3 get better, 1/3 get worse, and the rest stay the same. Dr. Squirrel has the same luck with the mixed grain and nuts diet of squirrels. Moral of the story: there is no one perfect diet. In spite of various noble efforts to categorize people based upon their blood type, their build, their nervous system type, their Ayurvedic status, or whatever...you need to ask the question: "What did my ancestors eat for most of the past thousands of years?" When I asked this question in one group of cancer patients, a person responded, "Then I guess I should be eating hog fat, like my grandpappy who was a farmer in Arkansas." I replied that, in order to give adequate credit to the adaptive forces of Nature, we need to go back further than 50 or 100 years.

HEALTHIER SEASONINGS

SUGAR: Americans consume over 140 pounds per year per person of refined sugar, which constitutes 20% of total calories. Excess simple carbohydrates in the gut can stimulate yeast overgrowth and lower immune functions, while causing a lengthy list of health hazards, like "tanning" blood proteins (glycation), constricting blood vessels, triggering cancer (via protein kinase C), increasing free radical damage to all body tissues, and more.

RECOMMENDATIONS: Cut back dramatically on intake of sweet foods. Cut white sugar intake by 90%. Change your taste buds to appreciate the real taste of the food, not having everything coated with sugar. Eat a small amount of fresh colorful fruit (i.e. blueberries, apricots, red grapefruit) after a meal containing fat, protein, and fiber. Do not eat large amounts of sweet foods by themselves (i.e. carrot juice). Use honey (Y.S. Bee Farms 800-654-4593), stevia, xylitol, and tagatose as acceptable sweeteners.

FAT: Americans eat about 90 pounds per year of fat, which constitutes around 40% of total calories. Excess fat or the wrong kind of fat (i.e. hydrogenated) or not enough fat-soluble antioxidants (i.e. vitamin E, lipoic acid) can lead to a fragile immune system, cancer-causing damage to the DNA, excess production of tumor-promoting hormones, and more.

RECOMMENDATIONS: Cut back fat intake by 50%, making fat only 20% of daily calories. Ask for your food to be broiled, baked, steamed, or grilled, rather than fried. Avoid gravies and high fat meats, like bologna and prime rib. If necessary, lose weight slowly to reduce excess body fat.

SALT: Americans consume 10 times the sodium compared to our ancestral diet and use mostly refined salt. While salt is an essential nutrient, too much salt (sodium chloride) may contribute to diseases. Deficiencies of calcium, magnesium, potassium, and fluid in conjunction with excess sodium probably lead to flaws in "cell membrane dynamics" or how the 60 trillion cells in your body take in nutrients and expel waste products. Every cell in the human body is an electrical battery, and these minerals contribute greatly to having the right charge for good health.

RECOMMENDATIONS: Use sea salt in cooking. Let people add their own sea salt or Celtic salt at the dinner table. Let your taste buds adjust to the real flavor of the food without the ever-present coating of salt.

SEASONINGS: Our ancestors were unknowingly practicing "herbal medicine" all day everyday in the kitchen--by seasoning foods with healthy herbs. Columbus discovered the Americas while in pursuit of the Spice Islands near India to allow wealthy people to flavor their foods with seasonings. Many herbal flavorings are not only delicious, but are very healthy for us.

RECOMMENDATIONS: Use healthy seasonings liberally. See chapter on "Nutritious and Delicious" for more information.

HEALTHIER SEASONINGS

SUGAR	FAT	SALT	SEASONINGS (use liberally)
pureed fruit xylitol honey fructose stevia unsweet fruit juice applesauce glycine tagatose	oil of olive, canola, flax, wheat germ, avocado, coconut, rice bran, sesame; butter from dairy, almond & cashew medium chain triglycerides, Pam	Morton Lite Salt, Salt Subst (KCl), Celtic Salt, Lawry's, lemon juice, vinegar, kelp powder, Spike, Mrs.Dash, Cajun salt, soy sauce	cinnamon, garlic, onion, cayenne, chili, paprika, salsa, rosemary, tarragon, thyme, sage, pumpkin pie spice, teriyaki, Gaylord's vegetable broth, allspice, bay leaves, caraway seeds, cardamom, celery seed, chives, cloves, oregano, mustard, dill, nutmeg, curry, almond, vanilla, Tabasco, Worcestershire, chocolate, cumin, ginger, carob, peppermint, spearmint, fennel, basil, hickory, liquid smoke

PATIENT PROFILES: MULTIPLE MYELOMA FROM 3 ANGLES

M.G.T. was diagnosed with advanced multiple myeloma. His doctors told him that chemo might extend his life to a year and without chemo he would succumb to the disease in much less time. Michael Gearin-Tosh pursued alternative cancer treatment aggressively, using diet, supplements (including ImmunoPower), intravenous vitamin C and detoxification. He went in to complete remission, considered impossible by his first oncologist, and remained disease free for eight years before writing LIVING PROOF: A MEDICAL MUTINY in 2002.

J.H. was a successful attorney and family man when he was diagnosed with multiple myeloma in 2002. He followed my recommendations for aggressive diet and supplement support while undergoing an autologous (using his own stem cells) then allogeneic (using his sister's stem cells) transplant procedure. His doctors were surprised at how well J.H. tolerated the rigors of a double stem cell transplant. James Huston is in good health as of 2005, enjoys his family, continues to fly (he was a former top gun Navy pilot), practice law, and write bestsellers like SECRET JUSTICE.

K.Q. was 39 when he was diagnosed with multiple myeloma. His oncologist told K.Q. that if he used any nutrition supplements during chemo that K.Q. would have to find another oncologist. K.Q. was given an assortment of chemo agents, plus decadron steroids, thalidomide and more. K.Q. died in intensive pain and on a ventilator 18 months later while his wife was pregnant with twins. K.Q. was my brother in law, Kevin Quinn. In my opinion, aggressive chemo or radiation therapy without aggressive protective nutrition therapy constitutes malpractice in medicine.

ENDNOTES

[1]. Jochems, R., DR. MOERMAN'S ANTI-CANCER DIET, Avery, Garden City, NY, 1990

[2]. Livingston-Wheeler, V., et al., THE CONQUEST OF CANCER, Waterside, San Diego, 1984

[3]. Gerson, M., A CANCER THERAPY, Gerson Institute, Bonita, CA 1958

[4]. Aihara, H., ACID & ALKALINE, George Ohsawa Foundation, Oroville, CA, 1986; see also Kushi, M., THE CANCER PREVENTION DIET, St. Martin Press, NY, 1983

[5]. Abdullah, TH, et al., Journal of the National Medical Association, vol.80, no.4, p.439, Apr.1988

[6]. Belman, S., Carcinogenesis, vol.4, no.8, p.1063, 1983

[7]. Kiukian, K., et al., Nutrition and Cancer, vol.9, p.171, 1987

[8]. Kroning, F., Acta Unio Intern. Contra. Cancrum, vol.20, no.3, p.855, 1964

[9]. You, WC, et al., Journal of the National Cancer Institute, vol.81, p.162, Jan.18, 1989

[10]. Ansher, SS, Federation of Chemistry and Toxicology, vol.24, p.405, 1986

[11]. Chihara, G., et al., Cancer Detection and Prevention, vol.1, p.423, 1987 suppl.

[12]. Kennedy, A., and Little, JB, Cancer Research, vol.41, p.2103, 1981

[13]. Messina, M., et al., Journal National Cancer Institute, vol.83, no.8, p.541, Apr.1991

[14]. Oreffo, VI, et al., Toxicology, vol.69, no.2, p.165, 1991; see also von Hofe, E, et al., Carcinogenesis, vol.12, no.11, p.2147, Nov.1991

[15]. Eaton, SB, et al., New England Journal of Medicine, vol.312, no.5, p.283, Jan.1985

CHAPTER 14

NUTRITIOUS AND DELICIOUS
★
RECIPES FOR HEALING
by Noreen Quillin

"Let food be your medicine and medicine be your food."
Hippocrates, father of modern medicine, 400 B.C

WHAT'S AHEAD?

Most healing begins in the kitchen and in the heart. Food for the body and food for the soul are crucial for a cancer patient to recover. Great tips follow for making your food nutritious, delicious, simple to prepare, and inexpensive:

-ideas for gaining or losing weight

-eating in restaurants and bulk cooking in your kitchen

-recipes for breakfast, snacks, lunch, dinner, and desserts

Eating should be fun! Just because you choose to eat healthy, does not mean you need to give up one of life's pleasures. You can not please everyone all the time. Some have felt the recipes in the other versions of this book were too strict or too lenient. Making food your enemy is not our purpose. We are trying to bring a balance to your dinner plate. The recipes listed are showing how you can get creative in the kitchen. Nothing is carved in stone here. If there are foods listed in this

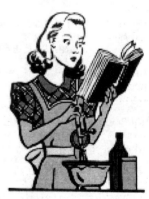

chapter that you don't enjoy, then cross it off your list. Make a meal appetizing. Think color. Instead of bland colors with the same look, (i.e. turkey, mashed potatoes and cauliflower), dress up the plate.

COMMONLY ASKED QUESTIONS:

Q) Many people are on the go and don't feel that they have time to plan healthy meals. Any suggestions?
A) Cook in bulk. Freeze leftovers in serving size packets. You can then make your own TV dinners. Crock pot cooking is good, because the food is ready when you arrive home hungry. Have fruits and vegetables on hand. Simplify cooking by leaving out heavy sauces and creams. Put foods that cook at the same temperature in the oven when arriving home. Plan ahead. Eat smaller portions throughout the day, then you won't be starving by dinner time and be tempted to pick up fast food.

Q) What is the best way to cook vegetables?
A) Cook to a crisp-tender stage. Steaming is much better than boiling. Do not microwave. Use spices to flavor, but not overpower the vegetable.

Q) Can you cut sugar in a favorite recipe?
A) Use concentrated fruit juices, unsweetened applesauce, crushed pineapple, and mashed bananas instead of sugar. Cinnamon or vanilla will enhance the sweetness. If a recipe calls for 1 cup of sugar, then instead substitute with one of the following:

Substitutes for 1 Cup White Sugar		Reduce Liquids in Recipe
Stevia equivalents:	1/3 to1/2 tsp. powder extract	
	1/2 to 3/4 liquid extract	
	1 1/2-2 Tbs. powder leaf	
Xylitol	3/4 cup	
Honey	1/2 cup	1/8 to 1/4 cup
Fructose	1/3 to 1/2 cup	1 to 3 Tbs.
Molasses	1/2 cup	1/4 cup
Unsweetened applesauce	3/4 cup	1/3 to 1/2 cup
Mashed ripe banana	1 cup	
Sucanat	3/4 cup	1 to 2 Tbs.
Maple sugar	1/2 cup	1/4 cup
Apple or other fruit juice	1 cup	1/4 cup

-Vanilla, cinnamon, cardamom – can be used to replace sugar in toppings and dessert sauces.

Q) How can a person cut back on salt?
A) Our taste for salty foods has been acquired. Gradually cut back on the use of highly processed foods and salty snacks. Cook with herb blends

instead of salt. Use more garlic, hot peppers, curry, cloves, and ginger, which are very healthy seasoning herbs. Use "Lite salt", which is made up of regular salt diluted with the helpful minerals of potassium, magnesium, and calcium, in your salt shaker.

Q) Do you have a helpful suggestion if someone eats too fast?
A) Make dining a separate experience. No watching TV while eating. Dine only while sitting at the dining table. Begin a meal with hot soup, or salad, or fresh fruit as an appetizer. This provides bulk. Never serve food "family style". After taking a bite of food, place utensil back on plate. Completely chew food to a liquid and swallow before putting more food on the fork.

Q) There are many studies on the benefits of garlic, but the taste is pretty strong, and bad breath would be a problem for me at work. Is there a way to prepare garlic that will "soften" the flavor?
A) Break a bulb of garlic into cloves. You don't need to peel them. Place in a coffee cup. Sprinkle on some olive oil. Add a bit of Spike, soy sauce, or your favorite low-salt seasoning. Stir until the cloves have been coated. Place a plate over the top. Roast in convection oven for 10 minutes or microwave for about 2 minutes. Your garlic will peel easily and taste somewhat like spring potatoes.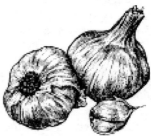

GARLIC MEASUREMENTS
1 fresh clove = 1/8 tsp. dried minced garlic or garlic powder
1 fresh clove = 1/2 tsp. bottled minced garlic
1 tsp. garlic salt = 1/8 tsp. garlic powder plus 7/8 tsp. salt

Q) We all know that breakfast is important but we don't have the time in the morning to cook a big meal. What can we do to nourish ourselves?
A) Americans eat 80-85% of the day's calories in just a few concentrated hours, usually in the evening. Some people skip breakfast, because they don't feel as hungry as they do if they eat breakfast. The reason for this unusual effect is that when you starve in the morning, the waste products (ketones) are released in the blood stream, depressing the appetite. But as soon as you eat, you will overeat. Some fast breakfast ideas are: hard boiled eggs prepared in advance; protein bar; hot instant cereals; whole grain cold cereals with apple juice for moisture; pancakes left over from the weekend; bowl of yogurt; whole wheat bagel with no-fat cream cheese or natural peanut butter; a mixed drink of fruit juice with protein powder.

Q) Are there any tips to be aware of when shopping for groceries?

A) Don't shop when you're hungry. Eat a variety of foods, which will improve nutrient intake and reduce exposure to toxins. Shop the perimeter of the grocery store. Read labels.

Don't eat heavily processed foods with a shelf life with a millennium time frame or that can glow in the dark.

FATS FOR COOKING
MCT
Olive Oil
Canola Oil
Coconut Oil
Flax Oil (not to be heated)

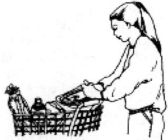

GOOD FATS
Kitchen: olive oil, canola, lecithin, vegetable spray oils (i.e. Pam), MCT oil, and better butter (1/2 butter & 1/2 canola or olive oil whipped together).
Therapeutic: fish, flax, borage, evening primrose, grape seed, hemp, black current, pumpkin

BAD FATS
oxidized (over used), hydrogenated, too much omega 6 from corn & soy

IDEAS TO REPLACE FAT
-Marinate without fat: lemon, orange, tomato, yogurt & juice with herbs, sauces - tomato with onions and garlic, vegetable stock
-Saute in: water, stock, vegetable bouillon, juice, liquid instead of oil or butter
-Steam vegetables
-Steam bake corn tortillas in oven instead of frying
-Crackers often contain large amounts of hydrogenated fats
-Use 2 teaspoons of canola or olive oil in place of 1 tablespoon shortening
-Use raised broiler pan in oven so the excess fat will drip away
-Avoid processed meats
Dairy: -low fat or nonfat plain yogurt vs. sour cream
-Salad dressings usually use fat as main ingredients
-Make your own (1/2 flax oil, 1/2 apple cider vinegar, 1 tsp. lecithin, and a packet of powdered Italian seasoning mix)
-Delicious low-fat garlic bread: coat bread with butter-flavor Pam and sprinkle with garlic powder. Bake 5-10 minutes at 350 degrees.
-Fried-like food: Dip chicken in egg. Then dip in sack with whole wheat cracker crumbs, oat flour, corn meal, and spices. Spray with Pam. Bake 400 degrees for 1 hour, turning every 20 minutes, spraying with Pam.

FOR GAINING WEIGHT

* -Try not to drink fluids or have soup or salad before the meal. It will fill you up on foods and fluids that are low in calorie density.
* -Eat on a large plate, thus avoiding food portions that appear overwhelming. Have small portions, knowing you can always have more.
* -People will eat more food when dining with groups than by themselves. Go to buffets. Eat with friends if possible.
* -Distract your mind. Rent a good video and have your meal in front of the TV. Have you ever sat down with a bowl of popcorn and realized you had eaten the whole batch and weren't aware of eating?

FOR LOSING WEIGHT

* -Eat six small meals a day. For example: a light breakfast upon rising; a small amount of fruit with a protein serving later in the mid-morning; a salad and half of a sandwich at lunch; and the other 1/2 of the sandwich at mid-afternoon. Even if you over-indulge at one meal, make sure you eat on schedule. This concept, called periodicity, trains the mind and body that food is constantly coming into the system, and there is no need to overindulge or become exceedingly efficient at storing calories.
* -Enjoy a warm fluid, like tea or soup, about 20 minutes before mealtime.
* -Use a smaller plate. It gives the illusion that you're eating more.
* Try not to eat after 7:30 pm.
* Time yourself to see how long a meal takes to eat. Make a meal last for at least 20 minutes. This is how long it will be before you start feeling full.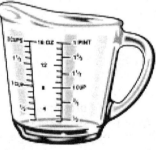
* -Drink plenty of purified water. It is good for weight loss, constipation, and wrinkles.
* -Adjust your bathroom scale to the exact weight you want to be. As you lose weight, you can readjust it closer to the zero, but always see your weight as you want it to be. This way, when you think about having that huge piece of cake, you will think to yourself, "A person of my weight wouldn't eat that."
* -Exercise within your ability. Make sure you enjoy it.
* -Eat more high-fiber foods, such as fruits, vegetables, beans, and whole-grain cereals.
* -Plan your meals and snacks instead of waiting until you are hungry.
* -When dining at a restaurant, ask for a carry out box to be brought with the meal. Then portion the amount before eating, so there will not be temptation to keep nibbling.

EATING OUT

- Skip the iceberg lettuce and enjoy the healthier greens, vegetables, and whole-grains from the salad bar. A good rule of thumb: the deeper the color of the vegetable, the more nourishing it is. Dark greens are better than pale greens, dark orange squash is better than pale squash, and so on. In nature, cauliflower is a dark green vegetable, until human intervention ties the leaves around the developing flower to deprive it of sunlight.

-Many restaurants offer low-calorie or light meals with gourmet versions.

-Instead of accepting that "fried" meal from a restaurant menu, most places will steam or broil your food.

-Airlines can be very accommodating in having a special meal ready for you. You need to give at least one week advance notice.

-Ask for the salad dressing to be served on the side of the plate.

-Have the rich sauces or gravies left out.

-Avoid foods that are deep-fried.

-Request a carry home box to be brought with your meal. Portion the food before you start to eat. You remove the temptation to keep eating.

Some Kitchen Hints

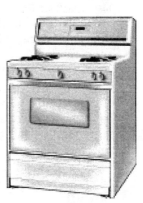

⇒ Hold a piece of bread in your mouth to absorb some of the strong vapors while peeling onions.

⇒ Most greens are interchangeable in recipes. Be aware that some have stronger in flavor than others.

⇒ Tomatoes' acidity reacts with certain metals (such as aluminum) and you end up with an off-taste. Cook in stainless steel, enamel, or some of the newer coated pans,

⇒ Overcooking ruins cabbage. It causes a mushy texture and a strong pungent taste.

⇒ Using spray vegetable oil on hands before cutting raw onions helps the odor wash off your hands.

⇒ Celery can be kept in the freezer until needed (for cooking only).

⇒ To restore crispness to fresh celery, trim the ribs and soak them in ice water for 10 to 20 minutes.

⇒ Salads should not be mixed ahead of time in wooden bowls.

⇒ Parsley flakes will cut down on the strong taste of garlic.

⇒ Scallions are excellent in stir-fries, because they cook quickly and stay green.

⇒ Use a few drops of vanilla in the coffee for sweetness.

⇒ Don't keep olive oil in a cabinet over the stove.

⇒ To ripen tomatoes, wrap green tomatoes in newspaper and store in a cool, dark place, and they will ripen

⇒ Cooked sweet potato can be used to thicken soups.

⇒ Dress up the plate with tomato peels. Take a ripe tomato and with a potato peeler, take off the peel in a continuous strip, then wind it into a pretty tomato rose.

⇒ Place sweet potatoes into water immediately after peeling to prevent discoloration.

⇒ Better Butter. Make Better Butter by whipping together: 1/2 cup olive oil and 1/2 cup butter. Refrigerate.

⇒ Make food ahead. You might have more energy on certain days to do this.

⇒ A pressure cooker is a great addition to the kitchen, especially when cooking in bulk, because it takes 1/4 the normal time required to cook foods. Good items to cook in bulk and have on hand are: beans, rice, refried beans, etc. Freeze in average size meal servings. This way you can make your own TV dinners.

⇒ A crock pot is very handy to have in the kitchen. You just place the ingredients into the pot in the morning and by evening, the meal is ready.

⇒ Using liquid lecithin. You can measure the amount by guessing. It's hard to get off a measuring spoon. If you do want to measure the lecithin, put a bit of oil on the utensil first. Liquid lecithin is a useful thickening agent. Too much lecithin can make bread dough gummy.

⇒ Look for lecithin in spray vegetable oil. There are some that have olive oil also (i.e. PAM).

⇒ When measuring honey, measure the oil first. The honey will just slide out of the measuring cup.

⇒ The garlic recipe is something to have as often as possible. If having garlic with dinner energizes you too much, switch to eating garlic at lunch.

⇒ Produce that will not be peeled needs to be soaked in a gallon of tepid water with 1-2 Tbs. cheap vinegar. Soak for about 5 minutes, then rinse off.

⇒ Leave peeled baby carrots in purified water in the refrigerator. This will make them sweeter.

⇒ Sweeten desserts by adding extra cinnamon and vanilla.

⇒ Grow alfalfa sprouts. It's fun to watch them grow, and you know they are organic. It only takes about a week.

⇒ Buy baking powder without alum in it.

⇒ You can add flax meal to salads and vegetables. Just sprinkle a bit on the top for a nice change of flavor.

⇒ Use leftovers for breakfast meals.

⇒ Sweeten desserts by adding extra cinnamon and vanilla extract.

⇒ Grow a pot of parsley in the kitchen. It's great to have on hand when you serve onions or garlic.

⇒ You can use unsweetened applesauce to replace 1/2 amount of oil in dessert recipes and add 1/4 to 1/2 tsp. lecithin.

⇒ Become a Label Reader. Check and see if that whole wheat bread lists "enriched flour" as first ingredient. Beware of "fat free". See if sugar was added. Limit saturated fat and sugar. Sugar can be listed as: maltose, dextrose, fructose, sucrose, corn syrup, date sugar, etc.

HEALTHY COOKING UTENSILS

AVOID TEFLON AND ALUMINUM. MINIMIZE MICROWAVE OVEN USE. Aluminum has been associated with Alzheimer's condition. Avoid using aluminum cookware. Teflon may give off a toxic gas. You want to cook healthy food in healthy containers using healthy heating techniques. It is well known among bird lovers and veterinarians that cooking with Teflon causes the out gassing of lethal fumes that can kill nearby indoor birds, a condition called polytetrafluoroethylene (PTFE) intoxication. Remember the canaries that miners would use to let them know when the air quality was poor enough to concern the miners. If birds can die from inhaling the vapors of Teflon, then we discourage its use.

Buy heavy duty stainless steel skillets, pots, and pans; then season them properly. Wash with soap and water and dry the pots. Coat the inside cooking surface of the pots with a liberal amount of peanut oil. Place pots on stove top on high for 4 minutes. There may be some smoking, so keep your kitchen ventilated to avoid causing the smoke detectors to go off. Once the pots have cooled, wipe them out with a paper towel. You now have non stick SAFE pots and pans. Do not wash with soap again, but rather use water and nylon scrub pads to clean.

Microwave ovens are convenient, yet are known to eliminate antioxidants in your foods. There are other lingering questions about the safety of cooking food in microwave ovens (Mercola.com). We do not cook meals in microwave ovens, but might occasionally warm up some food. We encourage you to warm up food on the stove top, or in a countertop convection oven (Walmart.com or Target.com), or the oven.

BULK COOKING

Cooking in bulk saves time and gives you the ability to make your own "TV dinners". You can cook a 20-25 pound turkey and freeze leftovers in serving size amounts. Pressure cook beans and rice and freeze leftovers in meal servings.. When grocery stores have a sale on banana bags for 99 cents, you can peel them and place in freezer bags and freeze. These are great for blender drinks.

ONE EASY WEEK MENU IDEAS AT A GLANCE

MONDAY
Brk:
Devil Eggs
Fresh plum
Mix greens w/ dressing
Lunch
Chicken with Pesto-Couscous Stuffing
Spinach Salad
Dinner
Tarragon Fish
Onion Soup w. Dulse
Spiced Beets

TUESDAY
Brk:
Spinach & Feta cheese Omelet
Blueberries
Lunch:
Shrimp Caesar Salad
Carrot & Celery sticks w/ Almond butter
Dinner:
Curry Chicken with Yogurt
Brussel Sprouts w/ Pine Nuts
Millet Cakes

WEDNESDAY
Brk:
Dragon Slayer
Orange
Lunch:
Hummus
Eggplant Dip
Vegetable Platter
Blue Corn Chips
Dinner:
Hearty Pot roast
Mix Salad Greens

THURSDAY
Brk:
Lean Ham Slice
Mixed Greens
Grapefruit

Lunch:
Mexican Beans
Whole Wheat Tortillas
Spinach Salad
Dinner:
Liver & Onions
Cabbage & Carrot Salad

FRIDAY
Brk:
Cottage Cheese Spread
Sprouted Bread
Strawberry slices
Lunch:
Tofu Burger
Sourdough Roll
Braised Leeks
Dinner:
Salmon Dinner
Miso Rice
Fresh plum
Carrot Soup
Delicious Garlic
Greek salad

SATURDAY
Brk:
Eggs scrambled w/ cheese
Tomato slices
Sausage
Papaya or kiwi
Lunch
Shrimp Salad w/ Nuts
Winter Squash w/Ginger
Dinner:
Lamb Roast
Yogurt
Italian Cauliflower Salad
Tomato Slices

SUNDAY
Brk:
Canadian bacon
Eggs
Apple slices
Lunch:

Crab & Avocado Salad
Black bean soup
Dinner:
Turkey Roast or Loaf
Sweet potato
Tomato & Red Onion Salad

RECIPES

BREAKFAST

It is a good idea to start the day off with some protein for the brain.
SOME FAST IDEAS:
-Avoid bacon. If you are really addicted to the taste of bacon, substitute fried (in coconut oil) lean ham or Canadian bacon.
-Yogurt, if not allergic to dairy.
-Hard boiled or deviled eggs are handy to eat with a muffin.
-Protein bar that is low in sugar
-Whole wheat bagel with natural peanut butter
-Oatmeal with powder protein or rice bran
-Leftovers, i.e. turkey sandwich
-Dragon Slayer drink
-Eggs scrambled and rolled in a tortilla with salsa

BEVERAGES

-Purified water
-Cafix
-Roma
-Herb tea
-dilute pure grape juice
-chicory
-Vitamin C powder & honey in hot water
-Ginger tea

-Hot natural apple juice with vitamin C
-Fresh orange juice

Rice Milk

1/4 cup brown rice
1 1/4 quarts of purified water
1/8 tsp. sea salt
1 1/2 Tbs. honey
1/2 Tbs. light olive oil or MCT oil

Bring the rice and water to a boil; then simmer for 45 minutes, or pressure cook for 5 minutes. Strain the rice, saving the liquid. Add back 1/4 cup of the liquid to the rice in a blender. Add the salt, honey, and oil. Blend on high. Add rest of the fluid and blend. You can make it as thick or thin by the amount of the fluid you choose to add. Chill. Shake before using.

Fast Rice Milk
1-2 cups cooked rice
1/4-1/2 tsp. salt
1/2 Tbs. any healthy oil you like the taste
1 1/2 Tbs. honey
6 cups water

Blend the first four ingredients with 3 cups water on high in a blender. Add the rest of the water and blend. For thicker milk, use less water. Chill.

Ginger Tea

1/2 to 1 tsp. grated ginger
1/4 tsp. vitamin C
1/2 to 1 tsp. honey
1 cup hot water
Mix all ingredients together.

If you miss the carbonated flavor of soft drinks, you might try this recipe. This is a good drink for nausea.

Ginger Ale

1/4 cup fresh ginger root (sliced)
1 lemon or lime (sliced)
4 cups water
1/3 tsp. Stevia extract
1 quart carbonated water

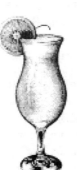

Peel and slice the ginger. Slice the lemon in 1/4 inch circles. Place both in the water and simmer for 25 min. Strain the liquid into a glass container. Stir in Stevia (to taste) and refrigerate. To serve, pour equal amounts of the ginger water and carbonated water into a glass. This will make 2 quarts.

Here are a few ideas for breakfast:

1) Spinach & feta cheese omelet
Dragon Slayer shake
2) Lean baked ham slice
Mix greens with Royal Dressing
Grapefruit
3) Eggs scrambled with diced onions, & mozzarella cheese
Tomato slices
Sausage, nitrate-free
Papaya or kiwi
4) Cottage cheese, 1/2 cup
Strawberry slices
English muffin, 1/2 oat bran or sourdough\
Celery sticks with almond butter
5) Eggs scrambled with diced onions, & mozzarella cheese
Tomato slices
Sausage, nitrate-free
Papaya or kiwi

6) Small lean steak,
Onion slices, fried
Whole grain bagel, small
Cherries
7) Sourdough toast with avocado
Salsa (opt.)
Egg any style
Apple Slices
8) Canadian bacon, slice
Oatmeal with cinnamon, vanilla & raisins
Orange
9) Spinach & feta cheese omelet
100-% Whole wheat toast with butter
Blueberries
10) Canadian bacon
Salsa (opt.)
Egg any style
Apple Slices

Power Oatmeal

3/4 to 1 cup hot water
1/3 cup old-fashioned oats, uncooked
2 Tbs. unsweetened apple juice
1 Tbs. raisins (opt.)
1/2 tsp. ground cinnamon
1/2 tsp. vanilla
1 tsp. flax meal
1 scoop protein power

Mix all ingredients together. Follow the directions for cooking oatmeal.

Hot Grain Cereal

1/3 cup bulgur
1/2 cup cornmeal
1-2 Tbs. dried fruit bits or raisins
1/4 cup toasted almond slivers
1/2 tsp. maple extract
cinnamon to taste
2 cups boiling water

Combine all of the ingredients with the boiling water in an uncovered pot; stir slowly. Return to a boil and lower to simmer for 10 to 15 minutes, or until ingredients reach desired consistency.

Granola
4 cups old-fashioned oats, uncooked
1/4 cup unprocessed rice bran
1/4 cup wheat germ
1/2 cup oat bran
1/4 cup extra light olive oil
2 Tbs. honey
1/2 to 1 cup sunflower seeds
1/3 cup raisins
2 tsp. vanilla

Heat oven to 300 degrees. Mix together the first six ingredients. Spread Preheat oven to 350 into a large, shallow pan. Bake for 45 minutes, stirring every 15 minutes. Add the sunflower seeds during the last 10 minutes of baking. Add the raisins and vanilla at the end of the baking time. Let cool.

Blueberry Rice Muffins
1 cup cooked brown rice, cold
1 cup unsweetened applesauce
3 eggs
2 Tbs. xylitol or honey
1 tsp. vanilla
1/4 -1/2 tsp. liquid lecithin
1/4 cup extra light olive oil or coconut oil
1/2 cup blueberries
1 1/4 cups whole wheat flour
1 Tbs. baking powder

Combine rice, milk, eggs, xylitol and vanilla. Add rest of ingredients and stir just enough to moisten. Pour batter into muffin tins that have been sprayed with oil. Bake at 400 degrees for 30 minutes or until golden brown on top.

Apple Bran Muffin
1 cup whole wheat flour
1/2+ cup wheat bran
1/4 teaspoon salt
1/2 teaspoon baking soda
1/4 teaspoon nutmeg
1/4 teaspoon cinnamon
1/2 cup finely chopped apple
1/4 cup raisins
1/4 cup chopped nuts
3/4 to 1cup buttermilk
1 beaten egg
1/4 cup molasses
1 tablespoon oil
1/2 teaspoon maple flavor

degrees. Grease a 12-cup muffin pan. Toss flour, bran, salt, soda, nutmeg, and cinnamon together with a fork.

Stir in apples, raisins, and nuts. Combine the liquid ingredients. Stir the liquid ingredients into the dry with a few swift strokes. Pour into greased muffin cups, filling them at least 2/3 full, and bake for 25 minutes. Makes 12.

Vegetable Scrambled Eggs
4 eggs, beaten
1/2 Tbs. water or rice milk
2 tsp. olive oil (or Pam)
1/2 cup chopped mushrooms
1/2 cup chopped onions
1/4 cup chopped green peppers (optional)

Beat the water into the eggs and set aside. Saute, in a frying pan, the mushrooms, onions, and peppers in the oil for about 5 minutes. Add the rest of the ingredients and cook like plain scrambled eggs.

Huevos Rancheros
eggs, fried
corn or whole wheat flour tortillas
mild or hot salsa, warmed
avocado slices
chopped green onion
grated cheese

Fry eggs and place on warmed tortillas. Pour 1/8 to 1/4 cup salsa over eggs and garnish with the avocado and onion. Sprinkle with cheese.

Mexican Omelet
2 eggs, beaten
1Tbs. olives, chopped
1 Tbs. canned green chiles
1/2 Tbs. onion, minced
butter, or spray vegetable oil

Melt a bit of butter or spray a frying pan with oil. Add all of the ingredients into the frying pan. As soon as the bottom begins to set, lift edges to let uncooked portion flow into contact with center of the pan. When eggs are set, turn omelet out of pan.

Sweet Potato Omelet
1 tsp. butter
1 Tbs. olive oil
2 sweet potatoes, peeled and diced
1 onion, diced
1/2 tsp. salt

1 tsp. parsley
6 eggs
2 Tbs. water
2 tsp. ground chile
1 4 oz. can diced green chile

Saute potatoes, onion, and chile powder in the butter and oil over medium heat. Cover and cook for 15 minutes or until potatoes are tender. Add the green chiles.

Combine the eggs, water, parsley, and salt in a bowl and beat with a fork. Pour over the potato mixture in the skillet and cook over low heat until eggs are set.

Egg Burrito
1 medium onion, diced
1 clove garlic, minced
1 Tbs. olive oil
6 eggs, beaten
1/2 cup salsa
6 olives, sliced
2/3 cup grated cheese
1 small tomato, diced
1 small avocado, diced
sour cream
salt to taste
warmed whole wheat flour tortillas

Saute onion and garlic in the oil until soft. Add the eggs and salsa. Scramble until done. Place some of the egg mixture in a tortilla and add some of the rest of the ingredients to taste. Roll into a burrito.

Deviled Eggs
4 hard-boiled eggs, peeled and cut in half lengthwise
1-2 tsp. mayonnaise or yogurt
1/2 tsp. prepared mustard
1 tsp. pickle relish
pinch dill (opt.)

Dash of onion powder
Salt and pepper to taste

Remove yolks from eggs and mash. Set aside egg white halves. Mix the yolks with remaining ingredients. Spoon mixture into egg whites. Garnish tops with a dash of paprika.

Mushroom Omelet

3 eggs
1 cup sliced fresh mushrooms
1/2 Tbs. olive oil
1/2 Tbs. water

Saute the mushrooms in oil in a frying pan. Scramble the eggs with the water. Add to the mushrooms. Cook over medium low heat covered. Flip over when the eggs are almost set. Cook the other side until done. Fold in half. Serve.

Scrambled Eggs with Rice

4 eggs
1 cup cooked brown rice or wild rice, (not hot)
2 Tbs. skim milk or water
1 tsp. Worcestershire or soy sauce
1/4 tsp. oregano
1 tsp. parsley
2 tsp. salsa

Combine all ingredients in a bowl. Beat ingredients until well blended. Lightly coat a nonstick skillet with better butter or spray oil; place over medium heat. Pour in egg mixture. Scramble the eggs until they are cooked. The mixture will still be moist. Serve with extra salsa.

Oat Raisin Scones

1 cup rolled oats
1 cup whole wheat flour
1 Tbs. xylitol or honey
1 1/2 tsp. baking powder
1/4 tsp. soda
1/8 tsp. salt
1/4 cup raisins
1/4 cup light olive oil or MCT oil
1/2 cup unsweetened applesauce
1/4 to 1/2 tsp. liquid lecithin
1 Tbs. lemon juice
1/4 tsp. cinnamon
1 egg

Blend together the dry ingredients. Add the raisins. Combine the rest of the ingredients. Mix. Turn dough out onto a lightly floured surface. Flour your hands. Dough might be a bit sticky. Don't add too much flour or it will toughen the scones. You can use a spatula to help in the kneading. Knead about 8-10 turns. Divide dough into two equal parts. Pat each part into a circle 1/2 inch thick. Cut into quarters. Transfer onto a baking sheet sprayed with vegetable oil or lined with oven paper. Bake until golden, about 20-25 minutes in 400 degree preheated oven. The scones can make a great dessert by serving warm and sprinkling a bit of Stevia or xylitol with cinnamon on the top. Can be served with yogurt or deviled eggs.

Alpine Barley

2 cups cooked barley
1 tsp. sesame oil
1/4 tsp. ground cumin
1/4 tsp. ground coriander
1/2 tsp. ground cinnamon
1/4 cup golden raisins

1/4 cup dried apricots, chopped
1/2 cup chopped, roasted almond, walnuts, or sunflower seeds (opt.)

Cook barley according to directions or use leftovers. Heat oil in pot. Quickly saute spices to bring out their flavors. Add dried fruit and 1 cup water. Cover and simmer 5 minutes. Add cooked barley; heat thoroughly. More water may be needed to reach desired consistency. Serve with chopped nuts.

Easy Pancakes

2 small to medium bananas
3 eggs
1 Tbs. baking powder (without alum)
1 Tbs. vanilla or maple extract
Oat flour

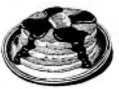

Blend the bananas, egg, and vanilla in the blender. Add the baking powder, and then add the oat flour until the whirlpool of the blending mix will no longer take any more flour (about a cup or less). Fry as normal in a frying pan sprayed with Pam. Cover while cooking on the first side only.

You can make your own oat flour by first blending rolled oats (i.e. Quaker Oats Oatmeal) in the blender and setting the flour aside.

Banana Bread

1 cup oat flour
1 1/2 cup whole wheat flour
1/2 cup honey
1/4 tsp. baking soda
3 1/2 tsp. baking powder
1 tsp. salt
3 Tbs. extra light olive oil
1 1/4 cups mashed bananas
1/3 cup soy milk, rice milk or apple juice
1 egg
1 cup chopped nuts

Heat oven to 350 degrees. Grease bottom only of loaf pan, 9x5x3 inches, or two loaf pans. Mix all the ingredients. Beat 30 seconds. Pour into pan(s). Bake until wooden pick inserted in center comes out clean, 9-inch loaf 55 to 65 minutes, 8-inch loaves 55 to 60 minutes. Cool slightly. Loosen side of loaf from pan; remove from pan. Cool completely before slicing. To store, wrap and refrigerate no longer than 1 week.

Breakfast Muffins

2 cups whole wheat flour
1 cup cornmeal
1 Tbs. baking powder
1 tsp. cinnamon
1/8 tsp. sea salt
1/4 cup xylitol or fructose
1/3 cup extra light olive oil
1/4 - 1/2 tsp. liquid lecithin
1/2 cup natural unsweetened applesauce
3/4 cup water
4 oz. tofu

Preheat oven to 375 degrees. Sift dry ingredients in large bowl. Puree tofu with the liquids in a blender until creamy smooth. Add wet ingredients to the dry ones; mix gently. (If batter is dry, add up to 1/4 cup extra water or applesauce.

Some flours absorb more liquid than others). Don't over-mix. Spray Pam in muffin pan or use paper muffin cups. Fill 2/3 full. Bake for 20 minutes or until done.
**Variations:
-add 1 cup washed blueberries
-add 1 cup cranberries and 1/2 cup chopped nuts
-1/4 cup bran, 1 cup raisins soaked in 3/4 cups orange juice. Omit water.
-Substitute whole wheat flour for cornmeal for a lighter muffin

Brown Rice Muffins
1 cup cooked brown rice, cold
1/3 to 1 cup unsweetened applesauce
3 eggs
2 Tbs. xylitol or honey
2 tsp. vanilla
1/4 -1/2 tsp. liquid lecithin
1/4 cup extra light olive oil
1 tsp. cinnamon
1 1/4 cups whole wheat flour
1 Tbs. baking powder
Combine rice, milk, eggs, xylitol, and vanilla. Add dry ingredients and stir just enough to moisten. Pour batter into muffin tins that have been sprayed with oil. Bake at 400 degrees for 30 minutes or until golden brown on top.

LUNCH IDEAS

If you are working out of the house and think you will "grab" something, chances are you won't find the time to eat out and will settle for vending machine fare. Packing a lunch the night before will make sure a meal is ready and saves time in the morning.

Own Mayonnaise
1 block soft tofu
3 Tbs. flax oil
3 Tbs. apple cider vinegar
salt to taste
your favorite seasoning (opt.)
Place the ingredients in a blender and puree until smooth. Use like peanut butter on bread or crackers.
You can also use the soy spread found in the snack section, as mayonnaise.

Bacon, Tomato, Spinach Sandwich
Turkey bacon or Canadian bacon, cooked
Tomato slices
Spinach leaves, cleaned
100% whole wheat bread, toasted
On toast, layer the bacon, tomato, and spinach leaves. You can spread toast with Royal Salad Dressing (found in the salad section) or mayonnaise.

Pita Bread Sandwich
Fill a pita pocket with some of the following and sprinkle with Royal Salad Dressing (found in the salad section) if appropriate:
Tomato slices
Grated carrot
Natural peanut or almond butter
Raisins
Mashed banana
Low-fat cheese
Sprouts
Avocado slices
Spinach leaves

Sliced mushrooms

Curry Eggs
4 hard-boiled eggs, peeled and cut in half lengthwise
1-2 tsp. yogurt or ranch dressing
1/2 tsp. curry powder
1/4-1/2 tsp. paprika
Dash of onion powder
1/4 tsp. garlic powder optional
Salt and pepper to taste

Remove yolks from eggs and mash. Set aside egg white halves. Mix egg yolks with remaining ingredients. Spoon mixture into egg whites. Garnish tops with a dash of paprika.

Egg Paste
Using the "Deviled Egg" recipe, add all the ingredients into a food processor and blend until a desired chunky texture is reached.

You can also use your favorite dressing instead of the mayonnaise.

Cottage Cheese Sandwich
This is a recipe for people who can eat dairy. The combination of cottage cheese and flax oil is very beneficial for cancer patients.
1/2 cup creamed cottage cheese
2 Tbs. flax oil
2 Tbs. wheat germ
1 Tbs. green chilies
1/4 tsp. oregano leaves
1/4 tsp. basil leaves
2 tsp. finely chopped onion
dash of sea salt or Lawry's salt w/o MSG
dash tabasco (opt.)
tomato slices

alfalfa sprouts

Mix first eight ingredients together. Spread on whole wheat bread or toast. Top with a tomato slice and sprouts. Can have as an open face sandwich or closed. You can also use pita bread as a sandwich or just spread the paste on top of the pita.

Avocado-Filled Pita Bread
1 large ripe avocado, peeled and diced
1 Tbs. lemon juice
1/2 tsp. garlic salt
1/4 tsp.spike
1/2 tsp Worcestershire sauce
homemade mayonaise (opt.)
4 whole wheat pita halves
1 tomato sliced
1 spring onion diced
salsa
alfalfa sprouts

Combine the first five ingredients. Lightly spread the mayonnaise if you choose. Fill pita halves with the mixture. Sprinkle the rest of the ingredients to taste. Four servings

Chicken Salad Sandwich
Finely diced cooked chicken
plain yogurt
chopped red or spring onion to taste
salt and pepper (optional)
diced celery (optional)
Spike to taste.

Mix chicken, onion, celery, and Spike. Add enough yogurt to make it the consistency you enjoy. Spread on whole wheat bread.

Vegetable Burgers
1 cup garbanzo flour (chickpea)

1 tsp. salt or 1 tsp. kelp
1/8 tsp. black pepper
1 tsp. parsley flakes
1 tsp. thyme powder
1 tsp. oregano
1 tsp. basil
1 tsp. Spike (or veg. seasoning)
dash of tabasco (opt.)
3/4 cup water
1/2 cup grated carrot
1/2 cup minced bell pepper or
1/2 cup chopped celery
1/4 cup finely chopped spring onions

Combine first 10 ingredients including water, and mix until free from lumps to make a thick batter. Add the carrots, peppers, and onion and mix well. Shape into patties. Place in a skillet that has been brushed with olive oil and cook on both sides until crisp. Serve on a whole wheat bun.

Barley Stew

1 1/3 cups raw barley, cooked
1/2 cup dry beans, cooked
3 Tbs. olive oil
1 large onion, chopped
2 cloves garlic
1/4 cup chopped fresh parsley
1 cup sliced carrots
1 cup fresh peas (or frozen)
6 cups vegetable stock
3 Tbs. miso
1 tbsp Gayelords vegetable broth powder
1 tsp. Spike
2 cups chopped tomatoes
pepper to taste

Saute the onion and garlic. Stir in the stock, and seasonings. Dissolve the miso in a small amount of hot stock.

Add miso to the pot. When the mixture has begun to simmer, add the rest of the ingredients. Simmer the soup, covered, for about 1/2 hour, stirring occasionally

Pita Pizzas

1 whole wheat pita bread
fresh tomato slices
thinly sliced onion rings
red or green pepper, diced
sliced mushrooms (opt.)
oregano
light olive oil, sprinkled over vegetables
grated low fat cheese (opt.)
2 to 3 Tbs. spaghetti sauce

You can use oven paper on a cookie sheet. Top bread with items listed. Baked in preheated 375 degree oven for about 8-10 minutes or until cheese is bubbly or the spaghetti sauce is hot.

SNACKS

Here are some ideas for easy and healthy snacks:
-Nuts: cashew, almond, walnuts, sunflower seeds, etc.
-Legumes: soynuts, peanuts, pinto beans, garbanzo beans (used in hummus)
-Grains: baked 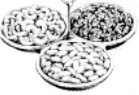 tortilla strips, Cheerios, shredded wheat, Grapenuts, whole grain bagels (low in sugar), pita bread, baked corn chips, wheat chips
-Protein: Natural beef or turkey or wild game jerky, hard boiled or

deviled eggs, plain non-fat or low-fat yogurt (can add fruit that is in season for sweetness) or as a dip with vegetables, peanut butter. You can spread peanut butter on baby carrots or a small frozen banana.

-Cottage cheese paste found in the lunch section used as a dip with vegetables.

-Vegetables: colorful, i.e.: red pepper, green pepper, broccoli, carrot, tomato, sweet potato chips with a dip or salsa

-String cheese

-Salsa with pita bread or other healthy food (i.e.: vegetables, whole wheat crackers, baked chips)

Your Own Trail Mix

100% shredded wheat
Cheerios
Grape Nut Flakes
Sunflower seeds
Almonds
Cashews
Raisins (opt.)
Papaya, dried (opt.)

Mix to your preference, keeping the fruit to a small amount. Can place in a sandwich bag to have handy.

Air Popcorn

With an air popcorn machine, you can eliminate all the hydrogenated fat and/or salt that is found in the microwave popcorn bags. Spray olive oil over the top and lightly season with onion salt or other favorite seasoning.

Roasted Nut Meal

1 cup toasted nuts of your choice or combination
1/4 cup toasted sesame or sunflower seeds
1 1/4 tsp. chili powder
1/2 tsp. cumin powder
1/8 tsp. garlic powder
1/8 tsp. onion powder
1/8 tsp. clove powder
2 Tbs. nutritional yeast (opt.)

Blend all ingredients in blender until nuts make a nut meal. Use to sprinkle on grains, vegetables, or salad dishes.

Dip Ideas:

Yogurt Dip

Using a container of plain yogurt, stir in a third to a package of dry soup, i.e. onion soup.

Easy Guacamole

One peeled and pitted avocado
1/4 to 1/3 cup medium salsa
1 Tbs. lemon or 1-2 Tbs. sun dried tomato vinaigrette

Place all ingredients into a food processor or a blender. Add salsa and lemon to taste. Blend until smooth.

Eggplant Dip with Sun-Dried Tomatoes

1 medium eggplant
1/3 cup sun-dried tomatoes
1/4 cup balsamic vinegar
1 Tbs. honey
1/2 to 1 tsp. garlic
1/4 tsp. sea salt
1/4 cup olive oil
Fresh basil to taste

Peel and dice the eggplant. Cook for about 10 minutes or until tender. Blend the above ingredients in a small food processor or blender. Spread on warm bread, toast, whole wheat crackers, or use as a dip.

Sesame Spread
3/4 cup sesame seeds
1 Tbs. honey
1/4 cup apple juice or water
1/8 tsp. salt

Toast sesame seeds and grind into a meal in a blender. Remove to a bowl and add honey, water, and salt. The mixture will thicken as it cools, so you may want to thin it by adding more juice

Basil Pesto
1 cup fresh basil leaves
1 1/2 cups spinach leaves
2 garlic cloves
1 Tbs. pine nuts or walnuts
2 Tbs. Parmesan cheese
1/2 Tbs. olive oil or MCT oil
2 Tbs. water

Add all ingredients together in a food processor or a blender. Process until a smooth paste. Use spatula and pulse on/off to help blend. If you don't want to add the cheese, cut the water to 1 Tbs.

Baked chips are sold in the grocery stores and make for an easy food to use with dips.

Bean Dip with Chips
1 (16 oz.) can kidney beans or black beans, drained
1/2 small jalapeno pepper, sliced
2 garlic cloves
1 dozen corn tortillas

Spike or seasoning salt without MSG

Blend first 3 ingredients in a blender or food processor until smooth. Cut tortillas into eight triangles. Place on a vegetable-sprayed or oven-paper-covered baking sheet and bake at 375 degrees about 5 minutes, or until crispy. Sprinkle with Spike seasoning . Serve with the dip.

Humus
1/2 onion, chopped
1 to 2 cloves garlic crushed
2 Tbs. olive oil
1 tsp. basil-2 tsp. Spike seasoning (opt.)
1 1/2 Tbs. soy sauce
1/2 tsp. oregano
2 Tbs. parsley, chopped fine
Dash cumin or dill weed (your choice)
1/2 Tbs. wet yellow mustard
1/4 cup basalmic vinegar or apple cider vinegar
Juice of 1 lemon
1/2 to 1 Tbs. honey
1/4 cup sesame seed tahini butter, almond butter, or peanut butter
2 cups cooked garbanzo beans
Sun dried tomatoes in olive oil
Sea salt to taste
Lemon pepper (opt.)

Saute the onion and garlic in olive oil until onion is transparent. Add cumin and cook until fragrant. Add herbs. Take off heat. You can use a food processor and blend all ingredients except the sun dried tomatoes. Stir in part of the tomato oil and use a scissors to cut the sun dried tomatoes into the paste. Stir. Or mash the beans and stir all ingredients together. You can use powdered onion and garlic and leave out the frying. You can grind fresh sesame seeds into meal instead of the butter form. If you want a bit of a kick to the paste, add chili power to taste.

Soy Spread

2 cups cooked, mashed soybeans
1 or 2 small red chili peppers
1 small chunk ginger
1/2 tsp. onion powder
1/4 tsp. garlic powder
1 Tbs. soy sauce
1/4 cup olive oil
1/2 cup lemon juice
1 cup water

Blend all ingredients in a blender. Use on top of pita bread or whole wheat crackers.

Whole Wheat Chips

Cut up whole wheat tortillas into strips and then cut in half to make bite size chips. Lay sections on a cookie sheet that is not greased. Bake at 350 degrees on the top rack in the oven for about 7 to 8 minutes or until slightly brown.

SALADS

The statement, "Eat as many colorful vegetables as your colon 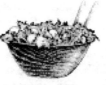 can tolerate", can seem like a challenge when you haven't been much of a green eater. It might seem to be a hassle to be fixing vegetables twice a day. One trick is to get a bunch of vegetables and greens and process them at once. Soak the vegetables that you won't be peeling in the kitchen sink full of water with about 1/4 cup of cheap vinegar. Then make a tray of bite size servings [example: baby carrots, broccoli flowers, cauliflower, cherry tomatoes, red bell pepper, snap peas, olives for color, etc.]. At the same time, cut enough vegetables to add to a large bowl of fresh greens. Now you have vegetables for most of a week.

Sprouting seeds, beans, etc.

You can use a glass jar (quart size or larger) with a large lid size, soft screen with small holes so the seeds don't spill out, and a rubber band to hold the screen in place. There are also commercial sprouting kits available in most health food stores. Place about one heaping tablespoon of seeds (alfalfa seeds are the easiest to try) in your glass container. Add the screen over the top and secure with the rubber band. The seeds will expand about tenfold as they sprout, so allow enough room for their expansion. Fill the container half full of purified water and let stand overnight. Next morning, drain and rinse the seeds. Let stand inverted at a 45 degree angle or so. A colander is one way to keep the angle for proper drainage. Rinse and drain twice each day for the next 6-7 days. Keep the jar away from heat or intense light.

Larger seeds, like peas, beans, and lentils take a shorter time to grow and should not be allowed to grow more than one half inch long or they will develop a bitter flavor. Mung bean sprouts can get up to one to two inches in length without a bitter flavor. Soak larger beans (pinto, chick peas, etc.) overnight in a large jar with a wide mouth and purified water. Enough to let beans swell 3-4 times their size. Drain the next day. Rinse, and let drain at an angle. Wheat, barley, oats, and other grass plants make terrific sprouts. Smaller seeds, like alfalfa, can grow to an inch in length without any bitter flavor. For some extra vitamin A, let the alfalfa sprouts sit by a sunny spot (not in direct heat) for the last day before eating. The green color indicates the welcome addition of chlorophyll, folacin, and beta-carotene.

In excess quantities, sprouts can blunt the immune system in humans. Do not eat more than two cups of sprouts daily.

Royal Salad Dressing
OPTION ONE
1/2 cup raw-unfiltered organic apple cider vinegar (i.e. Bragg's)
1/2 cup purified water
1 package dry Italian Salad Dressing Mix
1-2 tsp. liquid lecithin
1/4 cup olive oil
1/4 cup certified organic flaxseed oil or Essential Balance, which is a blend of organic oils from flax, sunflower, sesame, pumpkin, and borage by Omega Nutrition (Staywell 888-333-5346)

Add the first 3 ingredients together in a jar with a lid. Then add the oil and lecithin. Shake vigorously. Keep refrigerated.

OPTION TWO
Take your basic Italian dressing bottle from the grocery store. Pour half into a container for later use. With the other half, fill to the brim with equal quantities of:
Vinegar
Olive oil
Flax oil
MCT oil
Water
Extra seasonings if desired
Shake well before serving.
Other dressings: check labels for sugar quantity

Soup or Salad Seasoning
1 tsp. ground chili
2 tsp. onion powder
1 tsp. ground allspice
1 tsp. ground thyme
2 tsp. ground cinnamon
1 tsp. ground cloves
1/4 tsp. ground nutmeg
1/4 tsp. ground mace
1/2 tsp. garlic powder
1/2 tsp. pepper
1/2 tsp. salt
Mix the ingredients together and use in a salt shaker.

Shrimp Caesar Salad
1 clove garlic, peeled
8 anchovy fillets, cut up (opt.)
1/3 cup olive oil
1/4 cup lemon juice
1 tsp. Worcestershire sauce
1/4 tsp. salt
1/4 tsp. dry ground mustard
Fresh ground pepper
1 pound cooked, peeled, shrimp

1/2 sliced avocado (opt.)
Romaine lettuce, torn into pieces

Rub large wooden bowl with cut garlic. Mince the rest of the garlic and mix with the next seven ingredients in the bowl. Add the lettuce. Toss until coated. Toss in the shrimp. Place avocado on top.

Tangy Crab Salad
Mixed salad greens
1 small onion, thinly sliced
3/4 pound cooked crabmeat
1 tomato, chopped
1 carrot, peeled and grated
8 black olives, sliced (opt.)
1 lime

Dressing:
4 green Mexican chiles, roasted, peeled, seeded and chopped.
1/2 cup plain yogurt
2 Tbs. lime juice
1 tsp. horseradish sauce (opt.)

Combine the ingredients for the dressing. Refrigerate for an hour. Arrange the salad greens on four individual plates and arrange the onions and carrots on top. Next add the crab. Top with the tomatoes and olives. Serve the dressing on the side.

Greek Salad
4 cups mixed greens
1 small cucumber
2 ripe tomatoes
1 scallion
8 black Greek olives
1/2 cup feta cheese
fennel leaves, chopped (opt.)
1 Tbs. chopped fresh mint or 1/2 Tbs. dried

olive oil and vinegar
Sea salt and freshly ground pepper

Wash, dry, and break the lettuces into bite-size pieces. Peel and slice the cucumbers. (Seed if necessary.) Cut tomatoes into wedges. Chop the scallion. On each of the two plates, arrange the lettuces, then add the cucumbers, tomatoes, and olives. Sprinkle the scallions, mint, fennel leaves, and feta cheese. Add oil and vinegar. Top with salt and pepper.

Carrot and Cabbage Salad
2 cups grated carrots
2 cups grated cabbage
1 spring onion chopped (opt.)
1/4 cup raisins (opt.)
1/4 cup of pecans, walnuts or almonds chopped (opt.)

Mix together and cover with the Royal Salad Dressing found in the beginning of this section.

Grapefruit Salad
Peel and section grapefruit and arrange on top of spinach leaves or alfalfa sprouts. Can garnish with almond slices and or yogurt.

Colorful Salad
Spinach leaves
Alfalfa sprouts
Carrots, grated
Pickled beets, grated
Edible flowers (i.e. pansy) opt.

On a bed of spinach leaves, place some sprouts, carrots and pickled beets. Sprinkle with Royal Salad Dressing and place a flower on the top.

Spanish Tomato Salad
4 fresh tomatoes, cut into sixths

1/4 cup fresh cilantro, chopped
4 green onions, chopped
1 red bell pepper, finely chopped
3 Tbs. fresh lemon juice
1 Tbs. soy sauce
        Mix ingredients together. Allow flavors to blend.

Spinach & Bean Sprout Salad
8 ounces spinach
16 ounces bean sprouts or alfalfa sprouts
croutons (opt.)
Variations:
-grated carrots
-grated cheese
-cooked noodles
-diced egg
-chopped apples
-cut up dried fruit
-avocado
-nuts
-onions
-crushed bacon
-tomatoes
-any vegetables

Sesame Dressing
1/4 cup soy sauce
2 Tablespoons toasted sesame seeds
2 Tablespoon finely chopped onion
1/2 Teaspoon honey
1/4 Teaspoon pepper
        Mix all ingredients

Crisp Vegetable Salad with Lemon Dressing
1 cup julienne strips of carrot
1 cup julienne strips of zucchini
1 cup green beans, in 1 1/2-inch lengths
1/2 cup sliced mushrooms
salt and ground pepper to taste

        In a bowl, combine vegetables.

Lemon Dressing
1 Tbs. olive oil
1/4 cup lemon juice
2 Tbs. chopped fresh parsley
2 Tbs. chopped spring onions
1 clove garlic, finely chopped
        In a small bowl, combine oil, lemon juice, parsley, spring onions, and garlic. Mix thoroughly. Pour over vegetables and toss to mix. Add salt and pepper to taste. Cover and refrigerate.

Fruit Salad
Any fruit in season chopped into bite-size pieces and pour vanilla yogurt over the top.

Banana Delight
2 cups diced banana
1 1/2 cups diced apple
1 cup diced celery
1/2 cup chopped walnuts
1/2 cup raisins
1/2 cup yogurt
1 Tbs. lemon juice
        Use well-chilled fruit. Combine all ingredients. Mix well and serve on top of fresh spinach leaves or alfalfa sprouts. Yields six small servings.

Low-fat Cottage Cheese Tomatoes
Large tomatoes
Cottage cheese
Cinnamon to taste
        Cut tomatoes into quarters. Put a scoop of cottage cheese in the center and sprinkle with cinnamon.

Spinach Salad
Spinach leaves

Alfalfa sprouts
Carrots, grated
Grape tomatoes

On a bed of spinach leaves, place some sprouts, carrots and tomatoes. Sprinkle with Royal Salad Dressing (found in the beginning of this section).

Sprout Salad with Peaches
sprouts
peaches
almond slices

On a bed of sprouts, add some peaches. Sprinkle a few almond slices on top.

Tossed Avocado-Grapefruit Salad
1 medium grapefruit, sectioned
1 avocado, sliced
Mixed greens in bite-size pieces

Toss all ingredients and add Italian dressing.

California Spinach Salad
4 cups torn spinach leaves
1-2 cups alfalfa sprouts
1/4 pound mushrooms, sliced
1 large tomato, cut in chunks
2 spring onions, chopped

Toss ingredients together. Serve with avocado dressing or your favorite.

Avocado Dressing
1/2 large ripe avocado
1 tablespoon lemon juice
1/8 teaspoon salt
1/8 teaspoon chili powder
squeezed garlic
1/4 cup buttermilk (or milk substitute)

Mix all ingredients well. Serve over salad.

Healthy Gelatin
1 stick agar agar (can find in health food stores)
3 cups unfiltered apple juice
1-2 bananas, sliced
any other fresh fruit (optional)

Bring agar agar and juice to a boil, then simmer for 10-15 minutes until the stick has dissolved. Add fruit and chill until firm.

Variation: Can use any other fruit juice flavoring. If it isn't sweet enough to your taste buds, can add a bit of honey.

Banana Nut Salad
3 bananas
1 Tbs. sesame tahini
1 Tbs. honey
1 Tbsp. soy protein powder
chopped dates
chopped almonds

Mix tahini, honey, and soy protein powder together, and chop bananas into it. Mix in dates, and nuts. Chill.

Ginger Banana
4 bananas, sliced
juice of 2 lemons
2 tsp. grated ginger
1tsp. honey

Toss ingredients together.

Orange and Onion Salad
2 oranges
1 diced avocado (optional)
1 grapefruit
1 small red onion, thinly sliced and separated into rings
1/3 cup yogurt
2 Tablespoons chopped walnuts (optional)

salad greens or spinach leaves
salt and pepper to taste

Peel and section the fruit. Cut each section into two or three pieces and put in a salad bowl. Add all the juices from the oranges and grapefruit to the onion. Add avocado. Pour yogurt over mixture, toss and chill. Sprinkle with nuts, salt, and pepper, and serve on salad greens.

Tomato & Red Onion Salad
sliced tomatoes
thinly sliced red onion, separate rings

Alternate sliced tomatoes and onions. Can top with:
-grated parmesan cheese
-basil
-fresh herbs
-sunflower seeds
-Royal Salad Dressing (found in the beginning of this section).

Crisp Chop Suey
1/2 cup Chinese peas, sliced
1/4 cup each: green and red bell pepper (slice lengthwise thinly, then in half)
1/2 cup celery, diced
1/2 cup carrots, slivered
2 cups cabbage, bite-sized pieces
1 cup bean sprouts, cut
1 Tbs. sesame seeds
1/4 cup almonds, slivered
1 tsp. toasted sesame oil
Sweet 'n Sour Ginger Dressing

Cut vegetables Chinese style, cutting diagonally across the vegetable in bite size pieces. Add seeds and nuts.
Toss with last 2 ingredients.

Sweet 'n Sour Ginger Dressing
1 Tbs. soy sauce
1 Tbs. honey
3 Tbs. water
1 Tbs. grated fresh ginger
1/2 tsp. arrowroot

Mix ingredients for sauce in a small pot until arrowroot dissolves. Cook over medium heat, stirring constantly until thickened like a gravy sauce. Pour over salad and toss.

Cobb Salad
To your choice of amounts of portions:
Mixed Greens, then add:
Cooked chicken
Tomato, chopped
Avocado slices
Cooked turkey bacon, crumbled
Hard boiled eggs, sliced
Onions sliced fine or diced
olives, sliced
Royal Salad Dressing, or:
1-2 Tbs. honey
1/3 cup vinegar
1/4 cup olive oil or flax oil
1 tsp. tarragon
1/2 tsp. basil
1/2 tsp. dry mustard.

Mix the dressing well and pour over the other ingredients. Refrigerate.

SOUP

Add Dulse seaweed to soups for a healthier meal.

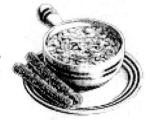

Black Bean Soup

6 jalapeno chiles, stems & seeds removed, chopped
2 medium onions, chopped
2 cloves garlic, minced
2 cups dried black beans
2 quarts water
1/2 to 1 pound cooked ham, cubed
1/4 tsp. allspice or cumin
8 cups chicken broth
1/2 cup dry red wine or 3 Tbs. lemon juice
1 can (8 oz.) tomato sauce
1 Tbs. parsley, chopped
1 Tbs. cilantro, chopped (opt.)

Rinse and sort beans, discarding any foreign material. Combine beans and water in a 5-quart pot and bring to a boil for 2 minutes. Cover and set aside for 1 hour. Drain off water and add the chicken broth, allspice, chiles, onion, parsley, and garlic. Bring to a boil and reduce to a simmer. Cook for about 1 1/2 hours. Add the tomato sauce and simmer for 1/2 hour. Puree the bean mixture, if desired, and add ham and put back to the pot. Add the wine and reheat soup. Freeze the extra soup if there is too much.

Gazpacho

2 medium tomatoes, chopped
1 small onion, diced
1/2 cucumber, peeled and diced
1/2 avocado, chopped
2 Tbs. canned mild green diced chiles
1/2 tsp. oregano leaves, crumbled
1/2 Tbs. parsley, chopped
2 Tbs. wine vinegar
2 Tbs. olive oil
4 cups canned tomato juice
2 limes

Put the first nine ingredients into a serving bowl. Stir in the tomato juice. Chill. Serve with lime juice to taste.

Fast Vegetable Soup

2 cups skim milk (or a milk substitute from soy or rice) or vegetable stock
1/2 Tbs. butter
1/2 Tbs. olive oil or MCT oil
2 Tbs. whole wheat flour
1Tbs. Gayelord's vegetable broth, "Better than Bouillon" or a vegetable broth powder
1 tsp. Spike or seasoning powder without salt
1/4 tsp. chili powder or pepper to taste
2 cups cooked vegetables (leftovers are great)

Put all ingredients in a blender in the order listed. Cover with the lid and blend until smooth. Pour into a saucepan. Cook over low heat, stirring occasionally until hot.

You can puree leftover vegetables from a previous meals and heat. Then add mini shredded wheat cereal to thicken.

Minestrone Soup

1/4 cup olive oil
1 cup diced celery
1/2 cup diced onion
2 cloves garlic
1 1/2 qts. water
1 to 2 tbs. flaky nutritional yeast (optional)
1 cup diced tomatoes
1/2 cup tomato paste
1 tsp. Spike

1/2 Tbs. Gayelord's vegetable broth powder
1 cup diced carrots
1 cup diced potatoes
1/2 cup diced green beans
1/2 tsp. basil
1 tsp. oregano
1 tsp. Worcestershire sauce
1 cup whole wheat noodles, broken up
1 cup cooked pink beans

Saute first four ingredients together. Put the rest of the ingredients except the beans in a pot and add the onion mixture. Blend the bean to a puree. Add the beans to the pot. Bring to a boil, then turn heat down and simmer for 20 minutes.

Lentil Soup

4 cups vegetable stock
2 cups dried lentils
1 onion, sliced
1 large carrot, sliced
1 large celery stalk, sliced
2 cloves, crushed
1/4 cup chopped celery
1 bay leaf
1/2 tsp. dried oregano
3 Tbs. tomato paste
2 Tbs. white wine vinegar or herbal vinegar
1 tsp. Spike unsalted (opt.)
2 tsp. sea salt
1 can (28 ounces) whole tomatoes
1/2 tsp. pepper
1/4 tsp. summer savory or oregano or thyme (opt.)

Saute in a large sauce pan, the onion, carrot, celery, and garlic until tender, about 10 minutes. Bring the stock to a boil in the pan. Rinse the lentils and add to boiling stock. Add all the remaining ingredients except the vinegar. Reduce the heat, cover and simmer until the lentils are very soft, about 1 hour. Remove the soup from heat and add the vinegar. Discard bay leaf. (If you want a creamier soup, puree half the soup. Return the puree back to the saucepan and reheat.) Or you can place all ingredients in a crockpot, (minus 1 cup fluid) in the morning and set on low for 9 to 10 hours.

Potato Celery Soup

4 cups water
4 medium-sized sweet potatoes, (peeled and diced)
1 medium stalk of celery, chopped
1/4 cup butter
1/4 cup nutritional yeast
2 Tbs. soy sauce
2 Tbs. nut or seed butter (sesame, almond, etc.)
Spike seasoning added to taste

Combine first four ingredients in a saucepan. Bring to a boil and simmer for 10 to 12 minutes or until tender. With slotted spoon, take out 2 cups of vegetables. Then combine remaining vegetables and soup stock in a blender with the last three ingredients and blend until smooth. Combine all ingredients and serve.

Winter Squash Soup

Dulse seaweed (to your taste level)
1 medium onion
1 medium winter squash, cubed
1/2 cup broccoli flowers (opt.)
1/4 cup parsley, chopped
Spike seasoning (opt.)
Miso to taste

Add the first five ingredients in a soup pot and cover with purified water. Simmer until squash is soft, 20 to 30 minutes. Puree miso with a bit of the broth. Add to pot.

Carrot & Ginger Onion Soup

1/2 medium onion, diced
2 cloves garlic, minced
1 Tbs. olive oil
1 lb. carrots, cut into 1-inch chunks, cooked
1Tbs. peeled & chopped ginger root
1 tsp. spike (seasoning) opt.
2 cups vegetable broth

Fry the onion & garlic in oil till soft. Add rest of ingredients and simmer 10 minutes. Puree in a blender and serve. Add salt and pepper to taste.

Onion Soup with Dulse

1/2 to 1 Tablespoon olive oil or sesame oil
2 lb. onions, thinly sliced
2 cloves garlic crushed
1/2-1 qt. stock (Gayelord's vegetable broth, or other vegetable broth)
1-2 Tbs. miso
1/4 cup chopped celery leaves (optional)
2 tsp. molasses
1-2 tsp. Spike

Saute onions and garlic in butter over medium heat in a large saucepan for about 10 minutes. Add the rest of the ingredients and bring to a boil. Reduce heat and simmer for 5 to 10 minutes. Serve with dulse.

Easy Cauliflower Soup

1 cup chopped white part of leeks
1 Tbs. butter or olive oil
3/4 to 1 lb. cauliflower flowers
1 cup plain yogurt
2 Tbs. fresh dill, chopped
chili powder (opt.)
Sea salt to taste

Cook leeks in butter until wilted, 5-10 minutes. Add broth and cauliflower. Cover and simmer over low heat for 10-20 minutes, until cauliflower is tender. Puree soup. Add the yogurt and spices. Warm (do not boil). .

Tangy Tomato Soup

2 tsp. MCT or olive oil
1 onion, diced
2 cloves minced garlic
1 Tbs. minced ginger (opt.)
3 cups tomatoes, cut up
2 cup vegetable stock
1 tsp. soy sauce
1 tsp. basil
1 tsp. Spike
1 Tbs. whole wheat or oat flour
pepper to taste

Fry onions and garlic in oil. Add the flour and cook the flour to remove the paste-like flavor. Don't burn. Add the rest of the ingredients and simmer until tomatoes are cooked.

VEGETABLES

Many people have a dislike for vegetables. If that is the case for you, an attitude

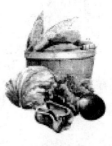

adjustment needs to take place. A short story might give you an idea of how to manage this feat. I had to start drinking "greens" for a health issue. Ugh! First thing in the morning on an empty stomach drinking dark green sludge caused shivers and disgust. Realized any benefits that the drink was suppose to have probably was hampered by this mental reaction. One day, I pretended that this beverage was "Shamrock Essence" and I was drinking down the magic of all the Irish tales associated with the Shamrock. (It might have helped to be a daughter of a Irishman. You can come up with a story referring to your own ancestry.) The drink even took on a better smell and was not as bitter. An example of how the mind can be a friend or foe.

Fresh Sliced Tomatoes
Slice down the stem parallel rather than across, you will lose less of the moisture.
Ideas:
-Slice the tomatoes and sprinkle with salt and your favorite herbs,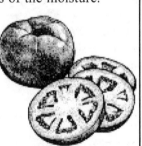
then drizzle with olive oil.
-Slice and top with fresh basil cut with scissors. Top with olive oil.
-Alternate tomato slices with thinly sliced mozzarella cheese. Can top fresh herbs (ie: basil, oregano, etc.) and sprinkle with olive oil.
-Alternate with thinly sliced sweet onion and sprinkle with herbs and salt and pepper.
-Sprinkle flax meal over the vegetables.

Italian Cold Vegetables
Using up leftover vegetables (i.e. broccoli, cauliflower, chile peppers, mushrooms, carrots, zucchini). Add beans that you like. Just make sure they haven't been overcooked.
Sprinkle with small amount of marinade from:
1/2 cup olive oil
1/2 cup apple cider vinegar
1/2 tsp. basil
1/2 tsp. oregano leaves
1/2 chopped onion
1 chopped clove garlic
1/4 tsp. sea salt
1/2 tsp. dry mustard
1 tsp. paprika
1 Tbs. honey
Chill in refrigerator.

Cabbage Pecan Salad
1 1/2 cups finely shredded green cabbage
1/4 cup red seedless grapes, halved (opt.)
1/4 cup red apple, diced
1/4 cup pineapple, diced (opt.)
1 Tbs. chopped pecans
Place the cabbage in a serving bowl. Add the rest of the ingredients. Toss. Serve with Royal Salad Dressing (found in the beginning of this section).

Vegetable Treat
1/2 Tbs. olive oil
1/2 cup broccoli flowerets

1/4 cup carrot, shredded
1/4 cup onion, chopped
1 Tbs. olives, minced
2 large eggs
1 1/2 Tbs. water or milk
1/2 Tbs. chopped fresh parsley
Dash of salt and pepper
Red pepper sauce (i.e. salsa) to taste (opt.)
1/2 cup shredded mozzarella (opt.)

Heat oil in frying pan over medium high heat. Cook the vegetables about 5 minutes, stirring frequently, until tender. Beat eggs and milk, parsley, salt and pepper. Pour mixture over vegetables. Sprinkle with cheeses, reduce heat and cover until set in center, about 10 minutes. Serve.

Spice Beets
2 cups cooked beets, grated
1/4 cup water
1/3 cup vinegar
1/2 to 1 Tbs. xylitol (opt.)
1/2 tsp. cinnamon
1/4 tsp. cloves
1/4 tsp. salt

Mix all ingredients together and simmer 7-10 minutes. Can add xylitol or Stevia to taste if desired.

Collard Greens with Eggs
1 bunch collards, washed and sliced
2 tsp. sesame or olive oil
1 onion sliced
2 cloves garlic, minced
1 tsp. soy sauce
2 hard cooked eggs, peeled and diced

Wash and slice collards. If stems are thick, slice thinly so they will cook faster. Steam until done. Meanwhile, heat oil in skillet; add onions and garlic and saute 2 to 3 minutes. Mix together with the collards. Gently toss in the eggs and soy sauce.

Tofu With Swiss Chard
1/2 lb. firm tofu
1 Tbs. sesame or olive oil
pinch of sea salt or soy sauce to taste
1 small bunch Swiss or red chard, washed and chopped
1 Tbs. fresh basil or dill (optional)

Press the fluid out of the tofu with a paper towel. Slice lengthwise. Heat oil and pan-fry tofu on one side until golden. Gently turn tofu with spatula. Sprinkle with sea salt or soy sauce. Place chopped chard and herbs on top of tofu. Cover and reduce heat. The greens will cook down in about 5 minutes. Add 1/4 cup water if needed to steam greens. Serve the tofu with greens on the side.

Vegetable Platter
Red and yellow bell peppers, sliced
Carrots cut into sticks
Celery cut into sticks
Radish, sliced
Broccoli cut in bite-size pieces

Arrange on a plate and serve or use to dip.

Delicious Garlic
1 bulb/head of garlic
Spike, or favorite seasonings
1 tsp. olive oil
soy sauce

Cut the garlic head through the fattest part in the center. Break up the pieces. Place in a dish and sprinkle with olive oil, soy, or teriyaki sauce. Cook covered in a microwave oven for 2 minutes or until tender.

Braised Leeks
2 cups chopped leeks
1 stalk celery, chopped (opt.)
Sea salt and pepper
1/2 to 1 Tbs. butter or olive oil
with juice of 1/2 lemon

Melt butter in saucepan and add leeks and celery. Stir and cover. Cook over low heat for 8-10 minutes, stirring occasionally. Season with salt and pepper.

Bright Broccoli
1 head broccoli
sunflower seeds (opt.)
Royal Dressing

Cut off outside part of stock. Dice stock and cut top into bit size pieces. Cut the top into small "flowerettes". Steam until tender, about 10 minutes. Sprinkle with seeds and dressing.

Carrots with Bean Sprouts
2 large carrots, shredded
2 cups alfalfa sprouts
1 cup bean sprouts
1/2 cup walnuts or pecans
1/4 cup sliced almonds
2 Tbs. white-wine vinegar
2 tsp. Dijon-style mustard (opt.)
1 Tbs. sesame oil
1 Tbs. olive oil
salt and pepper

2 tsp. chopped fresh coriander, parsley, or dill

Mix the carrots, sprouts, and nuts together and place in a serving dish. Blend the rest of ingredients together. Pour over the salad. Or you can use Royal Dressing.

Honey Baked Onions
2 large mild onions
2 Tbs. honey
1/6 cup water
1 Tbs. olive oil
1/2 tsp. paprika
1/2 tsp. ground coriander
Dash of Lite salt or sea salt
1/8 tsp. cayenne pepper

Peel and cut onions in half crosswise. Place cut side down in a baking dish just large enough to hold all the onions in one layer. Sprinkle with water. Cover with foil and bake at 375 degrees for about 20 minutes. Turn onions cut side up. Combine remaining ingredients and spoon half of the mixture over the onions. Return to oven and bake uncovered 15 minutes. Baste with remaining honey mixture and bake 10 more minutes.

Brussel Sprouts with Pine Nuts
1/2 lb. brussel sprouts
2 Tbs. butter
Juice of 1/2 lemon
Pine nuts or almond slices
Salt and pepper to taste

Trim and wash sprouts. Steam until barely tender. Halve each sprout lengthwise. Melt butter in a large saucepan, add sprouts and cook until heated through. Add lemon juice, nuts, and salt, and pepper to taste. Toss again before serving.

Stir-Fried Spinach with Ginger
1 lb. fresh spinach
1 small onion
1 Tbs. olive oil
1 clove garlic, minced fine
1/2 Tbs. ginger, finely minced
1 Tbs. soy sauce
1 tsp. honey

Wash and trim spinach and cut leaves into wide strips. Chop onion. Heat oil. Then add onion, garlic, and ginger. Stir-fry on high heat for 1 minute. Add spinach and stir for just a few minutes. Add soy sauce and honey; turn down heat and cook about 1-2 minutes longer.

Red Pepper & Zucchini Toss
1 lb. sweet red peppers
1 lb. zucchini
1 Tbs. olive oil or MCT oil
1/2 tsp. minced garlic
Salt & pepper to taste

Cut peppers into 1-inch pieces. Wash and trim the zucchini. Quarter lengthwise and then cut into 1-inch pieces. Salt, and then drain. Pat dry. Heat the oil and saute zucchini for 3-4 minutes, until lightly browned and barely softened. Stir in the garlic, cook 30 seconds, then add the peppers. Heat together for about 2 minutes. Season with salt and pepper to taste. Serve hot.

Ginger Steamed Squash and Apple
2 1/2 lb. winter squash
1 apple
1 quarter-size slice fresh ginger
1/2 to 1 Tbs. butter or olive oil
cinnamon, nutmeg, allspice to taste (opt.)

Trim squash and cut into 1 1/2-inch chunks. Cut apple coarsely. Put 1 inch water in steamer. Place squash, apple, and ginger in steamer basket. Bring to

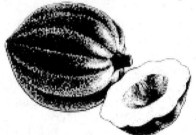

boil. Cover and steam 15-20 minutes. Season with butter and spices.

POULTRY

Turkey Feast
18 -20 pound turkey, thawed
Olive oil

Take out the parts and fat that are inside the turkey. Rinse. Pat dry. Tie the bird wings and legs together with cotton string. Place in roasting pan. Spread olive oil over the top of

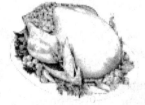

the bird. Cover with lid or foil. Take two pieces of foil and fold the two edges together lengthwise about 1/4 inch. Repeat the fold. When placing foil over turkey, go around the edge of pan and push gently on the foil so it fits below the rim on the inside of pan. (This will keep the juices from escaping and soiling the oven.) No basting is needed. Bake at 350 degrees for about 5-1/2 to 6 hours (less time if you like turkey very moist). Clean meat off the turkey bones while it's still warm. (The meat falls off easily). Divide in serving size portions and place in freezer baggies. Cool in refrigerator, then freeze what you will not eat in a few days.

Many people don't know what to do with the dark meat. A good sandwich paste can be made by using dark meat with your mayonnaise (recipe in the lunch section), mustard, onion powder, salt, and pepper. Blend in a food processor. Or use the meat in burritos, tacos, soups, and casseroles.

Savory Turkey Loaf

1 cup onion (large) diced
1/2 cup green pepper, diced
2 cloves garlic, minced
1/2 tsp. black pepper
1 piece whole wheat bread, cubed
1 egg
1 tsp. liquid lecithin
1 tsp. Worcestershire sauce
1/4 tsp. Tabasco
1 tsp. Spike, or dry poultry seasoning
1 tsp. dry oregano
1 Tbs. chopped parsley
12 ounces tomato sauce
1 pound raw ground turkey

Preheat oven to 425 degrees. Mix all ingredients, reserving 1/2 cup tomato sauce. Spray a 4 x 8 loaf pan with vegetable coating spray and place mixture in pan. Pat down until firm and top with remaining sauce. Bake at 425 degrees for 1 hour until lightly browned around edges.

Turkey Treat

1/2 medium size onion, finely chopped
2 tsp. finely chopped almonds
1 Tbs. olive oil
1 can (10 oz.) tomatillos
1/2 Tbs. cilantro, minced
1 1/2 Tbs. minced canned California green chiles, seeds removed
1 cup chicken broth
1 pound sliced cooked turkey
3 cups hot cooked wild rice or brown rice

Combine the onion, almonds, and oil in a pan over medium heat and cook, stirring, until onion is limp. Whirl tomatillos and their liquid in a blender until mixture is fairly smooth (or rub through wire strainer, using all liquid and pulp). Add to the onion mixture. Stir in cilantro and chiles. Add the chicken broth and boil rapidly, uncovered, until reduced to about 1 1/4 cups. Stir occasionally.

Arrange meat in a wide frying pan. Pour sauce over the meat and cover.
Warm over low heat until mixture begins to bubble slightly. Simmer for 5 to 10 minutes. Add salt to taste and serve on top of the rice.

Turkey with Creamy Salsa

1/2 to 1 Tbs. butter
1/2 pound turkey breast slices
1/8 tsp. sea salt
1/8 tsp. pepper

1/8 tsp. poultry seasoning (opt.)
1/4 to 1/2 cup salsa
1 tsp. soy sauce
1 tsp. lime juice
1 clove garlic, finely chopped
1/2 cup plain yogurt
1 green onion, sliced

Melt butter in skillet over medium high heat. Sprinkle both sides of turkey with poultry seasoning, salt, and pepper. Cook turkey in butter about 3 to 5 minutes, turning once, until no longer pink in the center. Remove turkey from skillet; keep warm in serving dish. Stir salsa, soy sauce, lime juice, and garlic into skillet. Heat to boiling, stirring constantly. Remove from heat. Stir in yogurt. Pour sauce over turkey. Garnish with onions.

the edge. Sprinkle the seasoning well. Cover with the thinly sliced mozzarella, onions, mushrooms, then top with the basil, parsley, oregano, and Parmesan cheese. Sprinkle a little olive oil over the top, and place in a preheated hot oven (450 degrees) for 20 minutes, or until the dough has cooked through and the cheese has melted. Serve.

Chicken with Pesto-Couscous Stuffing
Pesto-Couscous Stuffing
1/2 cup chicken broth
1/3 cup uncooked couscous
1/4 cup pesto
2 Tbs. chopped pecans or almonds
1-2 tsp. butter

Heat broth to boiling in 1-quart saucepan. Stir in couscous. Remove from heat. Cover and let stand 5 minutes. Fluff couscous with fork. Stir in pesto and nuts.
4 chicken breasts, boned
salt and pepper

Heat oven to 375 degrees. Grease pan, 9x9x2 inches, with vegetable spray. Place stuffing in bottom of pan. Lay chicken on top of stuffing. Spread butter over tops of chicken. Sprinkle salt and pepper on top. Bake uncovered about 45 minutes or until juice of chicken is no longer pink when centers of thickest pieces are cut.

Curry Chicken with Yogurt
2 pounds chicken breast
1 medium onion, chopped
1-2 Tbs. olive oil
1/4 tsp. season salt
2 Tbs. water
2 tsp. curry powder
1/8 tsp. ground cumin
1/2 cup plain yogurt

Place chicken in baking pan. Cut onion in wedges. Place around chicken. Sprinkle with oil. Sprinkle with seasonings. Bake in 375 degree oven for about 45 minutes or until chicken is cooked. Place a spoonful of yogurt on top of chicken.

Sesame Chicken
4 split chicken breasts, skinned and boned
1/2 Tbs. lemon pepper
1 tsp. basil
1/2 tsp. garlic, chopped
2 eggs lightly beaten
1/4 cup barley flour or whole wheat or oat flour

1/8 cup sesame seeds
Pam or other vegetable oil

Wash chicken and remove all visible fat. Place chicken in a zip lock bag with lemon pepper, basil, garlic and eggs, and coat the chicken. Mix the barley flour and sesame seeds together. Dip each piece of marinated chicken in the flour mixture and place meat side up in a baking dish that has been sprayed with Pam (or you can use oven paper). Spray the chicken with the vegetable oil. Bake at 350 degrees for 45-50 minutes, spraying the chicken with the oil 25 minutes into the cooking time.

Indian Spice Chicken
4 spring onions, sliced
1 Tbs. olive oil
10 whole cardamom pods, crushed
1/4 tsp. ground cumin
1/4 tsp. lemon peel, diced fine
1/4 tsp. ground cloves
1/4 tsp. cinnamon
1 tsp. ginger, minced
3 dried red chilis, stems & seeds removed, crushed
1 tsp. honey
2 cups water
1 whole chicken, cleaned
salt to taste

Saute the onion in oil in a pot and add the cardamom and toast for one minute. Stir in all the seasonings and add the water. Stir and bring to a boil. Add the chicken and cover. Simmer for 45 minutes, turning the chicken 3 times. Remove the cover and cook until the chicken is done, turning often to coat the chicken with the spices.

Apricot Chicken
1/2 pound chicken breast, cut into strips
2 tsp. cornstarch
2 tsp. apple juice or water
1 tsp. ginger, minced
2 tsp. garlic, minced
1 Tbs. white wine or unsweetened apple juice
2 Tbs. soy sauce
1 Tbs. hot bean sauce
5 dried apricots, cut in pieces and soaked in the wine
1 1/2 tsp. honey
1 Tbs. olive oil
5 small dried hot chiles

Combine the cornstarch and apple juice. Toss with the chicken in a zip lock bag and marinate for 15 minutes. Mix together the rest of the ingredients except the oil and chiles, then set aside. This will be the sauce. Heat a wok until hot and add the oil. As soon as the oil is hot, add the chiles and chicken. Stir-fry until chicken is almost done and add the sauce. Cook for another 45 seconds. Serve on top of cooked brown rice.

Simple Chicken & Sweet Potato Dinner
2-4 chicken breasts, washed
Onion powder
Spike seasoning or:
Lowry's seasoning salt without MSG
2-4 medium sweet potatoes or yams

Place sweet potatoes that have been pierced with a knife in a foil-lined pan. In a 375-degree preheated oven, cook the sweet potatoes for 30 minutes. Then add the chicken that has been placed in a foil-lined baking dish and sprinkled with the seasonings. Bake for 45 to 50 minutes

Mexican Oven Chicken
4 chicken breast halves, skinned
1 cup spiced tomato juice
1/2 cup crushed unsweetened corn flakes or wheat flakes
1/4 cup wheat bran
1 tsp. dried parsley
1/2 tsp. dried oregano
1/2 tsp. ground cumin
1/2 tsp. chili powder
1/2 tsp. paprika
1/2 tsp. minced onion
1/4 tsp. garlic powder
Vegetable spray (i.e. Pam)

Combine chicken and tomato juice in a baggie and marinate in the refrigerator 6 hours or overnight.

Combine the next nine ingredients. First drain the chicken, then dredge the chicken in the cereal mixture. Place chicken in a baking pan sprayed with the oil. Bake at 350 degrees for about an hour or until done.

BEEF/OTHER

It is preferable to use organic low fat beef or wild game (venison, etc.) whenever possible.

Hearty Pot Roast

About 3-lb. lean eye of round roast
2 carrots
2 wedges of red cabbage
1 onion, sliced thick
2-4 garlic cloves, peeled
dried fruit (opt.)
sun dried tomatoes (opt.)
1/2 – 2/3 cup red wine/water or water
2 Tbs. soy sauce
2 Tbs. dry onion soup (with out MSG)

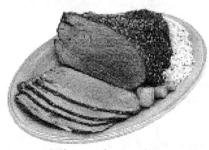

Mix the last three ingredients in a cup. On hot heat, brown the roast on all sides. Place the roast and then the next six ingredients in a slow cooking pot. Pour the fluid over the items. Cover and cook on low, 8 to 10 hours or until meat is tender. (If you are at home, you can add the vegetables 3 hours before serving for crisper vegetables.) Serve.

Herb Flank Steak
1 1/2 to 2 pound beef flank or round steak
2 Tbs. lemon juice
1/2 tsp. dried oregano leaves
1/2 tsp. sea salt
1/2 tsp. celery seed
1/2 tsp. onion powder
1/2 tsp. pepper
1 to 2 cloves garlic, finely chopped

Make cuts about 1/2 inch apart and 1/4 inch deep in diamond pattern on both sides. (This helps tenderize the beef.) Mix remaining ingredients; rub into beef. Can refrigerate up to 24 hours. Set oven control to Broil. Line pan with aluminum foil and place beef on rack in broiler pan. Broil beef with top 2 to 3 inches from heat about 5 minutes or until brown. Turn, broil about 5 minutes longer. Or you can fry in a skillet to your taste.

Ground Beef Stuffed Potatoes
2 hot baked sweet potatoes
1/4 cup hot skim milk or rice milk
1 green onion, minced
1 egg, beaten
2 tsp. butter or olive oil or MCT oil
1/4 tsp. salt
1/2 tsp. black pepper
1/2 cup diced tomato
1 pound ground beef, organic preferably, cooked

Cut a thin slice off the top of each baked potato, scoop out potato and combine with hot milk, green onion, the beaten egg and butter. Whip well. Add salt and pepper and gently stir in tomato and beef. Fill potato skins with this mixture, mounding it high. Place on baking sheet and cook at 400 degrees for 10-15 minutes.

Green Chili Stew
2 pounds boneless beef chuck, cut in 1-inch cubes
2 tsp. olive oil
2 cloves garlic, minced
1 medium onion, diced
2 cans (1 lb. 12 oz. each) tomatoes
1 can (7 oz.) California green chili, seeded and chopped
1/4 cup parsley, chopped
1/2 tsp. honey
1/4 tsp. ground cloves
2 tsp. ground cumin
1 cup red wine or beef broth
1 tsp. lemon juice
Salt to taste

Brown the meat on all sides in a large frying pan. Remove meat with a slotted spoon and set aside. Throw away drippings, add the olive oil, and cook the bell pepper, onion, and garlic until soft. In a large pot, pour in the tomatoes with the liquid. Break up tomatoes with a spoon. Add the chili, parsley, honey, cloves, cumin, lemon juice, and wine. Bring to a boil, then reduce heat to a simmer. Add all of the ingredients together, cover, and cook over low heat for 1 1/2 hours, stirring occasionally. Remove the cover and simmer for 1 more hour or until meat is tender.

Chili with Kidney Beans
2 cloves garlic
1 Tbs. oil
2 pounds lean ground beef
2-3 onions, chopped
2 green peppers, chopped
3 (1 pound) cans whole tomatoes
2 (1 pound) cans red kidney beans, drained
1 (6 ounce) can tomato juice
1/8 cup chili powder
1/4 tsp. cumin powder
1 Worcestershire sauce
1 tsp. vinegar
1 to 2 dashes red pepper

1 whole clove (spice) (opt.)
1 bay leaf
dash of sea salt & pepper

Place the onion, garlic, and crumbled beef in oil in a large heavy pot and cook 10 minutes, or until brown. Add the rest of the ingredients and cook, covered, over low heat, for about an hour. If it becomes dry, add more tomatoes or water. If it is too liquid, uncover and simmer longer. Serve with brown rice, if desired.

Spaghetti

1 pound lean hamburger
1 large onion, chopped
1 clove garlic, crushed
1 cup water
1 tsp. sea salt or Lite salt
1/2 tsp. xylitol or honey
1 tsp. dried oregano leaves
1 tsp. dried basil leaves
1/2 tsp. dried marjoram leaves (opt.)
1 bay leaf
8 ounces tomato sauce
6 ounces tomato paste
1/4 cup Italian dressing
cooked whole wheat spaghetti noodles

Cook and stir hamburger, onion, and garlic in a 10 -inch skillet until hamburger is light brown. Drain. Stir in remaining ingredients. Heat to boiling. Cover and simmer, stirring occasionally for 1 hour. Serve over cooked noodles.

Liver with Onions

1 Tbs. butter
1 Tbs. olive oil
2 to 3 cups thinly sliced onions
3/4 pound thinly sliced calves' liver
Whole wheat flour
Salt & pepper
Red wine (opt.)
Lemon wedges (opt.)

Cook onions in butter and oil slowly for about 20 minutes, stirring occasionally, until wilted and golden. Remove from pan. Lightly dust the liver in flour, salt, and pepper and sear over medium-high heat in pan until brown on both sides. Arrange the liver on a bed of the fried onions. Deglaze the pan with wine if desired, and pour over liver. Serve with lemon.

Lamb Roast with Yogurt

3-5 lbs. lamb roast
1 onion, sliced thick
4 garlic cloves, peeled
2 Tbs. dried fruit (opt.)
dried tomatoes (opt.)
mint leaves
1/2 tsp. cumin (opt.)
1/2 cup red wine or water
2 Tbs. soy sauce
2 Tbs. dry onion soup (with out MSG)

Mix the last 4 ingredients in a cup. On hot heat, brown the roast on all sides. Place the roast, and then the next 4 ingredients in a slow cooking pot. Pour the fluid over them. Add the mint on top. Cover and cook on low, 8 to 10 hours or until meat is tender. Serve.

Yogurt

1 cup yogurt
1/2 to 1 Tbs. flax meal
1-2 tsp. xylitol or honey
1 tsp. dill, chopped (opt.)

Mix all ingredients and serve with lamb.

FISH

While fish used to be one of the healthiest foods on the planet earth, we now have a problem with mercury and other pollutants accumulating in fish that are higher on the food chain. We recommend that you eat little or no fish high in mercury, consume the low mercury fish only once a week, and the very low mercury fish can be eaten as often as you wish.

HIGH MERCURY: tilefish, swordfish, shark, king mackerel

LOW MERCURY: red snapper, orange roughy, bass, marlin, tuna, lobster, grouper, brook trout, halibut, mahi mahi, can tuna

VERY LOW MERCURY: crab, catfish, scallops, salmon, oyster, shrimp, clams, sardines

For more guidelines about eating your local fish, visit: http://www.health.state.mn.us/divs/eh/fish/eating/safeeating.html

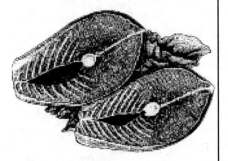

Creole Seafood Seasoning
1/6 cup salt
1/6 cup paprika
1/8 cup black pepper
1/8 cup garlic powder
1 1/2 Tbs. onion powder
1 Tbs. cayenne pepper
1 Tbs. oregano
1 Tbs. thyme

Combine all ingredients and mix. Keeps indefinitely in a tightly sealed glass jar. Makes one cup.

Easy Salmon Dinner
1-2 pound salmon filet or steak
Soy sauce or low sugar Teriyaki sauce

Turn on broiler. Place salmon on broiler pan sprayed with vegetable oil where you will be placing the salmon. Broil on one side for about 8 minutes. Flip. Spread the Teriyaki sauce on the top of salmon. Bake another 8 minutes or until done. You might have to move the fish to a lower shelf so the top doesn't burn. If you are broiling halibut or a less oily fish, you can put foil on the broiling pan to save on clean up time.

If you don't have access to fresh fish:

Salmon Cakes
1 can (14.75 oz) salmon
1 cup dry oatmeal cereal
2 eggs
1/2 Tbs. lemon juice
2 tsp. minced parsley
1 tsp. onion powder
olive oil

Drain salmon. Skim off skin and bones. Mix all ingredients. Make into patties. Fry in 2 tsp. olive oil. When brown, flip and brown other side.

Broiled Tarragon Fish
2-3 Tbs. olive oil

1 Tbs. lemon juice
1/2 tsp. tarragon
1/2 tsp. sea salt
1/8 tsp. pepper
2 pound fresh or partially thawed
cod, flounder, or other fish
1 lemon, cut into wedges
parsley sprigs (opt.)

Preheat broiler. In small bowl, mix first five ingredients. Place fillet fish in broiling pan and broil, basting generously with oil mixture occasionally. Broil 5 to 8 minutes until fish flakes easily when tested with a fork. Place fish on warm pan and garnish with lemon wedges and parsley.

BBQ Halibut
2 halibut steaks
Lowry's seasoning salt (without MSG)
Cooking oil
Juice of a lemon

Preheat your BBQ. Grease grill with oil. Place steaks on grill. Sprinkle with the salt. Cook 5 to 10 minutes on each side, depending on the thickness of the fish and how hot the grill is. You can serve it with lemon juice and a bit of melted butter on top.

Dill-Almond Cod
2 egg whites, beaten until foamy
2 Tbs. skim milk (or soy or rice milk)
1 1/2 pounds cod
1/4 cup wheat germ
2 Tbs. ground almonds
2 to 3 Tbs. Parmesan cheese (opt.)
1/3 cup wheat bran

1 tsp. fresh chopped dill or 1/2 tsp. dried dill
vegetable coating spray (i.e. Pam)

Combine egg whites and milk in a shallow bowl. Mix the rest of the ingredients in a shallow pan. Dip the fish in the egg mix and then the dry mix. Place the fish on a shallow baking pan sprayed with the oil. Bake at 350 degrees for 10 minutes or until fish flakes with ease. Broil one minute to brown. Serve with lemon, dill, or salsa.

You can substitute any similar fish: sole, sand dabs, mountain trout.

Tuna Cakes
6 ounces water-packed tuna, drained
6 whole grain crackers, finely crushed
1/4 cup oats
1/4 cup minced red bell pepper
2 Tbs. fresh, minced parsley
2 Tbs. minced onions
1 egg
2 tsp. yogurt or water
1 1/2 tsp. lemon juice
1 tsp. Worcestershire
1/8 tsp. ground red pepper or 1/4 tsp. chili powder
1-2 tsp. minced fresh basil
1/2 tsp. marjoram
1 clove garlic, minced
Non stick cooking spray

Spray a frying pan with the oil. In large bowl, gently mix all ingredients. Using a scant 1/4 cup mixture for each, make six cakes. Shape mixture into circle, pressing flat. (If they are too dry to hold a shape, add a bit more water.) Place in frying pan and fry on both sides until golden brown.

Tuna Stuffed Potatoes

2 large, hot baked sweet potatoes (can be cooked in the microwave)
1/4 cup hot skim milk or rice milk
1 green onion, minced
1 egg
2 tsp. butter or MCT oil
1/4 tsp. salt
1/2 tsp. black pepper
1/2 cup diced tomato
7 ounce can water-packed tuna, drained
2 tsp. Parmesan cheese, grated (opt.)

Cut a thin slice off the top of each baked potato, scoop out potato and combine with the hot milk, green onion, beaten egg and butter. Whip well. Add salt and pepper and gently stir in tomato and tuna. Fill potato skins with this mixture by mounding it high. Sprinkle with Parmesan cheese. Place on baking sheet and cook at 400 degrees for 10-15 minutes.

Crab Dinner

Fry in a small amount of olive oil and butter: Imitation crab (pollock fish), diced onions, garlic, sliced mushrooms, bell pepper, ginger. Sprinkle sunflower seeds or crushed almonds on top before serving.
Variations: bamboo shoots, olives, green chilis, Spike seasoning

Baked Scallops

1 lb. scallops, cut in half
1 oz wine, optional
2 Tbs. butter, melted
1/2 cup dry whole wheat bread crumbs

Arrange scallops in shallow buttered casserole dish. Sprinkle with wine. Pour half the butter over scallops. Cover with bread crumbs. Pour rest of butter over top. Bake at 375 degrees for 15 minutes.

SOY

Textured Tofu

(The day before, slice firm tofu and pat dry. Freeze separately.) Drop frozen tofu into boiling water. Take tofu out when it's been defrosted. When cool enough to touch, ring out and pat dry. Set aside. This will turn the tofu firm, almost like a sponge.

Tofu Steak

Firm tofu sliced 1/4 to 1/2 inch thick. Can use textured tofu.
In a baggie, mix:
1/4 cup water
1 tsp. vegetable broth
Dash Spike
Dash poultry seasoning

Add tofu to baggie and marinade. Dip tofu in a beaten egg. Then bread in equal parts of whole wheat flour and corn meal. Fry in small amount of olive oil.

Spicy Tofu with Cashews

3 Tbs. soy sauce
2 tsp. cornstarch
1/3 cup water or dry wine
1 tsp. honey
1 tsp. grated fresh gingerroot
1/2 tsp. crushed red pepper or 1/4 tsp chili powder
14 ounces tofu

1 Tbs. olive oil
4 green onions
1/4 to 1/2 cup cashews
1/2 cup orange sections, chopped
2 cups hot cooked brown rice or noodles.

Mix soy and cornstarch; stir in 1/3 cup water or wine, honey, red pepper, and ginger root. Set aside. Press moisture from tofu with paper towels or towel. Cube tofu. Stir-fry tofu in hot oil 3 to 4 minutes. Remove tofu. Stir fry nuts & onions for 1 to 2 minutes. Stir soy mixture into nuts. Cook and stir till bubbly; about 2 minutes. Add tofu. Cover and cook 1 minute. Stir in oranges. Heat. Serve over rice. You can use textured tofu (recipe in this section).

Soy Pilaf
1-2 Tbs. olive oil
1/8 tsp. black pepper
1 bay leaves, crumbled
1 pinch cloves
1/4 tsp. cinnamon
1 Tbs. minced fresh onion
1 clove minced garlic
1/2 tsp. grated fresh ginger
1/8 tsp. cayenne
1 cup diced celery
1/2 cup cooked brown rice
1 cup cooked soybeans

Toast first 10 ingredients. Add grain and beans and heat. Add vegetable salt or soy sauce to taste.

Tempeh a l' Orange
8 ounces tempeh (fermented soybeans)
3 Tbs. oil

1 large onion
1 stalk celery, chopped
1 carrot, grated
3 Tbs. whole wheat flour
2 cups boiling water
1/2 cup orange juice
1 1/4 tsp. salt
1 1/2 tsp. honey
1 orange peeled & finely chopped with juice
dash red pepper
1/4 cup chopped fresh parsley
1/2 cup white wine (or more orange juice)

Cut tempeh in 1/2 inch chunks and saute in 2 tablespoons oil for about 5 minutes. Drain on paper towels. Tempeh will soak up all the oil you give it, so save half the oil to saute the second side.

Saute onion and celery in remaining oil until celery is tender. Stir in flour and keep stirring over medium heat just a minute or so; then add boiling water gradually.

Cook, stirring, while mixture thickens. Add orange juice, salt, carrot, honey, orange, pepper, parsley, and wine. Stir, bring to a boil, and simmer 4 to 5 minutes. Add tempeh chunks and simmer a few minutes longer to let flavors be absorbed. Serves four, over brown rice, quinoa, or bulgur wheat.

Tofu Surprise
1/4 onion, chopped
1 tsp. olive oil
1 clove garlic, minced
1/2 tsp. minced ginger
1/4 green pepper
1 Tbs. natural peanut butter, or almond butter
1 Tbs. soy sauce
1/2 cup water (or more)

2 Tbs. celery leaves, chopped
1 Tbs. wakame (sea vegetable), soaked, rinsed and drained and diced
1 tsp. honey
1/4 pound firm tofu, cubed
2 Tbs. toasted cashew pieces

Saute onion in oil with the minced garlic. Add the ginger and pepper and cook a minute more. Stir in the peanut butter and soy sauce. Then add water, celery leaves, wakame, and honey. Stir and then simmer about 5 minutes. Add the tofu and cashews and heat through. Serve over steamed vegetables or noodles. Can use the textured tofu concept in this recipe.

BBQ Tempeh
1 lb. tempeh
2 Tbs. mustard
2 Tbs. miso
water to cover

Cut tempeh in "burger-size" portions. Place in a pot and cover with water. Dissolve miso and mustard in 1/4 cup water; add to tempeh and bring to a boil. Lower heat and simmer for 20 minutes. Remove from liquid. Place in frying pan with sauce (recipe below) and use the sauce to baste. Cook 5 to 10 minutes on each side. Serve on whole wheat bun or roll, with sliced onion, lettuce, and sprouts.

Sauce:
1/2 cup apple juice
1 Tbs. soy sauce
1/2 Tbs. lemon juice
1/2 Tbs. honey (opt.)
1 small piece ginger root, grated

1 tsp. arrowroot dissolved in a little water

Place apple juice, soy sauce, and syrup in a small saucepan. Simmer gently on a low heat to reduce volume slightly. Thicken with arrowroot. Add ginger. Adjust flavor.

Tofu Burger
1 pound tofu, drained and crumbled
1/2 cup finely-grated carrot
1/4 cup chopped scallions
6 Tbs. wheat germ
1 Tbs. chopped parsley
4 ounce alfalfa sprouts
1 Tbs. soy sauce
dash Tabasco sauce (optional)
1/2 tsp. Worcestershire sauce
1/4 cup whole wheat bread crumbs
olive oil

Put all ingredients, except wheat germ, in a bowl and mix well. Add just enough homemade mayonnaise to make the mixture hold together for shaping. Shape into 4 to 6 burger patties, coat with the reserved wheat germ, and pan-fry in a small amount of oil until browned and hot. Serve on a sourdough bun.

Soyburgers
4 cups cooked soybeans
1/2 cup water or tomato sauce
1/4 tsp. onion powder
1/4 tsp. garlic powder
2 Tbs. walnuts, minced fine
1/4 cup soy sauce
1/4 tsp. liquid smoke (opt.)
1 tsp. Spike
1/2 to 1 cup bran and/or rolled oats

Blend first 8 ingredients in a blender until smooth, using only 2 cups of soybeans. Pour into a bowl.

Grind remaining 2 cups of soybeans in blender without any liquid so they are coarsely chopped. Add to mixture in the bowl and add grains. Mix well and let sit 10 to 15 minutes so grains can absorb moisture. Shape 1/2 cup of the mixture at a time into patties and fry in a pan wiped with olive oil. Cook until brown, then flip and cook until brown on the other side. Serve with whole grain buns.

Ginger Tofu

1/4 cup soy sauce
1/4 cup honey
1/4 tsp. garlic
1/4 tsp. onion powder
1" to 1 1/2" chunk of fresh ginger grated
6 cups tofu, chunks or sliced

Blend first 4 ingredients together. Pour over slices or pieces of tofu that have been placed on a large baking dish sprayed with vegetable oil. Cover with foil and bake at 375 degree for about 20 minutes. Lift up corner of foil to make sure tofu is boiling and swollen. Remove foil and flip tofu over with a spatula. Bake 25-35 minutes or until sauce dries out and tofu is brown. Stir a few times in between.

SIDE DISHES

Apple Chutney

2 1/2 lbs. apples
1 to 2 Tbs. water
1 1/2 Tbs. butter
1/4 tsp. crushed chili pepper
1/2 Tbs. can California diced green chilis
1/2 tsp. nutmeg
1/4 tsp. allspice
1/2 tsp. ginger
1 tsp. cinnamon
dash nutmeg
1/2 cup honey

Peel, core, and chop apples into quarters. Steam apples in water until tender. When done, remove lid and cook off excess water, being careful not to burn. In a deep skillet, heat butter and toast spices. Add apples and chilis. Cook away excess liquid on high heat, stirring often. Add honey and cook on medium heat until jam-like, stirring frequently to prevent sticking and burning. Remove from heat. Allow to cool. Then refrigerate. Can be served warm, but it is better chilled.

Millet Cakes

2 cups cooked millet
2 eggs
2-3 Tbs. oat or whole wheat flour
1/8 tsp. cayenne pepper (opt.)
1/2 tsp. sea salt
1/4 tsp. pepper
1/2 medium onion, finely chopped
1Tbs. sun-dried tomatoes, finely chopped
1 Tbs. butter
1 Tbs. olive oil

Blend eggs with flour and seasonings. Add rest of the ingredients, except butter and oil. Form into patties and fry in the oil and butter until cooked through.

Spicy Mexican Beans

2 cups pinto beans
1 large onion, diced
4 cloves garlic, minced

1 to 2 dry red peppers, minced (can cut with scissors)
1 Tbs. chili powder
1 tsp. cumin powder
1/4 cup olive oil
2 tsp. sea salt
Purified water

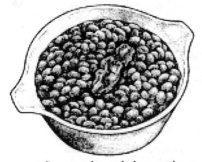

Sort and wash beans in a colander. Place beans in a pressure cooker and add enough water to cover the beans and then 4 cups more. Bring to a boil and boil for 2 minutes. Cover and leave for 1 hour. Drain and rinse beans. Place beans back into the pressure cooker and add water to just cover the beans. Add the rest of ingredients and close lid. Heat on high until the weight starts rocking. Turn down the heat, but keep the weight moving for 25 minutes. Turn off heat. Let the pressure cooker sit until the indicator shows that all pressure has been released. Remove lid and mash the beans with a beater until about 1/2 of the beans are mashed.

If you don't want to use a pressure cooker, follow the steps except when placing the beans with the rest of the ingredients, place the beans and ingredients in a large pot and let boil for about 90-120 minutes or until beans are tender. More water will be needed.

To give you a few ideas, these beans can be used to make: burritos, add ground cooked beef to tacos, a bean sandwich with a slice of onion on top, or a hot dip with baked corn chips.

Healthy Wheat Balls
3 cups water
1 1/2 cups cracked wheat
1/2 cup dry oatmeal
1/4 cup chopped parsley
1 Tbs. miso
1/4 tsp. each, nutmeg, thyme, basil
1/2 tsp. sage
1/2 cup sunflower seeds
1/4 cup sesame seeds
1 tsp. oil

Bring 3 cups water to a boil; stir in the wheat and oats. Lower the heat and simmer for 10 to 12 minutes until water is absorbed. Mix the rest of the ingredients, except the sesame seeds, into the hot mixture. Spoon into a bowl and allow to cool enough to handle. Moisten hands with water and form into walnut-sized balls; roll in sesame seeds. Place in oiled (or Pam sprayed) baking dish. Warm in 350 degree oven for 10 to 15 minutes. Serve with 100% whole wheat bread or pita bread.

Three Bean Salad
1 cup frozen green beans, cooked in microwave 1 to 2 minutes
1 cup cooked kidney beans
1/2 cup cooked garbanzo beans
1/2 cup cooked pinto beans
4 spring onions, chopped

2 cloves garlic, crushed
1/4 cup snipped parsley (opt.)
1/3 cup Royal Dressing
soy bacon bits or Turkey bacon (cooked and crumbled)(opt.)

  Mix all ingredients in a bowl. Cover and refrigerate, stirring before serving.

Couscous with Nuts
1 cup boiling water
1 tsp. olive or sesame oil (opt.)
1 cup couscous
1/3 cup chopped nuts or seeds
chopped parsley.

  Bring water to a boil. Add oil; pour couscous in gently. Cover and remove from heat. Allow grains to absorb water another 3 to 5 minutes. Add the nuts or seeds and parsley. Fluff with a fork.

Tabouli with Chickpeas
1 cup bulgur (cracked wheat)
1-1/3 cups water
1/4 to 1/3 cup olive oil
1/3 cup lemon juice
1 cup finely green onion
1 cup chopped fresh parsley
1/4 cup chopped fresh mint
2 tomatoes, diced
1/2 cup cooked chickpeas
1 cup chopped cucumber (optional)
2 tsp. soy sauce
dash of cayenne
ground pepper to taste

  To cook, combine water and cracked wheat and bring to a boil, then cover and simmer until done. Cool completely. Drain off any excess water. Mix the rest of the ingredients with the bulgur. Refrigerate

Spanish Rice
Cooked brown rice
Salsa to desired amount
Spring onions sliced
Chopped fresh parsley
Black olives, minced (opt.)

  Mix all ingredients together and warm in the oven.

Miso Rice
2 cups cooked brown rice
1 Tbs. miso mixed in 2 Tbs. warm water
1 tsp. Spike
1 Tbs. finely-chopped parsley
1 tsp minced spring onion

  Mix all ingredients together. Warm in the oven.

Brown Rice Delight
2 cups cooked instant brown rice or cooked brown rice
1 apple, diced
1-2 Tbs. walnuts or pecans, chopped
1-2 Tbs. raisins (opt.)
2 Tbs. celery leaves, chopped
1 tsp. poultry seasoning

  Mix all ingredients together. Add a few teaspoons of water if too dry. Warm in the oven.

Fettuccini
  This recipe is for people who do not have a dairy allergy.
5 ounces whole wheat or spinach fettuccini or linguini
1 Tbs. butter
1/2 cup organic whole milk or rice milk
1/4 cup grated Parmesan cheese
1/4 tsp. pepper (or chili powder)
1/8 tsp. nutmeg

Cook noodles according to package. Don't overcook noodles. Drain. Melt butter in a small saucepan and add milk. Heat just until hot. Do not boil. Place cooked noodles in a serving bowl. Add milk and 1/2 cheese. Toss. Add the spices and toss again. Add remaining cheese. Serve.

Spinach Linguini
12 ounces cooked whole wheat linguini
1/2 cup vegetable stock
4 garlic cloves, minced
1 to 2 cups chopped fresh spinach
1/3 cup Parmesan cheese (opt.)
1 Tbs. basil (or 1 1/2 tsp. dried basil)
1/2 tsp. pepper
Saute garlic in stock in large saucepan over medium heat for 2 minutes. Add spinach, basil and pepper. Cook over low until heated through. Remove from heat. Mix the ingredients together. Serve warm.

Fruited Bulgur Pilaf
1/2 Tbs. butter
1/2 Tbs. olive oil
1 medium onion chopped
1 cup bulgur uncooked
1/4 tsp. dill weed
1/4 tsp. oregano
1/2 tsp. salt (optional)
1/4 tsp. pepper
1 Tbs. parsley chopped
chopped apricots, dates and raisins to taste
2 cups water mixed with 1 Tbs. miso

Melt butter and oil in a large skillet. Add bulgur and vegetables. Stir constantly until vegetables are tender and bulgur is golden. Add the rest of the ingredients. Bring to a boil. Stir. Reduce heat and simmer 15 minutes.

Sweet Potato Delight
2 medium sweet potatoes, grated
1 medium onion, grated
1/3 tsp. sea salt
1-2 Tbs. olive oil
Add oil to frying pan. Add the rest of the ingredients and cook, covered, on medium heat. When brown on bottom, flip and cook with lid off until golden brown.

DESSERTS

Here is most people's favorite section: dessert. Sugar is a food that can be a craving, but is harmful to your health. "If you are not suppose to eat it, what are you

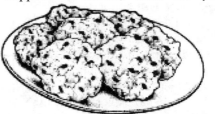

suppose to do?," is a question that has been asked frequently. Here are a couple of substitutions that are actually sweeter than sugar and healthier for you.

Stevia is easily found in health food stores. There is the herb, which is dark in color and more medicinal, then the clear color one you use in cooking and to sweeten drinks. Some people do experience a chemical after taste. Many companies have their own brand of Stevia products. Since it is touted as being 200+ times sweeter than sugar, less is used, which is a good thing since it is expensive.

Xylitol is harder to find, though you can locate it on the internet and in a few health food stores. It can be used like sugar. Patrick has a section on the benefits of this sweetener

We also need to take the taste bud reins back. Just because these sweeteners aren't harmful, the body still wants to be in a healthy balance. Not having everything look, taste, and smell sweet fills some people with a sense of denial. But the human race wasn't designed to live like hummingbirds. When you cut back on the intake of sugar and start tasting food in its natural state, a whole new culinary experience will begin.

For more information on sugar and sugar substitutes, see the beginning of this chapter.

In the summertime, frozen berries or a half of a frozen banana makes for a nice replacement for ice cream. Some of the better fruits are cherries, berries, apples, figs, kiwis, papaya, grapefruit, and pears. Limit dates and watermelon. A half of a teaspoon of honey cappings is a blast of sweetness. You chew it like you would gum and throw away the wax part when finished.

You can also replace milk, oil, and sugar in recipes with unsweetened applesauce.

Cocoa powder has no sugar. You can use this with the Stevia or Xylitol products in recipes for that chocolate taste

Watch out for foods that claim they are low fat or low in sugar. They can be loaded with corn syrup, honey, or other sweeteners that affect the blood sugar level

This sweet recipe section is controversial. Since sugar of any kind could possibly feed cancer, or throw off your blood sugar level, these recipes are to be used with discretion. Desserts should be eaten with meals to keep the blood sugar level stable. The amount of sweetener added to these recipes is minimal. The more you can use the herb Stevia or xylitol for your recipes instead of other sweeteners, the better. You can make desserts special by having them less often. Also, once you remove sugar from the diet, food starts tasting sweeter. A slice of bread will be noticeably sweet.

VARIATION OF PORTIONS

Sometimes the portion amount in a recipe will have a sliding scale. You need to feel the thickness of the dough or sauce and adjust it to what you feel would be your normal texture or desire. For example, some like a dense frosting, while other people appreciate a more fluffy texture. Have fun. Who is going to fire you if it doesn't make a cover of *Gourmet Magazine?*

Maple-Baked Pears

2 pears
1 Tbs. maple syrup
1/4 tsp. vanilla extract
2 tsp. wheat germ
1 tsp. flax meal
2 tsp. butter

Preheat oven to 350 degrees. Spray a nonstick baking dish with vegetable oil spray. Cut pears in half and core. Place in baking dish. Mix syrup and vanilla extract. Drizzle over pears. Sprinkle with wheat germ. Divide butter among pears. Bake 10 minutes or until tender.

Pear Bread Pudding

3 slices whole wheat bread, cubed
1 1/2 Tbs. chopped walnuts or pecans (opt.)
3 small ripe pears, peeled and chopped
1/4 cup unsweetened apple juice
3 eggs
3/4 cup non-fat plain yogurt or unsweetened applesauce
1/4 to1/2 tsp. lecithin
1/4 tsp. ground cinnamon
1 tsp. vanilla
Preheat oven to 350 degrees. Sprinkle bread cubes and walnuts into a square pan coated with non-stick cooking spray. Sprinkle with chopped pears; set aside. Beat together apple juice, eggs, yogurt, lecithin, cinnamon, and vanilla until smooth. Pour over bread and fruit in pan. Bake for 30 minutes. Press pears down into custard with spatula and bake an additional 20 minutes until custard is set. Serve warm or cold.

Apple Bread Pudding

3 slices whole wheat bread, cubed
1 1/2 Tbs. chopped walnuts or pecans (opt.)
3 small apples, peeled and chopped
1/4 cup unsweetened apple juice
3 eggs
3/4 cup non-fat plain yogurt or unsweetened applesauce
1/4 to1/2 tsp. lecithin
1/4 tsp. ground cinnamon
1/8 tsp. nutmeg (opt.)
1 tsp. vanilla

Preheat oven to 350 degrees. Sprinkle bread cubes and walnuts into a square pan coated with non-stick cooking spray. Sprinkle with chopped apples; set aside. Beat together apple juice, eggs, yogurt, lecithin, cinnamon, nutmeg, and vanilla until smooth; pour over bread and fruit in pan. Bake for 30 minutes. Press apples down into custard with spatula and bake an additional 20 minutes until custard is set. Serve warm or cold.

Fruited Gelatin

2 envelopes Knox unflavored gelatin
2 cups purified water
1 cup fresh or frozen fruit
1 tsp. Stevia
Sprinkle gelatin in 1/2 cup cool water for 1 minute. Add 1 1/2 cups hot water. Stir. Add fruit and the Stevia to the sweetness you desire. Stir once again. Refrigerate until set.

Oatmeal Raisin Delights

1 cup uncooked oatmeal
2/3 cup whole wheat flour
1/4 cup xylitol (opt.)
1 tsp. cinnamon

1/2 tsp. nutmeg
1/2 tsp. baking soda
1/2 tsp. salt
1 Tbs. flax meal
1/4 cup dry coconut
1/4 cup peanut butter (opt.)
about 1/2 cup unsweetened applesauce
1/4 cup extra virgin olive oil, coconut oil or butter
1/4 to 1/2 tsp. liquid lecithin (opt.)
2 tsp. vanilla
2 eggs
1/2 cup chopped nuts (opt.)
1 to 2 Tbs. raisins
1/4 cup water if needed

Heat oven to 375 degrees. Lightly spray cookie sheet with no-stick cooking spray or use oven paper. Combine dry ingredients, mixing well. Mix the rest of the ingredients, stirring until well mixed. Adjust the consistency with the applesauce or water to have a texture like cookie dough. Cook 1 or 2 spoons of dough to test for texture. Add either fluid or flour if necessary. Place rounded spoonfuls of mixture on the cookie sheet. Bake approximately 10 to 12 minutes until golden brown. If you want a sweeter taste, you could add some honey to the batter.

Blueberry Crisp
3 cups blueberries or 1 package (16 ounces) frozen unsweetened blueberries
1 Tbs. lemon juice (opt.)
1 to 2 Tbs. fructose or xyilotal
1/2 cup oat flour
1/2 cup quick-cooking oats
1/4 cup butter
1 tsp. cinnamon
1/4 tsp. salt

Heat oven to 375 degrees. Arrange blueberries in a square baking dish, 8x8x2 inches. Sprinkle with lemon juice. Mix the rest of the ingredients. Sprinkle on top. Bake until the topping is light brown and the berries are hot, about 25-30 minutes. You can use a variety of different fruits in this crisp recipe.
For example:
-For apple crisp: use 4 cups sliced tart apples and add 3/4 tsp. of nutmeg with the cinnamon.

Tofu Rice Pudding
1 1/2 cups brown rice, cooked
1 cup mashed tofu
1 egg slightly beaten
1/4 cup unsweetened applesauce
1 Tbs. honey, or xylitol
1 tsp. cinnamon
2 tsp. ground cloves
1/4 cup raisins
vegetable oil spray (i.e. PAM)

Combine ingredients and mix well. Place in a quart-size baking dish coated with the oil. Bake in a preheated, 350-degree oven for 45 minutes or until set.

Tofu Whipped Cream
10 ounces soft or silken tofu
1/4 tsp. Stevia
1 tsp. vanilla
1 Tbs. honey
1 Tbs. MCT or light olive oil (opt.)
pinch of salt

Blend all the ingredients in a blender until creamy.

Cherries Jubilee

1 qt. apple juice or cherry juice
1/3 cup agar flakes
1 lb. cherries, halved and pitted
1 tsp. vanilla
dash of cinnamon (optional)
pinch of salt

Pour the apple juice into pot and add agar. Stir and bring to boil over medium heat. Lower heat and simmer 15 to 20 minutes until agar is completely dissolved. While sauce is cooking, halve and pit cherries. After 20 minutes, add vanilla and cherries. Simmer 5 minutes; remove from heat. Pour into baking dish or bowls. Cool and place in refrigerator.

Easy Banana Pudding

1 ripe banana
1 packet Stevita or xyilitol to taste
1/2 tsp. lemon juice
1/2 cup of yogurt

Mash banana and add the rest of the ingredients. Can garnish with a few blueberries. Also is good on pancakes.

Rice Porridge

1 cup cooked brown rice, cold
1/2 cup apple juice
1/4 cup water
2 Tbs. raisins or other dried fruit
1/2 tsp. cinnamon
2 Tbs. chopped nuts

Place all ingredients in a saucepan. Bring to a boil. Reduce heat and simmer, covered, for 15 minutes, stirring frequently. Most of the liquid should be absorbed. Serve warm.

If creamier porridge is desired, puree half.

Baked Apples

4 large flavorful apples
1/4 cup toasted wheat germ
1/4 cup raisins
1/4 cup chopped walnuts
juice of 1/4 of a lemon
1/8 tsp. cinnamon
1 Tbs. xylitol or honey
pinch of salt
1 Tbs. whole wheat or oat flour
1/4 cup apple juice

Preheat oven to 350 degrees. Core apples and place in a greased baking dish with a cover. It's good if the apples are a snug fit. If not, cut up a fifth apple in quarters and pack it in. Mix the wheat germ, raisins, nuts, lemon juice, cinnamon, sugar, and salt, and press lightly into the apple cores. Mix the flour and apple juice. Pour over the apples. Bake 40 minutes, or until the apples are soft, but not mushy. Let cool slightly before serving for best flavor.

Broiled Apple Rings

4 small apples
1-2 tsp. honey
1/2 tsp. cinnamon

Wash, core, and slice apples into 1/2 inch rounds. In a cup, combine the honey and cinnamon. Place rings on a greased cookie sheet and broil for 8 minutes or until light brown. With a spatula, gently turn each ring. Sprinkle with the cinnamon mixture and broil for one more minute. Serve hot or cold.

Homemade Applesauce
6 apples
1/4 cup raisins (opt.)
1/2 cup water
1 tsp. cinnamon
1/4 tsp. nutmeg
1/4 tsp. allspice
1/4 tsp. cloves
Stevia to taste
lemon juice

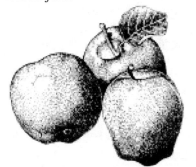

Core apples and cut into chunks. Add remaining ingredients. Bring to a boil and then simmer until tender. Mash with a fork or potato masher. Sprinkle with lemon juice.

Apple Crisp
2 lbs. apples, slices
1/2 tsp. cinnamon
1/6 cup apple juice
juice of one lemon
Crisp
2 cups rolled oats
1/2 cup whole wheat pastry flour
1/4 cup oil
2 Tbs. maple syrup
pinch sea salt
1/ tsp. cinnamon
1/3 cup brown sugar
1/2 cup chopped pecans

Toss the apples, lemon juice, and apple juice. Place apples in a deep baking dish. Mix crisp ingredients and crumble over apples evenly. Press down gently; bake for 20 to 25 minutes or till a wooden toothpick inserted in center comes out clean. Cool in pan on wire rack.

Spicy Ginger Snaps
1/3 cup molasses
1/4 cup extra light olive oil
2 Tbs. honey
1 1/4 cup whole wheat flour
1/2 tsp. salt
1/4 tsp. baking soda
1/4 tsp. baking powder
1/2 tsp. cinnamon
1/2 tsp. ginger
1/4 tsp. ground cloves
Dash of nutmeg
Dash of allspice

Measure out the oil first and then the molasses. (The molasses will slide out of cup). Mix the first 3 ingredients together. Mix in remaining ingredients. Cover and refrigerate at least 4 hours. Heat oven to 375 degrees. Shape dough into a log and roll dough into about a 3-inch log on wax paper or oven paper. Cut into 1/8 inch sections. Place on an cookie sheet and flatten out cookies with palm of hand. Bake until light brown, about 8 minutes. Thinner ones bake about 5 minutes.

Chewy Carrot Brownies
3/4 cup barley, oat, or whole wheat flour
1 tsp. baking powder
1 cup rolled oats
1/4 cup raisins
1 cup shredded carrots
1/4 cup honey
1/3 cup light olive oil or MCT oil

1/2 tsp. liquid lecithin
1/4 cup unsweetened applesauce
1 tsp. maple extract (opt.)

Preheat oven to 375 degrees. In a bowl, mix dry ingredients together. In separate bowl, stir together liquid ingredients, carrots, and raisins. Stir into dry ingredients until well moistened. Add a bit of applesauce if mixture is too stiff. Place in a greased 8x8 square pan. Bake for about 25 minutes until slightly browned. Can also make the dough into cookies and bake for 10-12 minutes or until golden brown on top. May add nuts or sunflower seeds when adding the raisins.

Cake Supreme
1/4 cup xyilitol or honey
1/4 cup extra virgin olive oil or other healthy oil
1 egg
2/3 cup unsweetened applesauce
2 tsp. vanilla
1/4 to 1/2 tsp. liquid lecithin
1 cup whole wheat flour
2 tsp. baking powder
1/4 tsp. salt

Beat together the first 6 ingredients. Add the remaining ingredients, stirring until smooth. If using honey, you might need to add an extra tablespoon of flour. Pour batter into a greased baking dish. Bake at 375 degrees for 20 to 25 minutes, until done.

Frosting
A frosting can be made with: mashed banana with peanut butter; a bit of honey and peanut butter mixed together; or frozen berries mashed and poured on top of the slices of cake.

Pumpkin Cake
1/2 cup dry 1-minute oat cereal
1/2 cup wheat germ
1/2 cup whole wheat flour
1/3 cup honey or xylitol
1 tsp. maple extract
2 tsp. cinnamon
1 tsp. pumpkin spice
1 tsp. baking powder
1 tsp. baking soda
1/2 tsp. sea salt
1/2 cup raisins
1 cup mashed cooked pumpkin (or canned)
2 eggs (unbeaten)
1/4 - 1/2 tsp. liquid lecithin
1/4 cup light olive oil
2/3 cup low-fat yogurt or unsweetened applesauce

In bowl, combine bran, flour, oats, honey, spices, baking powder, baking soda, salt, and raisins, and mix. Add rest of the ingredients and stir just until combined. Spoon batter into oil sprayed baking dish. Bake in a 375-degree preheated oven for 40 minutes or until firm to the touch and a toothpick stuck into the cake comes out dry.

Pumpkin Pie
Crust:
2 cups oat flour (can grind up "Old fashion" dry oat cereal in a food processor)
1/2 tsp. salt
Up to 1 stick of butter (if you need the calories)
4 to 5+ Tbs. Water

Blend. Press into a 9 inch pie pan.

Whole Wheat Piecrust

1 cup whole wheat pastry flour
1/2 teaspoon salt
3 Tbs. oil
1/4 cup water

Stir dry ingredients together. Mix in oil. Add enough of the water to make the dough form a ball. Roll flat between sheets of waxed paper and lift into pan. Make edge.

Filling:

Using the same processor bowl, add:

3 eggs – beat slightly
1 can pumpkin pie filling
1 tsp. cinnamon
1/2 tsp. ginger
1/4 tsp. cloves
1 tsp. pumpkin pie spice
1 cup unsweetened applesauce

Blend all the ingredients well. Pour into pie. Use a pie guard or aluminum foil to protect crust. Cook at 425 degrees for 15 minutes. Then cook at 350 degrees for 1 and 1/2 hours or until a toothpick comes out clean.

Healthy Cookies

1/4 cup light olive oil
1/4 cup MCT oil
1 tsp. liquid lecithin
1 egg
1 tsp. vanilla
1/3 cup honey
1/4 cup peanut butter

Beat ingredients together. Add:

1 cup quick oats
1 cup whole wheat flour (Or less. Stir in 3/4 cup and see how stiff dough is.)
1 tsp. baking soda
1 tsp. baking powder

Mix all together. Bake at 350 degrees for about 7-9 minutes, or until done.

Variations:

-1/4 cup coconut and 1/4 chocolate chips
-1/2 to 1 teaspoon almond extract and 1/2 to 1 teaspoon cinnamon
-1/2 to 1 teaspoon cinnamon and 1/4 cup raisins
-1/4 cup chopped dates, prunes

Peanut Butter & Coconut Treats

2 eggs
1/2 cup almond or natural peanut butter
1/2 cup honey
1/2 cup dry unsweetened coconut
1 Tbs. coconut oil (or butter)
2 Tbs. butter
1 to 1 1/4 cup oat flour or 1 cup whole wheat flour
1 Tbs. flax meal
1/2 tsp. baking powder

Preheat oven to 350 degrees. Mix all ingredients in a bowl. Spoon onto a baking dish. With a wet spoon, press down lightly onto top of cookie dough so cookies are flattened. Bake for 15 minutes or until lightly brown. Cool on wire racks.

Raspberry Couscous Cake

1 cup couscous
pinch sea salt
2 cups unsweetened apple juice
1/2 lemon juice
1/2 pt. raspberries
1-2 tsp. almond slivers
1 tsp. vanilla or almond extract

Bring apple juice and sea salt to a boil in a saucepan; then add lemon juice, couscous and nuts. Lower heat and stir until almost thick. Remove from stove; stir in washed berries. Pour cake into glass baking dish that has been lightly sprayed with vegetable oil. Allow mixture to cool. Cut into squares. Can serve as is or garnish with roasted nuts or own granola.

Frozen Fruit Slush

Puree frozen fruit (i.e.: blueberries, 1/2 banana, berries, pear, cantaloupe)
on high in a blender. Serve right away.

Chocolate Brownies

1/3 to 1/2 cup cocoa powder (depending on how rich you want the brownies)
3/4 cup oat or who wheat flour
1 Tbs. flax meal
1/2 tsp. baking powder
1 tsp. sea salt
1/2 cup xyilitol or honey
2 Tbs. coconut oil, MCT oil or butter
1/4 to 1/3 cup peanut butter (if you need the calories)
1 tsp. lecithin
1/3 cup applesauce
2 eggs
2-3 tsp. vanilla
1/4 cup warm water (more if batter is too stiff)
1/2 cup chopped nuts, or unsweetened coconut (opt.)
1/4 cup chocolate chips (opt.)

Heat oven to 350 degrees. Mix dry ingredients. Add and mix wet ingredients. The batter should be stiffer then cake batter. If the batter is too stiff, add more applesauce. Spread in greased pan. Bake until brownies begin to pull away from the sides of the pan, about 40 minutes. Don't overcook. For a more of a cake texture, add more baking powder.

Chocolate Cake

1/3 cup honey
1/4 cup butter softened
1 egg
2/3 cup yogurt
1-2 tsp. vanilla
1/2 tsp. almond extract (optional)
1 cup whole wheat flour
1 1/2 tsp. baking powder
1/4 tsp. salt

Cream together honey and butter; add egg, yogurt, and vanilla. Stir. Add remaining ingredients stirring until smooth. Pour batter into greased 8 or 9 inch round baking dish. Bake in a 350 degree oven for about 25 minutes or until done. Store covered until cool.

Chocolate Frosting

1/4 cup butter softened
1/4 cup honey
1-2 tsp. vanilla
1/2 cup yogurt
3 Tbs. cocoa powder
3 Tbs. carob powder (or a total of 6 tablespoons cocoa powder if you don't want to use carob)
dash of salt (optional)
1/4 cup chopped nuts (optional)

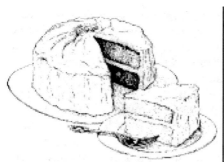

About 1 1/2 cups dry non-fat milk powder (or whey milk substitute)
dry pectin or powdered sugar (optional) for thickener

Mix first four ingredients until smooth. Stir in cocoa and carob. Sift or stir in the powder milk. Will be slightly lumpy if just stirred. Mix until slightly runny. Taste to see if mixture needs to be sweeter. Can add powder sugar. The frosting tends to thicken up, so wait a few minutes before frosting the cake for the right consistency. Sprinkle with nuts. Keep in refrigerator. Frosts 2 single layer cakes.

Oatmeal Cake with Chocolate Delight
1/4 cup butter
1/4 cup honey
1/4 cup xylitol or 1 Tbs. more of honey
2 eggs
2 tsp. vanilla
2 cups oatmeal flour
1 tsp. salt
1 Tbs. baking powder
1/4-1/2 cup chopped pecans (opt.)

Preheat oven to 350 degrees. Blend the first 5 ingredients together with a blender. Add the next 3 ingredients and blend. Stir in the nuts. Pour into a greased baking dish and cook at 350 degrees for about 25 minutes, until a toothpick comes out clean.

Chocolate Delight Frosting
1/4 cup cocoa powder
2 Tbs. flax meal
1/4 tsp. salt
1/4 cup natural peanut butter
1 Tbs. vanilla
1/3-1/2 cup whole yogurt
1/3 cup xylitol
1/2 cup shredded coconut (without sugar added)

Mix first 3 ingredients. Stir or blend in peanut butter and vanilla. Blend the yogurt and xylitol. Stir in coconut. Can let sit in refrigerator. The amount of yogurt will decide the consistency of the frosting.

Applesauce Cake
2 cups thick applesauce
1/3-1/2 cup fluid
1 Tbs. vanilla
3 eggs
1/2 tsp. salt
2 Tbs. flaxmeal
2 cups oat flour
1 Tbs. baking powder (without alum)

Blend the first four ingredients together. Mix in the next two. Blend in the flour and baking powder. Pour into a greased baking dish and cook at 350 degrees for about 40 minutes. The cake could "fall". "Chocolate Delight Frosting" will cover the any imperfections.

Coconut Power Balls

1/2 cup of natural peanut butter or almond butter
1-2 tsp. liquid lecithin
2 Tbs. chocolate chips
2 Tbs. honey
2 Tbs. ground flax meal
1 Tbs. wheat germ
1 Tbs. unsweetened coconut
2 Tbs. dry roasted soy nuts, or other nuts, chopped

Mix peanut butter, lecithin, chocolate chips, honey in a stainless steel pot. Warm until chocolate melts. Remove from heat and add remaining ingredients. Stir. Mixture should form a thick dough-like ball. If the dough is too crumbly, add a bit more peanut butter. If too moist, add more wheat germ. Make into small balls and place on a cookie sheet sprayed with vegetable oil or with oven parchment paper. Place in refrigerator.

Red Miso Power Balls

1/2 cup natural peanut butter
1/2 cup honey
1/4 cup carob or cocoa powder
1/4 cup whey protein
2 Tbs. wheat germ
1 Tbs. flax meal
1/4 cup chopped almonds or other nuts
1/4 cup sunflower or pumpkin seeds
1 Tbs. miso
1/2 tsp. cinnamon

Combine all ingredients and mix well. Roll into bite-size balls. Refrigerate. If dough is too tacky, just add more wheat germ.

Chinese Chews

1/4 cup butter
1 1/2 cups hulled sesame seeds (or: 3/4 cup sesame seeds, 1/4 crushed almonds, and 1/4 cup coconut)
1/4 cup natural peanut butter
3/4 cup whey protein powder
1 Tbs. wheat germ
1 Tbs. flax meal
1/2 cup honey
1 to 2 tsp. vanilla
2 tsp. brewers yeast (optional)

Melt butter in skillet. Add sesame seeds and lightly toast, stirring often. Stir in peanut butter, whey powder, flax meal, and wheat germ. Add honey and vanilla mixing well. Continue to cook until well blended, stirring constantly, about 3-5 minutes. Scoop out mixture into a greased pie pan and press down lightly with the back of a soup spoon. Cool and cut into squares.

Nut Clusters

1/2 cup chocolate chips
1/4 peanut butter
1 tsp. coconut butter (opt.)
1/2 Tbs. butter
1/4 tsp. sea salt
2 tsp. vanilla
1/2 cup coconut
1 Tbs. flax meal
2 Tbs. xylitol

In a heavy stainless pot, cook the first 4 ingredients until melted, stirring. Add salt and vanilla. Stir. Remove from the heat. Add flax meal and xylitol. Stir. Add coconut and mix. Add your favorite nuts. Start with 1 cup. Keep mixing in nuts until the nuts are coated, but there isn't much of the chocolate mixture by itself. Scoop spoonfuls (you decide how big you want the clusters) onto a non-stick cookie sheet or one covered with cooking parchment paper. Let set up in refrigerator. Place in storage bowels with lids and keep in refrigerator.

This dessert is calorie dense but still healthy. If your problem is too much lost weight, this dessert is for you. These clusters can become addictive, so don't overdo a good concept!

WHAT ABOUT ALCOHOL?

Alcoholic beverages are common with dinner in many countries. Moderate use of dry red wine may be somewhat protective of heart disease, but has no therapeutic impact on cancer. It is best to avoid alcohol while being treated for cancer. However, that said, I have worked with cancer patients who found that the stress of giving up their nightly ritual of a couple glasses of wine with dinner would have been worse that the theoretical value of giving up the wine. Use your own judgment.

FOOD AS MEDICINE

Most important, food should help to nourish the body, mind, and spirit. Have fun in the kitchen. Put love into the cooking process. Savor eating the food while making mealtimes a pleasant ritual. May food become a major portion of your healing journey and your enjoyment in life.

Noreen Quillin

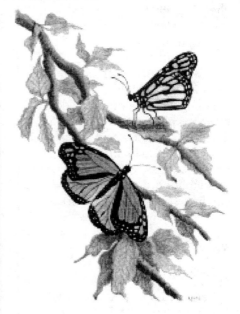

RECIPE INDEX

Red Pepper & Zucchini
Ginger Steamed Squash

POULTRY p.190
Turkey Feast
Savory Turkey Loaf
Turkey Treat
Turkey w/ Creamy Salsa
Chicken w/ Stuffing
Curry Chicken
Sesame Chicken
Indian Spice Chicken
Apricot Chicken
Simple Chicken
Mexican Oven Chicken

BEEF etc. p.194
Hearty Pot Roast
Herb Flank Steak
Beef Stuffed Potatoes
Green Chili Stew
Chili w/ Kidney Beans
Spaghetti
Liver w/ Onions
Lamb Roast w/ Yogurt

FISH p.197
Seafood Seasoning
Easy Salmon
Salmon Cakes
Tarragon Fish
BBQ Halibut
Dill-Almond Cod
Tuna Cakes

Tuna Stuffed Potatoes
Crab Dinner
Baked Scallops

SOY p.199
Textured Tofu
Tofu Steak
Spicy Tofu w/ Cashews
Soy Pilaf
Tempeh a l' Orange
Tofu Surprise
BBQ Tempeh
Tofu Burger
Soyburgers
Ginger Tofu

SIDE DISH p.202
Apple Chutney
Millet Cakes
Spicy Mexican Beans
Healthy Wheat Balls
Three Bean Salad
Couscous w/ Nuts
Tabouli w/ Chickpeas
Spanish Rice
Miso Rice
Brown Rice Delight
Fettuccini
Spinach Linguini
Fruited Bulgur Pilaf
Sweet Potato Delight

DESSERT p.205
Maple-Baked Pears
Pear Bread Pudding
Apple Bread Pudding
Fruited Gelatin

Oatmeal Raisin Delights
Blueberry Crisp
Tofu Rice Pudding
Tofu Whipped Cream
Cherries Jubilee
Easy Banana Pudding
Rice Porridge
Baked Apples
Broiled Apple Rings
Homemade Applesauce
Apple Crisp
Spicy Ginger Snaps
Chewy Carrot Brownies
Cake Supreme
Pumpkin Cake
Pumpkin Pie
Whole Wh.Piecrust
Healthy Cookies
Peanut Butt & Coco
Raspberry Couscous Cake
Frozen Fruit Slush
Chocolate Brownies
Chocolate Cake
Chocolate Frosting
Oatmeal Cake
Choc. Delight Frost.
Applesauce Cake
Coconut Power Balls
Red Miso Power Balls
Chinese Chews
Nut Clusters

CHAPTER 15

✴

SUPPLEMENTS AGAINST CANCER

"Individuals with special nutritional needs are not covered by the RDAs." National Research Council, RECOMMENDED DIETARY ALLOWANCES, pgs1&8, Washington, 1989

WHAT'S AHEAD?

Cancer patients probably need more nutrients than can be obtained even from a healthy diet. No supplement is a magic bullet against cancer. While nutrition products need to be taken with professional guidance, the risk-to-benefit ratio heavily favors the use of supplements for all cancer patients. Supplements can:

↪ stimulate immune function

↪ encourage "suicide" (apoptosis) in cancer cells

↪ improve cell-to-cell communication

↪ reduce the toxicity of chemo and radiation on the patient.

D o all humans or just sick humans need to take vitamin supplements? Are they safe? Are they cost effective? Should everyone taking vitamins work closely with a doctor on nutrient levels? Taking vitamins is a controversial subject. For decades, doctors and dietitians campaigned under the banner: "If you eat a good diet, then you do not need vitamin supplements." When you read the chapter in this book on "malnutrition among Americans", the question is asked: "Who eats a good diet?" The answer, according to extensive research from the United States Department of Agriculture, is that 92% of Americans DO NOT GET the Recommended Dietary Allowance (RDA, now called Reference Daily Intake, or RDI) for all listed essential nutrients. And there is compelling evidence that the RDA is a survival level for nutrient intake, not a level that allows for optimal health, nor recovery from cancer.

There are now over 20,000 scientific references that support the use of supplementing a good diet with vitamins, minerals, herbs, fatty acids, glandulars, probiotics, and food extracts.

For more information see:

DOCTORS' VITAMIN ENCYCLOPEDIA by Sheldon Hendler, MD, PhD
PDR FOR NUTRITIONAL SUPPLEMENTS, Medical Economics
DISEASE PREVENTION AND TREATMENT, Life Extension Media
ENCYCLOPEDIA NATURAL MEDICINE, Murray, ND & Pizzorno, ND
NUTRITIONAL INFLUENCES ON ILLNESS by Melvyn Werbach, MD

Notice the additional vitamins and minerals that are added to dog and cat food. Look at the amazing assortment of vitamins, minerals, herbs, etc; that are offered for horses. None of these products are sold due to the "placebo" effect, or simply because the animal believed in the product. Nutrients, like drugs, have a dose-dependent response curve. Meaning, the more you give, the greater the effect, until additional benefits taper off and toxicity becomes possible.

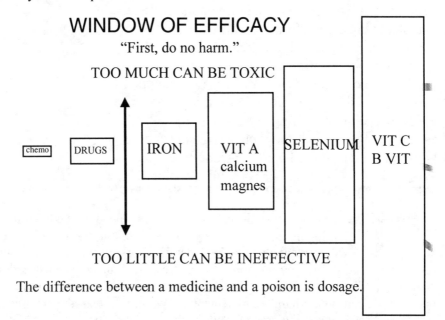

WINDOW OF EFFICACY
"First, do no harm."

TOO MUCH CAN BE TOXIC

| chemo | DRUGS | IRON | VIT A calcium magnes | SELENIUM | VIT C B VIT |

TOO LITTLE CAN BE INEFFECTIVE

The difference between a medicine and a poison is dosage.

For instance, at 20 milligrams of niacin per day, most adults have decent, normal health. At 100 mg/day of niacin, this B-vitamin becomes a powerful dilator of blood vessels and may improve circulation. At 2,000 mg/day, niacin becomes a potent agent at lowering cholesterol in the bloodstream of people with hypercholesterolemia. Most adults can survive on 20-40 mg daily of vitamin C. The RDA is 60 mg, while studies show that women can lower their risk for cervical cancer by 50% simply by taking 90 mg of vitamin C daily. At 300 mg/day, vitamin C has been shown to add 6 years to the lifespan of male supplement users. People with virus infections or cancer have benefitted by taking 1,000 to 20,000

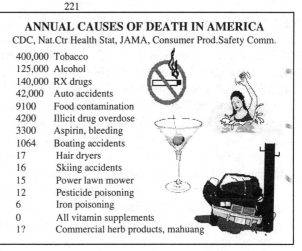

ANNUAL CAUSES OF DEATH IN AMERICA
CDC, Nat.Ctr Health Stat, JAMA, Consumer Prod.Safety Comm.

400,000	Tobacco
125,000	Alcohol
140,000	RX drugs
42,000	Auto accidents
9100	Food contamination
4200	Illicit drug overdose
3300	Aspirin, bleeding
1064	Boating accidents
17	Hair dryers
16	Skiing accidents
15	Power lawn mower
12	Pesticide poisoning
6	Iron poisoning
0	All vitamin supplements
1?	Commercial herb products, mahuang

mg of vitamin C daily. Show me a drug that you can take 100 times the normal prescription dosage and not have some serious harmful effect. The point is: "While nutritional supplements are far from cure-alls, they do rate very favorably on the risk-to-benefit-to-cost scale when compared to prescription medications.

All substances consumed--from chemotherapy to allopathic drugs to vitamins, minerals, herbs, and even food--all have a "window of efficacy". Above that level is too much and may cause damage. Below that level is probably ineffective. With drugs, the window of efficacy is much narrower and, hence, great caution must be used in administering prescription medication. All nutrients have a wider window of efficacy than all drugs. Yet some nutrients are more likely to harm than others. Iron, copper, selenium, and vitamins A and D are the nutrients that must be used with discretion. Most other nutrients are unlikely to harm.

DON'T TAKE YOUR VITAMIN C; UNLESS...

A couple of hundred thousand years ago, humans lost the ability to convert blood sugar (glucose) into vitamin C (ascorbic acid). Some scientists have called this evolutionary shift a figurative "fall from the Garden of Eden". All but a few creatures on earth produce their own vitamin C in massive quantities, with higher internal production when the creature gets sick. For instance, a 150 pound goat makes about 10,000 milligrams daily of vitamin C. Meanwhile, the Recommended Dietary Allowance for a 156 pound reference human is 60 milligrams per day.

Vitamin C is one of the more utilitarian nutrients in the human body, by assisting in the construction of connective tissue (the glue that keeps the body together), regulating the levels of fats in the blood, assisting in iron absorption, aiding in the synthesis of various brain chemicals for thought, and protecting against the damaging effects of free radicals. In a study done at the University of California at Los Angeles, men who took supplements of 300 mg daily of vitamin C (5 times the RDA) lived an average of 6 years longer than men who did not take supplements of vitamin C. Mark Levine, MD, researcher with the National Institutes of Health, finds evidence that 250 mg per day might be a more rational and healthy RDA for vitamin C.

Meanwhile, oncologists worry about the possibility that vitamin C might inhibit the free radical activity of chemotherapy and radiation in destroying cancer cells. While it might seem logical that an antioxidant (like vitamin C) might reduce the effectiveness of a pro-oxidant (like chemo and radiation), the opposite has been found in animal and human studies: antioxidants protect the healthy tissue of the patient while allowing the cancer tissue to become more vulnerable to the damaging effects of chemo and radiation.

In a study published in the *Proceedings of the National Academy of Science*, vitamin C always augmented tumor kill and never protected the cancer cells when scientists added various chemo and radiation therapies to cancer cells growing in a dish. In 2 major human cancer studies, adding vitamin C and other antioxidants to chemo and radiation improved patient survival, quality of life, and tumor kill.

Then an unpublished research project from Sloan Kettering Cancer Hospital in New York found that cancer cells are "gluttons" for vitamin C, absorbing more than their fair share. The researchers concluded, though they never proved, that cancer patients should avoid vitamin C supplements while undergoing chemo and radiation. Dr. David Golde, author of the study even speculated: "The cancer cell wants vitamin C because it wants antioxidant protection." If cancer cells are looking for protection, then why is vitamin C the only antioxidant that they absorb? What about the 20,000 bioflavonoids (like quercetin), the 800 carotenoids (like beta carotene), vitamin E, lipoic acid, glutathione, and other antioxidants in the human body? Why do cancer cells only absorb vitamin C and not the others? The researchers admitted that vitamin C was being selectively absorbed by tumor cells because cancer cells are "sugar feeders" and think they are absorbing their preferred fuel, glucose (which is nearly identical in structure to vitamin C), when in fact they are absorbing vitamin C, an "Elvis impersonator" of sorts.

Now let me weave all of this seemingly confusing data together to help make sense for the cancer patient. Any antioxidant can become a pro-oxidant in a given chemical soup. That is why Nature always gives us droves of different antioxidants to play "hot potato" with unpaired electrons until their destructive energy is dissipated. No food has just one antioxidant. No human cell wants just one antioxidant. Antioxidants can become pro-oxidants when in isolation, which is exactly what happens to cancer cells when they selectively absorb only vitamin C, hoping to get some fuel for growth. What really happens is the vitamin C quickly becomes a pro-oxidant, targeting its destruction exclusively for the cancer cells. Dozens of very well trained physicians have been giving high doses of intravenous vitamin C (10 to 100 grams daily) to thousands of cancer patients for decades with no side effects, and usually improved outcome. Intravenous vitamin C seems to have selective anti-cancer activity, according to an article in the *Annals of Internal Medicine* (Apr.6, 2004, p.533), authored by several doctors including researchers at the National Institutes of Health. Dr. Hugh Riordan has reported improved outcome in poor prognostic cancer patients who have been put in remission through use of high dose IV vitamin C.

Vitamin C supplements can be helpful in slowing cancer, while making medical therapy more of a selective toxin against the cancer and protecting healthy host tissue. Vitamin C protects against heart disease, lengthens life span, and more...when taken in conjunction with a wide assortment of other antioxidants along with a good diet.

A number of bright researchers have taken a tiny bit of knowledge out of context (vitamin C thickens artery walls, is selectively absorbed by tumors, can become a pro-oxidant), then ASSUMED a sequence of unproven conclusions, without consulting the "prior art" in this field. Don't take your vitamin C supplements--unless you want to live longer.

VITAMIN E SUPPLEMENTS CAUSE PREMATURE DEATH?

In January 2005, researchers published a meta-analysis in the *Annals of Internal Medicine* (vol.142, p.1) of the literature on vitamin E supplements and concluded: "vitamin E supplements may cause early death." Though none of the 11 trials that these researchers analyzed came up with the same conclusion, when pooled together and using an unproven statistical model developed by these authors, they found a 5% increase in death among the vitamin E users. Dr. Miller, lead author of the study, admitted that only very sick people were analyzed, including people who were the institutionalized elderly, smokers, recent heart attack, Alzheimer's disease, etc. I have been conducting a study, too. I go to the local health food store and find primarily older sicker people, some with walkers and oxygen tubes up their nose. Then I go to a nearby swinging night club and find young attractive healthy people who smoke and drink and stay out all night. My conclusion is that health food stores are hazardous to your health and that drinking and carousing all night is good for you. Which is as ridiculous as saying that fire engine trucks should be banned because they are always at the scene of a fire or accident.

The authors of this study, which received international publicity, further stated that they examined malnourished populations, that there were considerable differences in the biological activity of the vitamin E forms used (DL vs natural D). In fact, dozens of studies have demonstrated the safety and efficacy of vitamin E in such conditions as heart disease, Alzheimer's disease, immune dysfunctions, and diabetes. Even the conservative and prestigious PHYSICIAN'S DESK REFERENCE FOR NUTRITIONAL SUPPLEMENTS finds considerable merit in vitamin E supplements. It is strange how the safe, cheap, and effective use of vitamin E was ignored by the international publicity from this dubious study.

RISKS OF NUTRITION THERAPY

In an extensive review of the literature found in the New York Academy of Sciences textbook BEYOND DEFICIENCIES (vol.669, p.300, 1992), Dr. Adrienne Bendich found the following data on nutrient toxicity:

⇨ B-6 can be used safely for years at up to 500 mg (250 times RDA)

⇨ Niacin (as nicotinic acid) has been recommended by the National Institute of Health for lowering cholesterol at doses of 3,000-6,000 mg/day (150-300 times RDA). Time-release niacin is more suspect of causing toxicity as liver damage.

⇨ Vitamin C was tested in 8 published studies using double-blind placebo-controlled design. At 10,000 mg/day for years, vitamin C produced no side effects.

⇨ High doses of vitamin A (500,000 iu daily) can have acute reversible effects. Teratogenecity (birth defects) is a possible complication of high dose vitamin A intake.

⇨ Vitamin E intake at up to 3,000 mg/day (300 times RDA) for prolonged periods has been shown safe.

⇨ Beta-carotene has been administered for extended periods in humans at doses up to 180 mg (300,000 iu or 60 times RDA) with no side effects nor elevated serum vitamin A levels.

In MICRONUTRIENTS AND IMMUNE FUNCTION (NYAS, vol.587, p.257, 1990), John Hathcock, PhD, a Food and Drug Administration toxicologist, reported the following data on nutrient toxicity:

⇨ Vitamin A toxicity may start as low as 25,000 iu/day (5 times RDA) in people with impaired liver function via drugs, hepatitis, or protein malnutrition. Otherwise, toxicity for A begins at several hundred thousand iu/day.

⇨ Beta-carotene given at 180 mg/day (300,000 iu or 60 times RDA) for extended periods produced no toxicity, but mild carotenemia (orange pigmentation of skin).

⇨ Vitamin E at 300 iu/day (30 times RDA) can trigger nausea, fatigue, and headaches in sensitive individuals. Otherwise, few side effects are seen at up to 3,200 iu/day (320 times RDA).

⇨ B-6 may induce a reversible sensory neuropathy at doses of as low as 300 mg/day in some sensitive individuals. Toxic threshold usually begins at 2,000 mg for most individuals.

⇨ Vitamin C may induce mild and transient gastro-intestinal distress in some sensitive individuals at doses of 1,000 mg (16 times RDA). Otherwise, toxicity is very rare at even high doses of vitamin C intake.

⇨ Zinc supplements at 300 mg (20 times RDA) have been found to impair immune functions and serum lipid profile.

⇨ Iron intake at 100 mg/day (6 times RDA) will cause iron storage disease in 80% of population. The "window of efficacy" on iron is probably more narrow than with other nutrients.

⇨ Selenium can be toxic at 1-5 mg/kg body weight intake. This would equate to 65 mg/day for the average adult, which is 812 times the RDA of 80 mcg. Some sensitive individuals may develop toxicity at 1,000 mcg/day.

CHOOSING YOUR VITAMIN SUPPLEMENTS

There are many vitamins, minerals, botanicals (herbs), fatty acids, food extracts, glandulars, and other nutrient compounds that can be of benefit to the cancer patient. You may take all of these "a la carte" at a cost of $1,500-$2,000 per month and 200+ pills per day, or you may consider using the ImmunoPower supplement (ImmunoPower.com or toll free 800-247-6553, which is a mixture of 87 nutrition factors, in pill and powder form, that is much more convenient, complete, and cost-effective than the usual "life and death scavenger hunt" that cancer patients have embarked upon. For people who are limited in their budget and what they can take in pill and powder form, ImmunoPower EZ may be worth considering.

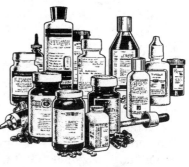

Vitamins can be expensive, especially since these are "out of pocket" expenses, meaning not reimbursable by insurance companies. Odd how insurance and Medicare will pay $3,000 per day for a cancer patient in intensive care, but neither will pay for nutrition supplements that might prevent the patient from developing malnutrition (cachexia) and ending up in the intensive care unit of a hospital. Other multi-vitamin supplements worthy of your consideration include Life Extension Mix (lef.org or 1-888-741-5433). Choose the supplement regimen that best suits your ability to tolerate vitamins and your ability to pay for them.

IMMUNOPOWER INGREDIENTS

PILLS		POWDER	
Serving size: 1 packet (10 pills)		serving size 23 grams=3 T.	
Servings per container	15	servings per container	15
Calories	40	Calories	50
Calories from fat	35	Calories from fat	10
Total Fat	4 gm	Total fat	1 gm
Vitamin A	2000 iu	Sodium	260 mg
Vitamin C	30 mg	xylitol	2 gm
Vitamin D	250 iu	Protein	7 gm
Kyolic aged garlic	1000 mg	Vitamin A (mix carot)	25,000 iu
Cod liver oil	1000 mg	Vitamin C	2500 mg
Borage oil	1000 mg	Vitamin D	667 iu
Shark liver oil	1000 mg	Vitamin E	400 iu
CLA (in safflower oil)	720 mg	Vitamin K	100 mcg
Oligomeric proantho	50 mg	Thiamin	10 mg
Silymarin	140 mg	Riboflavin	10 mg
Echinacea	80 mg	Niacin	450 mg
Curcuminoids	333 mg	Vitamin B-6	50 mg
Ginkgo biloba	40 mg	Folate	200 mcg
Astragalus menbran	167 mg	Vitamin B-12	1000 mcg
Panax ginseng	167 mg	Biotin	50 mcg
Green tea	100 mg	Pantothenic acid	20 mg
Diindolylmethane	75 mg	Calcium	300 mg
Rhodiola rosea	200 mg	Iron	4 mg
Maitake d-fraction	33 mg	Phosphorus	90 mg
L-glutathione reduced	100 mg	Iodine	50 mcg
Thymus (BSE free)	300 mg	Magnesium	150 mg
Spleen (BSE free)	300 mg	Zinc	10 mg
Coenzyme Q-10	100 mg	Selenium	200 mcg
Lipoic acid	33 mg	Copper	1 mg
Lycopene	3 mg	Manganese	1.7 mg
Ellagic acid	100 mg	Chromium	200 mcg
Quercetin	167 mg	Molybdenum	167 mcg
L-carnitine	100 mg	Potassium	490 mg
MSM (methyl sulf)	250 mg	Vanadium	33 mcg
Resveratrol	20 mg	Aloe vera	167 mg
Probiotic blend	500 mg	Trimethylglycine	16.7 mg
Proprietary enzymes	300 mg	Bovine cartilage	3000 mg
Exclzyme enzymes	500 mg	DNA (nucleic acid)	500 mg
Lactoferrin	13 mg	RNA (nucleic acid)	500 mg
Isoflavones	13 mg	Tocotrienols	20 mg
		Lecithin	1000 mg
		Calcium-d-glucarate	500 mg

CHAPTER 16

✳

HERBS

"Behold, I have given you every green plant, and it shall be food for you."   *Genesis 1:29*

WHAT'S AHEAD?

Many herbs (botanicals) contain powerful healing ingredients for cancer patients. No herb is a magic bullet for all cancers. Herbs may help by:
↪ stimulating immune functions
↪ detoxifying the liver and body
↪ directly killing yeast and other cancer-causing microbes

O ur ancestors used to practice botanical medicine all day every day--in the kitchen. While we have a tendency to think of herbs as mysterious plant concoctions blended up for a very sick person by some eccentric older woman (the quintessential herbalist), in fact, our ancestors ate potent anti-cancer herbs in their diet and as seasonings each day. Columbus set sail in a mad suicidal adventure over the edge of the Earth in the unlikely event that he might find the Spice Islands, near India. Spices (a.k.a. seasonings, herbs, botanicals) have been used throughout history to cover the rotting stench of unrefrigerated food. As an unintentional by-product of using these seasoning agents, such as

HERBAL MEDICINE

AS SUPPLEMENTS:	AS FOODS:	AS SEASONINGS:
echinacea	soy	garlic
astragalus	green & orange	onion
Cat's claw	dandelion greens	hot peppers
Pau D'arco	citrus	cinnamon
ginseng	tomato	ginger
grape seed extract	green tea	real licorice
aloe vera	broccoli/cabbage	turmeric (curry)
red clover	beets	parsley
milk thistle	sprouts	sage
Essiac	flaxseed meal	chicory
Hoxsey	sesame seeds	thyme
Flor-Essence	Maitake mushrm	basil

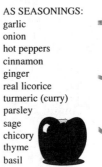

cinnamon, garlic, hot pepper, ginger, and curry, our ancestors were able to keep the cancer incidence well below what we currently have. While this section pays homage to the scientific data using botanical extracts as anti-cancer medicines, I would strongly encourage you to use the herbs listed as foods and seasonings on a regular basis.

The list of scientific references presented here is only representative of the peer-reviewed data on the use of nutrition supplements as part of comprehensive cancer treatment.

BOTANICAL (best form for absorption) suggested daily dosage
Primary functions in human body and anti-cancer activities

Oligomeric proanthocyanidins (OPC) 50 mg
Potent antioxidant, supports vitamin C functions, penetrates the blood-brain barrier, reduces capillary fragility, enhances peripheral circulation, protects DNA from damage by radiation and chemotherapy

---

Scurvy (deficiency of vitamin C) has played a huge role in human history. Humans roamed the oceans of the world throughout the 15th through the 19th centuries, often losing up to half the people on board ship due to scurvy. The English physician, James Lind, discovered that limes cured scurvy in 1747 and began to wind down the death toll from scurvy, while also labeling the English sailors as "limeys". In 1930, Nobel prize winner, Albert Szent-Gyorgy, MD, PhD, isolated pure vitamin C. Ironically, the pure white crystalline vitamin C that Dr. Szent-Gyorgy isolated would not cure bleeding gums, whereas the crude brown mixture of citrus extract would. The difference between these two mixtures was "bioflavonoids", which include over 20,000 different chemical compounds that generally assist 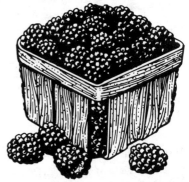 chlorophyll in photosynthesis and protect the plant from the harmful effects of the sun's radiation. The rainbow colors of fall foliage are Nature's art exhibit of bioflavonoids and carotenoids.

Some of the main categories of bioflavonoids include:
- anthocyanins; deep purple compounds found in black grapes, beets, red onions, and berries
- catechins and epigallocatechin, which are polyphenols found in apples and green tea
- ellagic acid, a true anti-cancer compound found in cranberries, raspberries, and other berries

- flavones, found in citrus fruit, red grapes, and green beans
- flavanols, such as quercetin, myricetin, found in kale, spinach, onions, apples, and black tea
- flavanones, such as hesperidin and naringen, found in citrus fruits of grapefruit, oranges, and lemons.
-

Some of the better-known bioflavonoids include rutin, which is defined in the DORLAND'S MEDICAL DICTIONARY as capable of "preventing capillary fragility." Hesperidin, quercetin, pycnogenol from pine bark, and proanthocyanidins are other popular bioflavonoids. While bioflavonoids are known to be essential in the diet of insects, bioflavonoids are not yet considered essential in the human diet.

As the science of nutrition matures, we are finding that some of the "star" nutrients of the past may be just "supporting actors" for the real star nutrients. For instance, tocotrienols and coenzyme Q may be more important than vitamin E in human health. Eicosapentaenoic acid (EPA from fish oil), though not considered essential, may be more important than alpha-linolenic acid (ALA from flax oil), which is considered essential. And bioflavonoids may be more important than vitamin C. OPC bound to phosphatidylcholine (lecithin) has been shown to improve absorption and cell access to OPC.

Animals with implanted tumors lived longer when given anthocyanin from grape rinds.[1] Flavonoids administered in the diet of rats helped to reduce DNA damage from benzopyrene carcinogens.[2] Bioflavonoids are potent chelators, helping to eliminate toxic minerals from the system.[3] Bioflavonoids in general help to reduce allergic reactions, which create an imbalanced immune attack against cancer and infections. OPC traps lipid peroxides, hydroxyl radicals, delays the onset of lipid peroxidation, prevents iron-induced lipid peroxidation, and inhibits the enzymes that can degrade connective tissue (hyaluronidase, elastase, collagenase), which then helps to prevent cancer cells from "knocking down the walls" of surrounding tissue for metastasis. Bioflavonoids may inhibit tumor promotion.[4] Bioflavonoids enhance the activity of T-lymphocytes.[5] Various flavonoids have produced striking reductions in cancer incidence in animals, sometimes up to almost total inhibition of tumorogenesis.[6]

Silymarin (milk thistle) 140 mg
Stimulates liver detoxification and tissue regeneration, may also augment immune functions

---

Silybum marianum, or milk thistle, is a stout annual plant that grows in dry, rocky soils in parts of Europe and North America. Its seeds, fruit, and leaves are widely prescribed medication in Europe for most diseases affecting the liver. Silymarin has been shown to help regenerate liver tissue, protect the liver against toxic chemicals, and increase the production of glutathione (GSH), which is fundamental in the cell protecting itself against hydrogen peroxide that the cell produces.[7]

Since the liver is the primary detoxifying organ of the body and automatically becomes involved in the internal cancer battle, metastasis to the liver complicates cancer treatment. Among other functions, the liver also stores many vitamins and minerals, produces bile salts for fat digestion and absorption, and is generally one of the more versatile and essential organs in the body. For recovery from cancer to be possible, the liver must be healthy.

Echinacea (purpurea) 80 mg
  Immune stimulant

Echinacea species consist primarily of E. angustifolia, E. purpurea, and E. pallida. Native American herbalists used echinacea more than any other plant for medicinal purposes. There are over 350 scientific articles worldwide on the immune-enhancing effects of echinacea, including the:
- activation of complement, which promotes chemotaxis of neutrophils, monocytes, and eosinophils; "gearing up" the immune cells
- solubilization of immune complexes
- neutralization of viruses.[8]

One of the components of echinacea, arabinogalactan, has shown promise as an anti-cancer agent in vitro.[9]

In patients with inoperable metastatic esophageal and colorectal cancers, supplements of echinacea (as Echinacin) provided modest improvements in immune functions, slowed the growth of some tumors, and increased survival time.[10] Outpatients with advanced colorectal cancers were given echinacea as part of therapy, with some patients experiencing stable disease, reduction in tumor markers, increases in survival time, and no toxicity reported.[11]

Curcumin (Curcuma longa) 50 mg
  Potent antioxidant, protector of DNA

Curry is an Indian spice mixture that includes turmeric as one of the flavoring agents. The active component in turmeric appears to be a bright yellow pigment, curcumin (a.k.a. Curcuma longa), which helps to enhance the immune system by protecting immune cells from their own poisons (pro-oxidants) used to kill cancer cells. Mustard is a good source of curcumin.

Curcumin appears to be a potent inhibitor of cancer.[12] In animal experiments, curcumin was shown to be directly toxic to tumor cells.[13] In a study with smokers, turmeric tablets were able to dramatically reduce the excretion of urinary mutagen levels (indicators of the possibility of cancer).[14] In patients with skin cancers (squamous cell carcinomas) who had failed therapy with chemo, radiation, and surgery, supplements or ointment of turmeric were able to provide significant reduction in the smell, size, itching, pain, and exudate of the lesions.[15]

Ginkgo biloba (24% heteroside) 40 mg

Improves circulation, augments the production of healthy prostaglandin PGE-1, immune stimulant, and adaptogen (helps to regulate many cellular functions)

The ginkgo tree is one of the oldest living species on earth, having been around for over 200 million years. The ginkgo tree is an incredibly adaptable and tenacious plant. One ginkgo tree survived the near-ground zero nuclear blast in Hiroshima, Japan. Millions of these cone-shaped evergreen trees survive amidst air pollution, drought, and poor soil throughout the world. A ginkgo tree may live as long as 1,000 years. The leaves and berries contain a wide assortment of phytochemicals (collectively called "ginkgoflavonglycosides"), which have been a pivotal medicine in China for 5,000 years. There are now over 1,000 scientific studies published during the past 40 years demonstrating the medicinal value of ginkgo, with ginkgo extract becoming one of the more widely prescribed medications in Europe today. In 1989, over 100,000 physicians worldwide wrote over 10 million prescriptions for ginkgo.

There are several ways in which ginkgo may help the cancer patient:

- Vasodilator which expands the tiny capillaries that nourish 90% of the body's tissues, thus bringing oxygen and nutrients to the cells. In doing so, ginkgo improves depression[16] and general circulation to the organs.[17]
- Inhibits platelet aggregation, or the stickiness of cells. Stroke, heart attacks, and cancer metastasis are fueled by sticky cells that are generated by platelet activating factor (PAF). Ginkgo inhibits PAF.[18] By modifying PAF, ginkgo helps to reduce inflammation and allergic responses.[19]
- Antioxidant of exceptional efficiency.[20] Slows down free radical destruction of healthy tissue, therefore protects immune cells in their semi-suicidal quest to kill cancer cells and also protects the favorable prostaglandin, PGE-1. This antioxidant activity also helps to stabilize membranes, where the lipid bi-layer is vulnerable to lipid peroxidation.

♦ This protection extends to the DNA, which is why Chernobyl workers were given ginkgo to protect them from further damage via radioactivity.

Astragalus (membranaceus) 167 mg
    Adaptogen and immune stimulant

Adaptogens are a small and elite group of herbal compounds, including garlic and ginseng, which coordinate and regulate a broad spectrum of biochemical processes, including prostaglandins, cell membranes, blood sugar levels, etc.. "Adaptogen" is the term coined in 1957 by the Russian pharmacologist I. Brekhman. Criteria for an adaptogen are that it must be:[21]

♦ innocuous, causing minimal harm in reasonable quantities

♦ non-specific in activity, that is, able to influence a wide range of physical, chemical, and biochemical pathways in the body

♦ a normalizer of functions, meaning that it will lower or raise a bodily measurement, depending on what needs to happen for improvement in overall health to occur, such as raising blood pressure in hypotensive individuals and lowering blood pressure in hypertensive individuals.[22]

Astragalus has also demonstrated anti-viral activity as it was able to shorten the duration and severity of the common cold in humans.[23] Researchers at M.D. Anderson Hospital in Houston found that astragalus was able to enhance the immune capacity using the cultured blood of 14 cancer patients,[24] as well as augment the anti-tumor ability of Interferon-2.[25] In a study of 176 patients undergoing chemotherapy for cancers of the gastrointestinal tract, astragalus and ginseng were able to prevent the normal immune depression and weight loss that occurs.[26] In a variety of human studies, astragalus has been shown to stimulate various parameters of the immune system, has anti-tumor activity, and inhibits the spreading (metastasis) of cancer.[27]

Panax ginseng (8%) 167 mg
    Adaptogen, immune stimulant, anti-tumor activity, inhibits metastasis[28]

Ginseng is one of the oldest, most widely used, and scientifically studied of all the world's herbs. The original proponents of ginseng were Chinese physicians several thousand years ago, using it to treat nearly every conceivable ailment. Given the known "adaptogenic" qualities of ginseng, the enthusiasm of these ancient Chinese doctors may have been well placed. Ginseng is a plant species term (Panax), which is further subdivided into

Panax quinquefolium (American ginseng), Panax japonicum (Japanese ginseng), Panax pseudoginseng (Himalayan ginseng), and Panax trifolium.[29] Eleutherococcus senticosus, a relative newcomer to this category, contains some ginseng-like compounds (triterpenoid saponins), but is not considered true ginseng. Panax ginseng C.A. Meyer is the best studied in the scientific literature and is referred to in the followed studies.

The wide disparity in outcome of clinical studies using ginseng probably stems from the lack of active ingredients in many substandard ginseng products sold today. Ginseng's therapeutic value comes from the 13 different triterpenoid saponins, collectively known as ginsenosides, which are found in various concentrations in various types of ginseng grown on various soils and experiencing various drying and storage techniques. While most ginseng is about 1-3% ginsenosides, better products will offer 8% concentration. In one study published in 1979, of the 54 ginseng products analyzed, 60% were worthless and 25% had no ginseng at all![30] It is the regularly-formed root from wild Panax ginseng that is most highly prized. Nearly 60,000 people are employed in Korea for the raising and processing of ginseng.

Ginseng may help cancer patients for the following reasons:

♦ **Adaptogenic qualities**. Ginseng is nearly unsurpassed in the plant kingdom for its ability to bring about biochemical adjustments in whatever direction is necessary.

♦ **Central nervous system stimulant**.[31] In various animal and human studies, ginseng provides both calming and stimulating effects simultaneously. It allows people to better adapt to stressful situations, including cancer. It also provides for energizing effects and improvement of moods and alertness.

♦ **Blood glucose regulator**. While ginseng will lower blood glucose levels in the diabetic individual or the one fed a high sugar diet, it will not lower blood glucose in the healthy individual fed a normal diet.[32] Since cancer is a sugar feeder, keeping blood glucose levels in check is a crucial job of ginseng.

♦ **Immune-stimulating effects**. Ginseng has been shown to stimulate the reticuloendothelial system, which means getting more macrophages ("big eaters") to gobble up (phagocytosis) cancer cells and cell debris.[33] In animals, ginseng was shown to prevent viral infections.[34] Ginseng can dramatically bolster host defense mechanisms in animals and humans.

♦ **Liver cleansing, protection, and stimulation**. Ginseng activates the macrophages in the liver, known as Kupffer cells, which are responsible for removing cellular debris from the body's most important detoxifying organ, the liver. Macrophages in the liver help to "take out the trash". Ginseng also helps to improve protein synthesis in the liver[35], reverse diet-induced fatty liver, and protect the liver from chemically-induced damage.[36]

♦ **Anti-clotting and metastatic**. Cancer spreads by adhering to blood vessel walls. Hence reducing the stickiness, or platelet aggregation, of cells is a major plus. Ginseng reduces platelet aggregation.[37]

♦ **Anti-cancer properties**. Ginseng is a potent inhibitor of cancer in animals[38] and humans.[39] Ginseng has the unique, paradoxical, and nearly miraculous ability to control cell growth, or hyperplasia. In healthy cells with adequate nourishment, ginseng encourages cell division. Yet under adverse conditions, ginseng helps to suppress abnormal cell division.[40] Ginseng helps to repair damaged DNA.[41]

In tumor-bearing mice, 8 days of ginseng administration brought about a 75% reduction in average tumor size.[42] Oral administration of ginseng in tumor-bearing mice inhibited the growth of liver cancer (solid ascites hepatoma), while inhibiting metastasis to the lungs.[43] Panax ginseng was able to enhance the uptake of mitomycin (an antibiotic and anti-cancer drug) into the cancer cells for increased tumor kill.[44] Ginseng was able to slow tumor growth and improve survival time in rats with chemically-induced liver cancer.[45]

SAFETY ISSUES
Ginseng and estrogen

Of the many supplements that may be useful for cancer patients, 2 of them contain estrogen-like compounds: soy and ginseng, which merit a special discussion. There is some controversy in the scientific community regarding the use of estrogen-like compounds in the treatment of breast or ovarian cancer patients.

First, it is critical to set the record straight regarding the importance of estrogen. Estrogen is an essential hormone produced by women throughout their menstruating years as part of fertility. Estrogen has 260 different functions in the human body, including antioxidant, maintenance of bone structure, and protection against cardiovascular diseases. Estrogen does not cause breast or ovarian cancer, but it is a growth hormone and can accelerate the growth of anything, including hormone-dependent cancers.

There are 4 primary categories of estrogen-like compounds:

♦ **Estrogen**, which actually refers to a family of hormones, including estradiol, estriol, and estrone, manufactured in the female body for specific bodily functions.[46]

♦ **Phytoestrogens**, which are estrogen-like compounds in plants, which have about 0.05% (1/2000) the strength of estrogen and have demonstrated beneficial effects both pre- and post-cancer diagnosis. These compounds compete with estrogen for binding to estrogen receptor sites.[47]

- **Xenoestrogens**, which are estrogen-like compounds in herbicides, pesticides, and other commercial chlorinated hydrocarbons. These have been shown to have disastrous consequences of antagonizing all the negative aspects of estrogen.[48] Women with breast cancer have been found to have more chlorinated hydrocarbons, or xenoestrogens, in their bloodstream. These xenoestrogens are creating havoc in the wild, where male animals end up with dramatically deformed genitals, and females have reduced fertility and increases in birth defects.

- **Estrogen-receptors**, which are compounds that escort estrogen from the body, hopefully after it has performed its essential functions. The human body makes estrogen-receptors through the PGE-1 prostaglandin pathways when blood sugar levels are kept low and essential fatty acids (EPA, ALA, GLA, LA) are sufficient.

Tamoxifen is an estrogen binder that can be of value in short-term use to slow down breast cancer, but in long term use elevates the risk for heart attack,[49] eye,[50] and liver damage[51] and INCREASES the risk of endometrial cancer.[52]

Researchers, like Stephen Barnes, PhD at the University of Alabama, find that soy is able to inhibit the growth of hormone-dependent tumors, including breast and prostate. Soy and ginseng are Nature's "kinder, gentler" forms of Tamoxifen.

Adding all this complex biochemistry together and trying to make the recommendations simple, there are several reasons why the 4 above-mentioned categories of estrogen-like compounds are not equal. Soy products and ginseng have been used both to prevent and to reverse cancer. The macrobiotic diet, which uses soy as a pivotal source of protein, has not been shown to accelerate the course of breast or ovarian cancer. While soy and ginseng products can reduce the symptoms of menopause by working as phytoestrogens, they do not increase the risk for breast or ovarian cancer nor do they accelerate the disease once present.

Green tea polyphenols 100 mg
     Antioxidant, protector of DNA, immune stimulant

America was founded upon a tea revolt. The American colonists decided that, rather than pay the English King's taxes on tea without representation in the British Parliament, the colonist would rather go into caffeine "cold turkey" by throwing the tea into Boston harbor. While the British have brought "high tea time" into its revered limelight, tea was first introduced to England in the 17th century via trade with China, where it had been a favorite beverage for over 3,000 years. Of the 2.5 million tons of dried tea produced each year worldwide, most is grown and consumed in the Orient.

Tea comes from the plant Camellia sinensis, an evergreen shrub in which the young leaves can be either:

◆ lightly steamed to produce **green tea** or
◆ air dried and oxidized to produce **black tea**.

The potent polyphenols are maintained in green tea, since steaming denatures the enzymes that would normally convert the polyphenols to less beneficial ingredients. Green tea is healthier than black tea. While both forms of tea have caffeine, only 20% of tea produced annually comes as green tea.

Green tea contains a variety of polyphenolic compounds, including catechin, epicatechin, and the reputed chief active ingredient, epigallocatechin gallate. One cup of green tea contains 300 to 400 mg of polyphenols and 50 to 100 mg of caffeine. Green tea works as an antioxidant, perhaps even more potent than vitamins C or E.[53] In animals, green tea was able to induce major improvements in antioxidant and detoxifying enzymes in the body.[54] In human studies, green tea users have about half the cancer incidence of non-tea drinkers.[55] In test tube studies, green tea shut down the tumor promoters involved in breast cancer.[56] Green tea inhibits the formation of cancer-causing agents in the stomach, including nitrosamines.[57]

The anti-cancer properties of green tea include:[58]

◆ Immune stimulant
◆ Inhibits platelet adhesion
◆ Antioxidant that protects immune cells for a higher tumor-kill rate, while protecting the valuable prostaglandin PGE-1
◆ Inhibits metastasis
◆ Inhibits the breakdown of connective tissue via collagenase, which is the primary mechanism for the spreading of cancer cells[59]

Aloe powder 100-200 mg
Immune stimulant, aids in cellular communication

For 5,000 years, many cultures and herbalists around the world have been using aloe vera as a primary medicinal plant. King Solomon used it as his favorite laxative. Hippocrates, the father of modern medicine 2,400 years ago, used at least 14 different medicine formulas containing aloe. Alexander the Great conquered an island in order to have aloe for his soldiers. As I write this section, I am looking at one of many aloe plants that we keep in our house. Aloe thrives on neglect. All the plant needs is decent soil and a little water and sun, then you get to harvest one of Nature's most versatile and impressive healers. Fresh aloe gel applied topically may be the greatest skin cream on the planet earth. The yellow bitter part of the plant leaf is a proven laxative that has brought relief to many of my patients. And whole-leaf extracts have the ability to gear up the immune system, reduce swelling, improve healing, kill bacteria and viruses, and improve communication between cells (intercellular) and within the cell (intracellular).

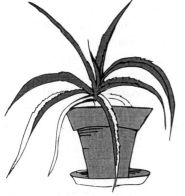

Of the 300 species of aloe, it is aloe vera that has received the most attention. Aloe certainly typifies the complexity of understanding the healing properties of plants. There are over 200 biologically active ingredients in aloe vera, including prostaglandins, essential fatty acids (including GLA), vitamins, minerals, anthraquinones, and polysaccharides (longer chains of sugar-like molecules).[60]

In the movie, MEDICINE MAN, a doctor (Sean Connery) discovered a cure for cancer from a plant in the Amazon forest, which was rapidly being levelled by bulldozers and fire. But now he cannot reproduce his original concoction from the same plant. To ruin the suspense and tell you the ending, the active ingredient in his original cancer cure was from the spider feces that was found in the sugar used to dilute the herbal concoction. Moral of the story: We are still neophytes when it comes to understanding just what is the active ingredient(s) in medicinal plants, which is why using low-heat processing of the whole leaf aloe is crucial for preserving the active ingredient.

While once discussing the merits of aloe with a noted researcher on the subject, I commented: "It seems as if aloe cures almost everything[61], as if it were an essential nutrient that we are not getting in our diet!!" He grinned and commented: "You may be right. For most of the millions of years of human history, our ancestors ate food that was not refrigerated, hence our food supply had all sorts of mold (yeast) growing on it. I think that we have an essential need for the unique collection of sugar-like molecules (mannans) that come from the cell wall of yeast and the aloe plant."

Indeed, there are receptor sites on immune cells (macrophages) for D-mannose (one of the sugars in aloe) just like a key fitting a keyhole.[62]

Aloe may help the cancer patient in many ways.

♦ **Antibacterial & antifungal**. Aloe vera applied topically to burn regions of animals was superior to the common antibacterial medication used, silver sulfadiazine.[63]

♦ **Antiviral activity**. Feline leukemia is a form of cancer contracted by cats and caused by a virus. This disease is invariably fatal, with 70% of cats dying within 8 weeks of early symptoms. Most cats are euthanized as soon as the diagnosis is made. In one study, acemannan from aloe was injected weekly for 6 weeks into the cats, with a followup 6-week waiting period. After this 12 week study, 71% of the cats were alive and in good health.[64] Acemannan has also demonstrated a potent ability to fight the flu virus, measles, and the HIV virus, while also reducing the dosage required of the drug AZT.[65]

♦ **Anti-inflammatory**. Drugs, such as cortisone, that are effective at reducing inflammation also shut down wound recovery. Aloe has the ability to reduce swelling, while also enhancing wound recovery.

♦ **Immune stimulant**. Aloe has been shown to increase the activity of the immune system.[66] Aloe seems to provide neutrophils with more "bullets", or toxic substances to kill cancer and invading organisms.[67] Aloe (acemannan) increases the production of nitric oxide, a potent anti-cancer "napalm" used by immune cells.[68]

♦ **Anti-cancer activity**. Various fractions of aloe (mannans and glucans) have been found to have potent anti-neoplastic activity.[69]

♦ **Radio-protective**. Some forms of mannan are bone marrow stimulants and can protect mice against cobalt-60 radiation.[70] In my experience with cancer patients, those who took aloe before and during radiation therapy had minimal damage of healthy tissue while still getting an impressive anti-cancer effect from the radiation. Generalized radiation to the pelvic region for prostate or colon cancer can be particularly nasty in harming the bladder and gastrointestinal tract. I remember one cancer patient who used aloe throughout 40 rounds of pelvic radiation and suffered no burns and only mild GI distress.

♦ **Cell communication**. Many forms of carbohydrates, called glycoproteins, may play a key role in promoting healthy communication within the cell and between cells. Aloe may contribute an important carbohydrate (mannan) that becomes part of this crucial "telegraph system", which prevents or slows down cancer.[71] Given the 8 monosaccharides used in the body and the 18 configurations used to arrange these molecules, the possible number of "words" in this complex "telegraph" system works out to 18 to the 8th power, or over 11 billion "messages". No doubt, more important breakthroughs will come out of this new and exciting field of cell communication.

Cat's claw, 3:1 concentrate 200 mg
Immune stimulant, anti-inflammatory, DNA protector, antioxidant

Cat's claw, or Uncaria tomentosa, is a relative newcomer to Western botanical medicine. It has been used therapeutically for centuries by Native South Americans in the higher elevations of the Peruvian Amazon rain forest. Cat's claw is a woody vine that grows to 100 feet by wrapping around nearby trees. The root and inner bark are used to prepare herbal concoctions that have demonstrated some effectiveness at cleansing the gastrointestinal tract of parasites and re-establishing a favorable environment for healthy microflora bacteria.

Cat's claw may be able to:

♦ Inhibit free radicals[72]
♦ Stimulate the immune system[73]
♦ Cleanse and strengthen the intestinal tract
♦ Inhibit auto-immune diseases, such as Crohn's and rheumatoid arthritis
♦ Protect the DNA from damage[74]
♦ Slow down cancer growth[75]

Rhodiola rosea root extract, standardized to 4% Rosavins and 1% salidrosides; 200 mg
    Adaptogen, cardio-protective, mood enhancer, energizer, hormonal regulator, immune enhancement

---

Rhodiola is an extremely tenacious herb that grows at high elevations in colder climates, such as Siberia. Rhodiola was a secret herb that was well researched by the Russians and used by Russian military and athletes in secrecy. At the end of the Cold War and the fall of the Berlin Wall, secrets from Russia began to trickle out to the rest of the world. One of those valuable secrets was Rhodiola.

Rhodiola was first mentioned in the medical herb text DE MATERIA MEDICA by the Greek physician Dioscorides in 77 AD. Chinese emperors would regularly send expeditions to Siberia to retrieve the "golden root" Rhodiola for energy enhancement and libido.

Rhodiola has generated considerable enthusiasm among herbalist who find compelling scientific evidence that Rhodiola can act as an:

✓ adaptogen, enhancing many bodily functions in a non-specific fashion
✓ increase energy and improve moods[76]
✓ protect DNA from mutagens that can trigger cancer[77]
✓ protects the body from the damaging effects of certain chemo agents (cyclophosphamide)[78]
✓ increase endurance[79]
✓ elevate mental concentration and clarity[80]
✓ stress reliever, such as used by Russian cosmonauts in space
✓ cardioprotective effects during oxygen deprivation[81]

✓ anti-depressant, relieving depression in 64% of patients in a Russian study[82]

✓ hormone balancer, without triggering hormone-related cancers[83]

Rhodiola appears safe in doses up to 20,000 mg per day for adults. Recommended dosages range from 100 to 500 mg per day.[84]

OTHER BOTANICALS: There are literally thousands of botanical agents that hold promise in cancer treatment. The above list offers some of the better studied and more widely available herbal agents to help the cancer patients. Herbal combinations worthy of consideration include:

♦ Tianxian herbal concoction (tianxian.com) that has been clinically studied in China, but no scientific papers yet available in English.

♦ Hoxsey formula, available as Herbal Veil Tonic from Lenox Labs 800-256-2253

♦ Essiac formula available in raw herb form (Herbal Healing Academy 501-269-4177) or in finished form at a higher price from Essiac Intl. (613-820-0503)

♦ Goldenseal

♦ Licorice

♦ Pau D'Arco

There are thousands of herbs commonly used in the Orient that are not widely available in the U.S.. These herbs can be very helpful when recommended by a qualified herbalist. Among the more promising Oriental herbs for cancer patients are Codonopsis available from China Herb Co. (800-221-4372) or Frontier Herbs (800-669-3275).

PATIENT PROFILE: BEAT COLON CANCER

D.M. was 48 years of age when he was diagnosed with stage 4 colon cancer that had spread to the liver. His doctor used chemotherapy with little hope of any benefit from this therapy, much less a cure. D.M. began using the principles in this book including proper diet and ImmunoPower supplements to reverse his cancer. Within 6 months he was disease-free and has remained so for 2 years. D.M. writes "I really believe your book helped to save my life."

SKIN CANCER. A special note about basal cell and squamous cell carcinoma. These cancers are extremely common, with about 800,000 medical office procedures done annually to remove minor skin cancers. Surgical excision is about 90% effective as a long term cure. Melanoma is a much more lethal and rare form of skin cancer that requires professional attention. For those people interested in treatment options for routine non-malignant skin cancer, you may consider the herbal escharotics (selectively burn away abnormal tissue when applied topically) of Cansema (800-256-2253 or AltCancer.com or BloodRootProducts.com).

ENDNOTES

[1] . Koide, T., et al., Cancer Biotherapy & Radiopharmaceuticals, vol.11, p.273, Aug.1996

[2] . LeBon, AM, et al., Chem.Biol.Interactions, vol.83, p.65, 1992

[3] . Havsteen, B, Biochem Pharmacol., vol.32, p.1141, 1983

[4] . Fujiki, H., in Plant Flavonoids in Biology and Medicine, vol.1, p.429, Liss Publ., NY, 1986

[5] . Berg, P, in Plant Flavonoids in Biology and Medicine, vol.2, p.157, Liss Publ., NY, 1988

[6] . Wattenberg, L., et al., Cancer Research, vol.30, p.1922, 1970

[7] . Werbach, M., et al., BOTANICAL INFLUENCES ON ILLNESS, p.30, Third Line, Tarzana, CA, 1994

[8] . Werbach, M., IBID, p.189

[9] . Luettig, B., et al., J. Natl.Cancer Inst., vol.81, p.669, 1989

[10] . Lersch, C., et al., Tumordiagen Ther., vol.13, p.115, 1992

[11] . Lersch, C., et al., Cancer Invest., vol.10, p.343, 1992

[12] . Nagabhushan, M., et al., J. Am.Coll. Nutr., vol.11, p.192, 1992

[13] . Kuttan, R., et al., Cancer Lett., vol.29, p.197, 1985

[14] . Polasa, K., Mutagen, vol.7, p.107, 1992

[15] . Kuttan, R., et al., Tumori, vol.73, p.29, 1987

[16] . Schubert, H., et al., Geriatr Forsch, vol.3, p.45, 1993

[17] . Kleijnen, J., et al., Br. J. Clin.Pharmacol. vol.34, p.352, 1992

[18] . Kleijnen, J., et al., Lancet, vol.340, p.1136, 1992

[19] . Koltai, M., et al., Drugs, vol.42, p.9, 1991

[20] . Pincemail, J., et al., Experientia, vol.45, p.708, 1989

[21] . Shibata, S., et al., Econ.Med.Plant Res., vol.1, p.217, 1985

[22] . Siegel, RK, JAMA, vol.243, p.32, 1980

[23] . Chang, HM, et al., Pharmacology and Applications of Chinese Materia Medica, vol. 2, World Scientific Publ., Teaneck, NJ, p.1041, 1987

[24] . Sun, Y, J. Biol Response Modifiers, vol.2, p.227, 1983

[25] . Chu, DT, et al., J. Clin.Lab.Immunol., vol.26, p.183, 1988

[26] . Li, NQ, et al., Chung Kuo Chung Hsi I Chieh Ho Tsa Chih, vol.12, p.588, 1992

[27] . Boik, J., CANCER AND NATURAL MEDICINE, p.177, Oregon Medical, Princeton, MN, 1995

[28] . Boik, J. CANCER AND NATURAL MEDICINE, p.180 Oregon Medical, Princeton, MN, 1995

[29] . Murray, MT, HEALING POWER OF HERBS, p.265, Prima Publ., Rocklin, CA 1995

[30] . Ziglar, W., Whole Foods, vol.2, p.48, 1979

[31] . Samira, MMH, et al., J.Int.Med.Res., vol.13, p.342, 1985

[32] . Ng, TB, et al., Gen.Pharmacol., vol.6, p.549, 1985; see also Yamato, M., et al., Proceedings of the 3rd Intl Ginseng Symp, p.115, 1980

[33] . Jie, YH, et al., Agents Actions, vol.15, p.386, 1984; see also Gupta, S., et al., Clin.Res., vol.28, p.504A, 1980

[34] . Singh, VK, et al., Planta Medica, vol.51, p.462, 1984

[35] . Oura, H., et al., Chem.Pharm.Bull., vol.20, p.980, 1972

[36] . Hikino, H., et al., Planta Medica, vol.52, p.62, 1985; see also Oh, JS, et al., Korean J.Pharmacol., vol.4, p.27, 1968

[37] . Yamamoto, M., et al., Am.J.Chin.Med., vol.11, p.84, 1983

[38] . Yun, TK, et al., Cancer Detect.Prev., vol.6, p.515, 1983

[39] . Yun, TK, et al., Int.J.Epidemiol., vol.19, p.871, 1990

[40] . Lee, KD, Jpn.J.Pharmacol., vol.21, p.299, 1971; Fulder, SJ, Exp.Ger., vol.12, p.125, 1977

[41] . Rhee, YH, et al., Planta Medica, vol.57, p.125, 1991

[42] . Hau, DM, et al., Int. J. of Oriental Med., vol.15, p.10, 1990

[43] . Yang, G., et al., J. of Trad. Chin. Med., vol.8, p.135, 1988

[44] . Kubo, M., et al., Planta Med, vol.58, p.424, 1992

[45] . Li, X., et al., J. Tongji Med Univ., vol.11, p.73, 1991

[46] . Murray, RK, et al., HARPER'S BIOCHEMISTRY, 24th ed, p.550, Lange, Stamford, CT 1996
[47] . Boik, J., CANCER AND NATURAL MEDICINE, p.44, Oregon Medical, Princeton, MN 1995
[48] . Davis, DL, et al., Environmental Health Perspectives, vol.101, p.372, Oct.1993
[49] . Nakagawa, T., et al., Angiology, vol.45, p.333, May 1994
[50] . Pavlidis, NA, et al., Cancer, vol.69, p.2961, 1992
[51] . Catherino, WH, et al., Drug Safety, vol.8, p.381, 1993
[52] . Seoud, MAF, et al., Obstetrics & Gynecology, vol.82, p.165, Aug.1993
[53] . Ho, C., et al., Prev.Med., vol.21, p.520, 1992
[54] . Khan, SG, et al., Cancer Res., vol.52, p.4050, 1992
[55] . Yang, CS, et al., J. Natl., Cancer Inst., vol.85, p.1038, 1993
[56] . Komori, A., et al., Jpn.J.Clin.Oncol., vol.23, p.186, 1993
[57] . Stich, HF, Prev.Med., vol.21, p.377, 1992
[58] . Boik, J., CANCER AND NATURAL MEDICINE, p.178, Oregon Medical, Princeton, MN 1995
[59] . Beretz, A, et al., Plant Flavonoids in Biology and Medicine II, p.187, Liss Publ., 1988
[60] . Haller, JS, Bull.NY Acad.Sci., vol.66, p.647, 1990
[61] . Danhof, IE, REMARKABLE ALOE, Omnimedicus Press, Grand Prairie, TX 1987
[62] . Lee, YC, Adv.Exp.Med.Biol., vol.228, p.103, 1984
[63] . Robson, MC, et al., J.Burn.Care Rehab., vol.3, p.157, 1982
[64] . Sheets, MA, et al., Mol.Biother., vol.3, p.41, 1991
[65] . Kahlon, JB, et al., Mol.Biother., vol.3, p.214, 1991
[66] . t'Hart, LA, et al., Planta.Med., vol.55, p.509, 1989
[67] . t'Hart, LA, et al., Int.J.Immunopharmacol., vol.12, p.427, 1990
[68] . Karaca, K., et al., Int.J.Immunopharmacol., vol.17, p.183, 1995
[69] . Kamasuka, T., et al., Gann, vol.59, p.443, 1968
[70] . Tizard, IR, et al., Mol.Biother., vol.1, p.290, 1989
[71] . Murray, RK, et al., HARPER'S BIOCHEMISTRY, p.648, Lange Medical, Stamford, CT 1996
[72] . McBrien, DC, et al., LIPID PEROXIDATION AND CANCER, Academy Press, NY 1982
[73] . Wagner, H., et al., Planta Medica, vol.12, p.34, 1985
[74] . Rizzi, R., et al., J. Ethnopharmacol., vol.38, p.63, 1993
[75] . DeOlivera, MM, et al., Anals Acad.Brasil Ciencias, vol.44, p.41, 1972
[76] . Spasov, AA, Phytomedicine, vol.7, no.2, p.85, 2000
[77] . Saratikov, AS, Stimulative Properties of Rhodiola Rosea, in RHODIOLA ROSEA IS A VALUABLE MEDICINAL PLANT, Tomsk, Russia, Izdatelstvo Tomskogo Univ., 1987
[78] . Udintsev, SN, European J.Cancer, vol.27, no.9, p.1182, 1991
[79] . Seifulla, RD, Sports Pharmacology Source Book, Moscow, Mosovskaya Prauda, 1999
[80] . Shevtsov, VA, Phytomedicine, vol.10, no.2-3, p.95, 2003
[81] . Afanasev, SA, Biokhimiia, vol.61, no.10, p.1779, 1996
[82] . Krasik, ED, New data on the therapy of asthenic conditions: clinical prospects for the use of golden root extract, Kemerov, Riussia, Russian Academy of Medicinal Sciences, p.298, 1970
[83] . Eagon, PK, abstract from American Association of Cancer Research meeting, 2003
[84] . Brown, RP, THE RHODIOLA REVOLUTION, Rodale Press, 2004

CHAPTER 17

✷

GLANDULARS

"Health begins on the farm, not the pharmacy."Dr. Alan Gaby's uncle

---

WHAT'S AHEAD?
↪ The thymus gland and spleen are valuable parts of the immune system that can sometimes be "worn out".
↪ Taking thymus and spleen glandular concentrates sometimes improves immune functions.
↪ Melatonin is a valuable antioxidant and anti-cancer agent.

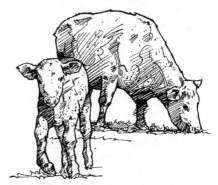

Glandular therapy has been practiced, at least inadvertently, since the dawn of mankind. A gland is an organ in the body that secretes or excretes something. For instance, the pineal gland in the brain secretes melatonin, which acts as an antioxidant, regulator of our biological clock, anti-aging hormone, and works to prevent and slow cancer. There are many other organs that we will discuss in this chapter. Essentially, as we age or are exposed to toxins, stress, and malnutrition, our glands do not perform their jobs ideally. This is where glandular therapy can be of benefit. One of the more commonly practiced forms of glandular therapy is the use of synthroid or thyroid extract to treat people with underactive thyroid glands. We are merely replacing what Nature is not making. Glandular therapy can be a rate-limiting step in the cancer patient getting well and oftentimes requires professional assistance in determining which gland is not working up to par and how to fix the problem.

In the seminal book, NUTRITION AND PHYSICAL DEGENERATION, Weston Price, DDS, relates that Native Americans in the cold regions of northern Canada avoided scurvy in the winter by first eating the raw adrenal gland from any animal captured. Adrenal glands provide the most concentrated depot of vitamin C in the body. Our hunter-gatherer ancestors would offer the liver and heart of the captured animal to the slayer. Liver and heart are among the organs that are rich in CoQ, carnitine, lipoic acid, trace minerals, and a variety of nutrients that are missing in our diets.

Today, there are millions of people taking prescription supplements of thyroid gland from animals to bolster a failing thyroid gland. This is glandular therapy. We now use gelatin extracts (which are from connective tissue of hooves and hides) of glucosamine sulfate and chondroitin sulfate to improve connective tissue diseases, such as osteo and rheumatoid arthritis. There are peptides in each gland that are specific to that gland, such as thymus and spleen, which will be targeted to that gland once consumed.

As we mature, many of our glandular functions deteriorate.[1] Although our biochemistry textbooks would have us believe that polypeptides, such as those found in glandular extracts, are all hydrolyzed in the digestive processes of the gut, in fact, many peptides survive this chemical gauntlet. How else do we explain the passage of Immunoglobulin A from mother's milk to bolster the newborn infant's immune system, or the food proteins that pass directly into the bloodstream and trigger allergic responses? Glandular replacement therapy, such as thymus and spleen, may be essential for many people who are struggling with life-threatening diseases.

GLANDULAR (best form for absorption) suggested daily dosage
Primary functions in human body and anti-cancer activities

Thymic concentrate 500 mg
Bolsters functions of thymus gland, which is crucial to the maturation of immune cells into T-cells

---

The thymus gland in humans usually atrophies with aging. Anyone over 30 years of age probably has a thymus gland that is well below optimal in size and functional capacity. There are thymus-derived factors with hormone-like activity, called thymosins, that have long been recognized for their potential at stimulating immune functions.[2] An extract of thymus, thymosin 5, was able to stimulate immune functions in mice with induced tumors.[3] Other researchers found that thymus extract is more of an immune regulator than an immune stimulant. In human lung cancer patients receiving chemotherapy, thymus supplements provided for longer survival time.[4] Other researchers found that thymus extract (TP-1) was able to increase lymphocyte counts in incurable gastrointestinal cancer patients treated with chemotherapy.[5] Other researchers followed over 1,000 patients who had been treated with thymus extract (TFX) over the course of 15 years and found the thymus to be extremely helpful in normalizing immune panels and improving outcome in a wide variety of immune suppressive disorders.[6] Researchers at the University of California isolated a fraction of thymus (thymic protein A), which improved immune parameters in mice.[7] Probably a wide variety of subsets of peptides and glycoproteins in thymus work to improve differentiation of bone marrow (B-cells) lymphocytes into active T-cells that can recognize and destroy cancer cells.

Spleen concentrate   500 mg
     Bolsters functions of the spleen gland, a storage and filtering organ for the blood and immune system

---

The human spleen oftentimes atrophies with aging. Supplements of spleen extract have been used in conjunction with ginseng as a clinically tested immune stimulant for cancer and AIDS patients in Europe.

Melatonin 3-20 mg at bedtime
     Regulates circadian rhythm, enhances immune system (IL-2) against tumor, antioxidant, stimulates thymus (immune enhancement), inhibits several different tumor lines, reduces toxicity (myelodysplasia) from chemo and radiation, may reduce lean tissue wasting (cachexia), stimulates immune system to become more toxic against tumors

---

There is a pea-sized gland in the center of the human brain called the pineal gland. This gland has been the source of intense research and interest since it was first called "the third eye" by scientists two centuries ago. There is evidence that our toxic world full of light at night, alcohol, and an invisible sea of electrical emissions all dampen down the normal effectiveness of the pineal gland. Studies in other creatures find that melatonin is the "juvenile" hormone, which is directly responsible for the effects of aging. Melatonin may be one of the master hormones in the human body, coordinating and regulating growth and aging, and very essential for optimal health.

Melatonin is now being used around the world as part of comprehensive cancer treatment. Only side effects noted are drowsiness upon awakening. If so, reduce or discontinue dosage. Do not use melatonin in conjunction with other psychotropic drugs, such as Prozac, Lithium, or monoamine oxidase inhibitors.

♦ Tumor regressions were found in 36% (5 out of 14) patients studied with liver (hepatocellular carcinoma).[8]

♦ Melatonin was effective as sole therapy in refractory cancer patients (have not responded to other conventional therapies), with improvement in quality of life and control of cancer growth.[9]

♦ Melatonin was effective against metastatic lung cancer (non-small cell) in patients who had failed first-line therapy (cisplatin).[10]

♦ Melatonin prevented the common side effect from IL-2 therapy of thrombocytopenia (low platelet numbers in the blood).[11]

♦ Melatonin was shown effective in patients with relapsed melanoma.[12]

♦ In cancer patients who had failed all other cancer therapies, melatonin provided a 39% response rate (stopped tumor progression) with no side effects, and nearly all patients reported an improved sense of well being.[13]

♦ Melatonin along with Tamoxifen produced better results in metastatic breast cancer patients than Tamoxifen treatment alone.[14]

PATIENT PROFILE: BEAT ADVANCED BREAST CANCER
R.T. was diagnosed with stage 4 breast cancer. R.T. had surgery and was bald from the chemo when a friend presented her with BEATING CANCER WITH NUTRITION. R.T. followed the diet and supplement recommendations in this book and went into complete remission. That was 7 years ago. She has since written a book ONE, TWO, OR THREE BREASTS for other women battling breast cancer.

ENDNOTES

[1] . Klatz, R., et al., STOPPING THE CLOCK, Keats, New Canaan, CT, 1996

[2] . Oats, KK, et al., TIPS, p.347, Elsevier Press, Aug.1984

[3] . Wada, A., et al., J.Nat.Cancer Institute, vol.74, no.3, p.659, Mar.1985

[4] . Chretien, PB, et al., NY Acad Sci, vol.332, p.135, 1979

[5] . Shoham, J., et al., Cancer Immunol. Immunother., vol.9, p.173, 1980

[6] . Skotnicki, AB, Med. Oncol. & Tumor Pharmacother., Vol.6, no.1, p.31, 1989

[7] . Hays, EF, et al., Clin Immun. & Immunopath., vol.33, p.381, 1984

[8] . European J.Ca., vol.30A, p.167, 1994

[9] . Oncology, vol,48, p.448, 1991

[10] . Oncology, vol.49, p.336, 1992

[11] . J.Biol.Regul.Homeostat.Agents, vol.9, no.2, p.52, 1995

[12] . J. Pineal. Research, vol.21, p.239, 1996

[13] . Anticancer Research, vol.18, p.1329, 1998

[14] . British J.Cancer, vol.71, p.854, 1995

CHAPTER 18

✳

LIPIDS (FATS)

"May you make lots of money--and spend it all on doctor bills."

anonymous

WHAT'S AHEAD?

- Human health is highly dependent on the quality and quantity of our fat intake.
- Americans eat too much fat and the wrong kind of fat.
- Therapeutic fats, such as fish oil, can stimulate immune functions and help to slow cancer.

Fat is both essential for human health and potentially toxic. Most Americans eat too much fat, the wrong kind of fat, AND do not get enough of the essential fatty acids that should be in our diet, hence the need for supplements and dietary changes.

Not all fat is created equally. Fat-phobic Americans have lost sight of the fact that there are good, bad, and ugly fats.

DIETARY FATS		
THERAPEUTIC	**GOOD**	**BAD**
fish,primrose,borage, MCT,lecithin,hemp, sesame,CLA,sharkoil, rice bran, wheat germ, black currant	olive, safflower, soy, walnut,almond,pecan, avocado, cashew, coconut,palm, butter,pumpkin,canola	hydrogenated (trans), or oxidized (from fast food deep fryers), or not enough vit.E, olestra

Cod liver oil 1-6 grams, including Vitamin A & Vitamin D
 Augments immune system, improves production of favorable prostaglandin PGE-1, prevents metastasis of cancer cells by changing the stickiness of cells, improves cell membrane dynamics to augment nutrient absorption and toxin elimination

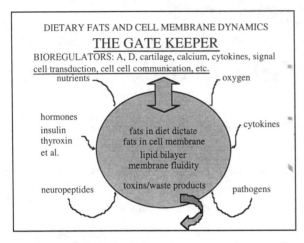

DIETARY FATS AND CELL MEMBRANE DYNAMICS

THE GATE KEEPER

BIOREGULATORS: A, D, cartilage, calcium, cytokines, signal cell transduction, cell cell communication, etc.

nutrients — oxygen

hormones
insulin
thyroxin
et al. — cytokines

fats in diet dictate
fats in cell membrane
lipid bilayer
membrane fluidity

neuropeptides — toxins/waste products — pathogens

When the Senate Diet Goals were released by a blue ribbon panel of nutrition experts in 1977, they included the recommendation to decrease fat intake from 40% of calories to 30%. Yet, experts then looked at the Greenland Eskimos, who get 60% of their calories from fat and practically no dietary fiber, yet mysteriously had little cancer or heart disease. Three factors saved these people from an otherwise disastrous diet:

1) genetic adaption, at least 40,000 years to adjust to this uniquely skewed diet

2) fish oil, which contains a very special and highly unsaturated fat, eicosapentaenoic acid (EPA)

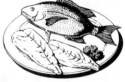

3) no sugar in the diet, which helps the body make PGE-1, a healthy prostaglandin

EPA is, essentially, Nature's anti-freeze. In the Arctic regions of the world, the ocean temperature drops to below freezing, yet water-based life will explode at that temperature, like leaving out a water balloon on a sub-freezing night. So Nature provides the algae in the ocean with this special fat, EPA, which prevents freezing and bursting at low temperatures. Smaller fish eat the algae, and bigger fish eat the smaller fish, until we have major concentrations of

EICOSANOIDS: lipid mediators in mammalian cells
medically important, pharmaceutically profitable

*100+ eicosanoids include: prostaglandins, prostacyclins,
*thromboxanes,, leukotrienes, HPETE, etc.
*prostaglandins are formed by most cells in our body and
*act as autocrine and paracrine lipid mediators
*half life of seconds
*regional (not systemic) mediators, insignificant in bloodstream
*nanomolar concentrations
*the eicosanoids possess a vast array of biological actions
*in many different cell types
*vasodilation, bronchodilation, inflammation, vascular permeability,
*immunity, bone repair, pain are all influenced by eicosanoids

Funk, CD, Science, 294, 1871, Nov.30, 2001
Innis, SM, in PRESENT KNOWLEDGE IN NUTRITION, p.58, ILSI, 1996

EPA in cold water fish, like cod, salmon, mackeral, tuna, and sardines. Much of the fat in seals and whales that were consumed by the Greenland Eskimos was rich in EPA, which provided these people with extraordinary protection against many diseases. EPA is so valuable against cancer that the National Library of Medicine has created a special report on the hundreds of scientific studies found in their data base on the therapeutic benefits of EPA.

IS FISH OIL AN ESSENTIAL NUTRIENT?

Convincing evidence that fish oil and fish can reduce[1]:

- ❖ heart disease
- ❖ sudden heart attack
- ❖ infant development abnormalities
- ❖ autoimmune disorders (i.e. lupus and multiple sclerosis)
- ❖ Crohn's disease
- ❖ cancer of breast, prostate, colon
- ❖ hypertension
- ❖ rheumatoid arthritis

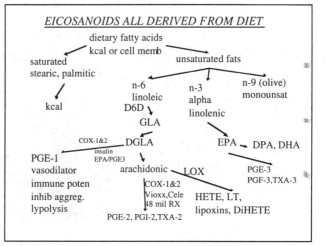

EICOSANOIDS ALL DERIVED FROM DIET

EPA may help the cancer patient:

♦ **Changes membrane fluidity.** Cell membranes contain fats that are a direct reflection of our diet, including the unnatural hydrogenated fats found in Crisco and Pop Tarts. When we are talking about dietary fats, the old saying is literally true, "you are what you eat." Cell membranes that are fluid and flexible and allow the proper nutrients to pass into the cell will improve

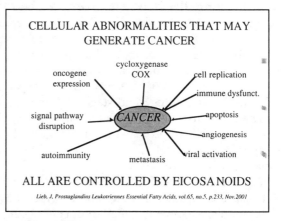

CELLULAR ABNORMALITIES THAT MAY GENERATE CANCER

ALL ARE CONTROLLED BY EICOSANOIDS

Lieb, J, Prostaglandins Leukotriennes Essential Fatty Acids, vol.65, no.5, p.233, Nov.2001

overall wellness, thus discouraging abnormal cell growths, like cancer. Cells that are flexible with EPA can squeeze down narrow capillaries to feed the distant tissue. Cells that are rigid with too much saturated or hydrogenated fat or having been "tanned" from too much sugar in the blood will not be able to move down narrow capillaries, like a car trying to get down a hotel hallway.

♦ **Increase prostaglandin E-1**, (PGE-1), which favors reducing the stickiness of cells for less risk of metastasis.[2] PGE-1 also bolsters immune functions, dilates blood vessels, elevates production of estrogen receptors, and provides other benefits for the cancer patient.

♦ **Slows tumor growth in animals.**[3] Slows tumor growth by altering protein synthesis and breakdown.[4]

♦ **Augments medical therapies.** EPA improves tumor kill in hyperthermia and chemotherapy by altering cancer cell membranes for increased vulnerability.[5] Increases the ability of adriamycin to kill cultured leukemia cells.[6] Tumors in EPA-fed animals are more responsive to Mitomycin C and doxorubicin (chemotherapy drugs).[7] EPA and GLA were selectively toxic to human tumor cell lines while also enhancing the cytotoxic effects of chemotherapy.[8]

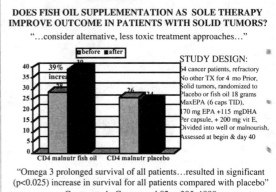

DOES FISH OIL SUPPLEMENTATION AS SOLE THERAPY IMPROVE OUTCOME IN PATIENTS WITH SOLID TUMORS?

"...consider alternative, less toxic treatment approaches..."

STUDY DESIGN: 4 cancer patients, refractory No other TX for 4 mo Prior, Solid tumors, randomized to Placebo or fish oil 18 grams MaxEPA (6 caps TID), 170 mg EPA +115 mgDHA Per capsule, + 200 mg vit E, Divided into well or malnourish, Assessed at begin & day 40

"Omega 3 prolonged survival of all patients...resulted in significant (p<0.025) increase in survival for all patients compared with placebo"

Gogos, et al., Cancer, vol.82, p.395, 1998

♦ **Reduces initiation, promotion, and progression of hormonally driven cancers**, such as breast, prostate, and ovarian. An EPA-rich diet significantly lowered the levels of estradiol, a marker for breast cancer, in the 25 women studied who were at risk for breast cancer.[9] Modulates estrogen metabolism for reduced risk and spreading of breast cancer.[10]

Fish oil may be as effective as any cancer treatment available. In a study examining end-stage refractory cancer patients who have exhausted all chemo and radiation options, fish oil supplements provided a substantial improvement in length of life and immune functions compared to placebo.

CAN FISH OIL IMPROVE OUTCOME IN CANCER TREATMENT?

- anti-cachectic; prevents and reverses wasting syndrome[11]
- induces apoptosis (suicide) in cancer cells[12]
- upregulates immune function[13]
- reduces stickiness of cells to slow metastasis[14]
- improves insulin sensitivity, lowers blood glucose, impairs tumor angiogenesis (making of blood vessels)[15]

Flax oil is rich in alpha-linolenic acid (ALA), which is a precursor to EPA. While flax oil is cheaper and more palatable than fish oil, it requires enzyme conversion steps in the body to turn flax oil (ALA) into fish oil (EPA). Flax oil is used in several recipes in the "Nutritious and Delicious" chapter in this book. Flax meal (whole ground flax seeds) may be even more effective against cancer than flax oil. One study found that the more flax meal was fed to lab animals, the fewer and smaller were the metastatic tumors spreading from the implanted melanoma cancer.[16]

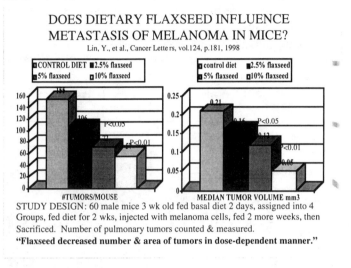

DOES DIETARY FLAXSEED INFLUENCE METASTASIS OF MELANOMA IN MICE?
Lin, Y., et al., Cancer Letters, vol.124, p.181, 1998

#TUMORS/MOUSE   MEDIAN TUMOR VOLUME mm3

STUDY DESIGN: 60 male mice 3 wk old fed basal diet 2 days, assigned into 4 Groups, fed diet for 2 wks, injected with melanoma cells, fed 2 more weeks, then Sacrificed. Number of pulmonary tumors counted & measured.
"Flaxseed decreased number & area of tumors in dose-dependent manner."

Borage or Evening primrose oil   1-6 grams (of which 9-20% is GLA)
Improves production of PGE-1, selectively toxic to tumor cells.

Our ancestors consumed a diet of range-fed animals who grazed on wild grain, nuts, and seeds. In these foods is a wide assortment of valuable fatty acids, including gamma linolenic acid (GLA), which is richly concentrated in the evening primrose and borage plants. Intake of GLA in modern Americans has dropped off substantially with the consumption of corn-fed beef, which is rich in linoleic acid that generates the tumor-promoting

D6D (delta 6 desaturase): rate limiting step in arachidonic
MAKING THE CASE FOR GLA SUPPLEMENTATION

PRODUCTION OF GLA VIA D6D REDUCED VIA:
→aging
→stress (catecholamines)
→insulin resistance
→diabetes
→high glycemic diet
→alcohol
→viral & other infections
→trans fatty acids (partially hydrogenated oils)

supplementation with GLA (borage, primrose) may be warranted in arthritis, CAD, cancer, autoimmune diseases, mental illness

Horrobin, DF, Prog.Lip.Res., vol.31, p.163, 1992

eicosanoid of arachidonic acid. The reason why range-fed lean buffalo was good for Native Americans, yet corn-fed high fat beef is not so good for modern Americans, is primarily the quality and quantity of fats in these two animals. A ratio of approximately 4:1 of EPA to GLA is very favorable for host defense mechanisms to fight off cancer.

We are able to make less GLA internally as we age, are exposed to stress and toxins, become compromised by disease, and eat hydrogenated fats--which describes millions of Americans. GLA in the diet helps to drive PGE-1, mentioned above, while also being selectively

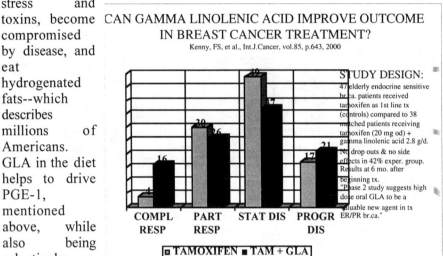

CAN GAMMA LINOLENIC ACID IMPROVE OUTCOME IN BREAST CANCER TREATMENT?

Kenny, FS, et al., Int.J.Cancer, vol.85, p.643, 2000

STUDY DESIGN: 47 elderly endocrine sensitive br ca. patients received tamoxifen as 1st line tx (controls) compared to 38 matched patients receiving tamoxifen (20 mg od) + gamma linolenic acid 2.8 g/d. No drop outs & no side effects in 42% exper. group. Results at 6 mo. after beginning tx. "Phase 2 study suggests high dose oral GLA to be a valuable new agent in tx ER/PR br.ca."

COMPL RESP | PART RESP | STAT DIS | PROGR DIS

□ TAMOXIFEN ■ TAM + GLA

toxic to tumor cells.[17] GLA was selectively toxic to cultured human breast cancer cells.[18] In 21 human cancer patients with refractory (failed medical treatment) and untreatable malignancies, GLA was able to provide measurable benefits, including weight gain and reduction in tumor mass based on radiological evidence.[19] When healthy and cancer cells are cultured with EPA and GLA, the healthy cells begin to outgrow the cancerous cells.[20]

One study found that when GLA was given to women with breast cancer in conjunction with Tamoxifen therapy, there was a 400% increase in the number of women who achieved complete response when compared to women just receiving Tamoxifen.

Shark oil 1-6 grams (20% alkylglycerols)
Improves the production of white (immune) and red (erythrocyte) cells from the bone marrow. Protects against the damaging effects of radiation therapy.

While it may be true that "sharks don't get cancer", it is more than cartilage that works in the shark's favor. Shark liver oil is rich in a compound called "alkoxyglycerols" or "alkylglycerols". The highest concentration of alkoxyglycerols in Nature are found in mother's milk, bone marrow, and shark liver oil, which is an indication of the importance of this fatty compound. Bone marrow seems to derive the greatest benefit from alkoxyglycerol administration by nourishing the "cradle of all blood cells". Bone marrow is responsible for manufacturing red blood cells (hemopoiesis, or hematopoiesis) and white blood cells for the immune system.

Shark oil may help cancer patients:

♦ **Reversing anemia.** Many cancer patients become anemic, or deficient in red blood cells, which leads to weakness and increased risk for infections. Shark liver oil encourages normal production of red blood cells, which is a much better strategy than giving high dose iron supplements. See the section on "iron" in the chapter on minerals. I have found significant improvement in red blood cell (hemoglobin) and white blood cell (lymphocyte) counts in patients taking shark liver oil capsules.

♦ **Protecting healthy tissue** from radiation damage. In cancer patients given shark oil capsules before, during, and after radiation therapy, there was a 67% reduction in radiation-induced injuries.[21] Administration of shark oil capsules prior to radiation provided a 47% reduction in both severe (such as fistulas) and less harmful injuries from radiation therapy for cervical/uterine cancer.[22]

♦ **May slow cancer growth.** Shark oil was able to reduce cancer mortality in a human clinical trial.[23] Patients with uterine cancer who were given alkylglycerols throughout their cancer treatment had regression of tumor growth.[24]

Conjugated linoleic acid (CLA) 1-3 grams
Improves cellular communication to prevent and reverse cancer, stabilizes blood glucose, antioxidant and immune regulator.

CONJUGATED LINOLEIC ACID (CLA)
a promising anti-cancer nutrient

☞ isomers of linoleic acid produced by bacteria in gut of ruminants
☞ only dietary sources are milk and meat of ruminants
☞ anticarcinogenesis (50%⇓ br.ca. animals), ⇑apoptosis
☞ immunomodulation: ⇓cachexia, ⇑cell mediated response
☞ body composition alteration: ⇑lean mass, ⇓fat mass
☞ antiatherosclerosis
☞ normalizes impaired glucose tolerance in diabetic rats
☞ antioxidant? reduced malondialdehyde, lipid peroxides
☞ ⇑vitamin A status

Whigham, LD, Pharmacological Research, vol.42, 6, p.503, 2000
Kelly, GS, Alternative Medicine Review, vol.6, no.4, p.367, 2001
Kritchevsky, D, British Journal Nutrition, vol.83, p.459, 2000
McDonald, HB, J.American College Nutrition, vol.19, no.2, p.111S, 2000

Recently, I had to find a cable to connect my computer to my monitor. This was no easy task. In describing my needs to the salesperson, we got into a spirited discussion of how many pins in how many rows for each end of the cable. "Close" is not good enough in either computer cables or fatty acid requirements in the human body. Americans often consume fats that are unhealthy, like hydrogenated fats, and are deficient in valuable fats, like CLA. A tiny difference in molecular structure, just like computer cables, can make a huge difference in whether this fat will help or hinder your cellular machinery.

CLA is a collection of unique "18 pin" fatty acids found primarily in the meat and milk of grazing animals, like beef and dairy. CLA is one of the more exciting recent developments in anticarcinogenic fats. There is 300-400% more CLA in spring and summer milk and most Australian dairy products due to the availability of fresh green pasture land, which augments CLA content in the milk and fat of grazing animals.[25]

CLA is just another example of my first axiom of nutrition: "Nature knows best." Scientific studies in the past have come up with some conflicting results regarding diet and cancer. While most studies find that a high fat diet increases the risk for cancer, one recent study found that milk fat may protect women against breast cancer.[26] While most nutritionists argue that beef, in general, increases the risk for cancer, one prospective epidemiological study found that people consuming meat along with green or yellow vegetables on a daily basis had up to a 75% reduction in colon cancer incidence compared to those who consumed either meat or vegetables alone.[27]

CLA makes a good argument for humans consuming an omnivorous diet, since there is far more CLA, carnitine, EPA, taurine, and lipoic acid in animal foods than in plant foods. Dr. Weston Price was a dentist and, in my humble opinion, one of the more important nutritionists in history. He toured the world in the 1930s with his nurse-wife visiting numerous cultures and found many different diets. But he never found a group of people who were complete vegans...all of our ancestors ate some animal food. Maybe CLA is one of the nutrients that we need from a healthy mixed diet.

CLA is a unique fat, derived from linoleic acid, which is one of the two essential fatty acids in human nutrition, along with alpha-linolenic acid. CLA has unsaturated bonds in either the 9 & 11 position or the 10 & 12 carbon position. It comes in both "cis" (looks like a horseshoe) and "trans"

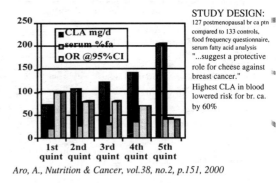

DOES DIETARY CONJUGATED LINOLEIC ACID (CLA) PREVENT BREAST CANCER in humans?

STUDY DESIGN: 127 postmenopausal br ca ptn compared to 133 controls, food frequency questionnaire, serum fatty acid analysis "...suggest a protective role for cheese against breast cancer." Highest CLA in blood lowered risk for br. ca. by 60%

Aro, A., Nutrition & Cancer, vol.38, no.2, p.151, 2000

(looks like a lightning bolt) isomers. Bacteria in the gut of ruminants, like cows, sheep, deer, and buffalo, can produce CLA. Yet there is more CLA in grilled beef than raw beef, so the cooking process also enhances CLA content.[28] Of all the nutrition factors studied, CLA is one of the more impressive at arresting cancer cells in animal and test tube studies.[29]

CLA may be able to help the cancer patient through:

♦ Cellular communication. Healthy cells know when to grow and when to stop growing and when to die. Cancer cells lose this crucial "knowledge". There is evidence that CLA assists in "signal transduction" pathways that tell cancer cells to commit suicide (apoptosis).

♦ Protection from toxins. CLA provided major cancer protection against toxins (like DMBA) in animal studies.[30] CLA may protect us from cancer by encouraging detoxification pathways.[31]

♦ Antioxidant. There is a large and growing list of non-essential dietary antioxidants, including CLA, ellagic acid, curcumin, quercetin, and epicatechin, which have shown remarkable abilities to slow down the oxidative damage, or the "rusting" that occurs constantly in all human beings.[32] Antioxidants can provide immune cells with a protective shield as they dowse the cancer cells with potent free radicals. Antioxidants can protect the healthy tissue of the patient, while the chemotherapy and radiation become more selective at destroying tumor tissue that does not absorb antioxidants as effectively as do healthy cells. However, other researchers found that if CLA is an antioxidant, then it does not protect cells in the usual antioxidant fashion, as shown by protection of cell membranes in culture.[33]

♦ Inhibitor of the cancer cascade. Cancer results from a series of deterioration steps in the cells. Cancer results after the stages of initiation, promotion, and progression have occurred. Hyperplasia (rapid cell growth) can worsen into metaplasia (above normal cell growth), can further deteriorate into dysplasia (abnormal cell growth), which can become neoplasia (new form of cell growth, or cancer). There are numerous pre-cancerous

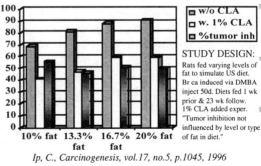

DOES CONJUGATED LINOLEIC ACID (CLA)
PREVENT BREAST CANCER in animals?

tumor incidence

Legend: w/o CLA; w. 1% CLA; %tumor inh

STUDY DESIGN:
Rats fed varying levels of fat to simulate US diet. Br ca induced via DMBA inject 50d. Diets fed 1 wk prior & 23 wk follow. 1% CLA added exper. "Tumor inhibition not influenced by level or type of fat in diet."

10% fat 13.3% fat 16.7% fat 20% fat

Ip, C., Carcinogenesis, vol.17, no.5, p.1045, 1996

conditions, including fibrocystic breast disease, diverticulosis (colon), oral leukoplakia (mouth), cervical dysplasia (cervix), and benign prostatic hypertrophy (prostate), which all need more attention from both patient and physician. CLA seems to prevent this cancer cascade or avalanche from occurring. CLA also reverses cancer in animals even when they possess a genetic predisposition for cancer.[34]

♦ Neutralizing the potential damage from other fats. Animals fed varying levels of fat (10-20% by weight, similar to American diet) in the diet and different types of fat (corn oil vs lard) were protected against breast cancer when fed only 1% of the diet as CLA.[35]

♦ Generating unknown but valuable fatty acid by-products from the liver. In animal studies, CLA in the diet generated a unique collection of fats in the liver and outside of the liver.[36] Maybe CLA also provides the raw ingredient for the liver to make something very valuable in the body.

♦ Shuts down abnormal cell growth. CLA in test tube studies (in vitro) has shown a remarkable ability as a cytotoxic (kills cancer cells) and cytostatic (stops or slows cancer growth) agent in a wide variety of human cancers, including melanoma, colorectal, prostate, ovarian, glioblastoma (brain), mesothelioma, leukemia, and breast.[37]

♦ Some studies have found that CLA enhances immune functions[38] while another study showed no effect on the immune system while feeding the animals a diet that was 50% sucrose.[39] As I have stated repeatedly, a high sugar diet will encourage cancer growth beyond the inhibitory effect of any single anticancer nutrient, including CLA. A high sugar diet is a much more powerful "vector" than micronutrients.

♦ Improve glucose and insulin levels. CLA manages to also make cells more sensitive to insulin, thus lowering insulin requirements and blood glucose levels. These researchers from Penn State and Purdue boldly state: "CLA may prove to be an important therapy for the prevention and treatment of non-insulin dependent diabetes mellitus."[40] Controlling blood glucose can provide the cancer patient with major assistance in slowing cancer growth.

♦ Timing is crucial. Studies with animals show that when CLA is fed to animals from post-weaning through puberty, it can prevent breast cancer from occurring even when a potent carcinogen is injected in the animals. However, if animals are deprived of CLA until the breast cancer occurs, then CLA must be fed to the animal for the remainder of its life in order to prevent a recurrence of cancer.[41] Apparently, CLA in young animals helps to ensure proper maturation of the mammary glands and to prevent the initiation and promotion phases of cancer.

Basically, CLA is one of the more promising, non-toxic, inexpensive, anti-cancer, anti-heart disease, anti-diabetes nutrients to come along in the history of nutrition science.

FAT CONSUMPTION IN AMERICA

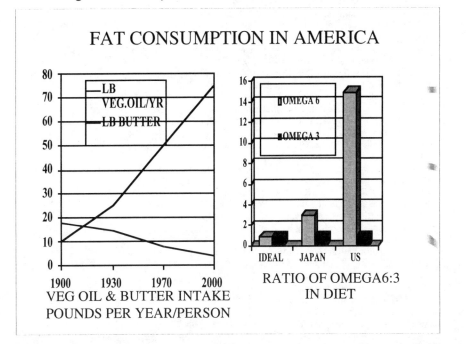

VEG OIL & BUTTER INTAKE
POUNDS PER YEAR/PERSON

RATIO OF OMEGA6:3
IN DIET

PATIENT PROFILE: REVERSING COLON CANCER
B.D. was diagnosed with stage 4 colon cancer metastasis to the liver, spleen, stomach, and intestines. Surgeons said the tumor was inoperable. Wife purchased this book and began using principles of food and supplements. Tumor on liver has shrunk from the size of a large grapefruit to half that size. Patient gained back 20 of 50 pounds that he had lost. Tumor markers dropped from 75 to 20 in 2 months. Patient and doctor are confident that a cure is in sight.

ENDNOTES

[1] . Connor, W., Am.J.Clin.Nutr., vol.71, no.1, p.171S, Jan.2000
[2] . Gorlin, R., Archives Intern. Med., vol.148, p.2043, Sept.1988
[3] . Karmali, RA, J. Nat. Cancer Inst., vol.73, p.457, 1984
[4] . Wan, JM, et al., Fed. Amer Soc Exper Biol., vol.A350, p.21, 1988
[5] . Burns, CP, et al., Nutrition Reviews, vol.48, p.233, June 1990
[6] . Guffy, MM, et al., Cancer Research, vol.44, p.1863, 1984
[7] . Cannizzo, F., et al., Cancer Research, vol.49, p.3961, 1981
[8] . Begin, ME, et al., J.Nat.Cancer Inst., vol.77, p.1053, 1986
[9] . Karmali, RA, J.Internal Med. suppl, vol.225, p.197, 1989
[10] . Osborne, MP, et al., Cancer Investigation, vol.6, p.629, 1988

[11] . Ross, JA, Curr.Opin.Coin.Nutr.Metab.Care, vol.2, no.3, p.219, May 1999

[12] . Hardman, WE, J.Nutr., vol.132, no.11 supp, p.3508S, Nov.2002

[13] . Kelley, DS, Nutrition, vol.17, no.7, p.669, Jul.2001

[14] . Woutersen, RA, Mutat.Res, vol.443, no.1, p.111, Jul.1999

[15] . Rose, DP, Nutr.Cancer, vol.37, no.2, p.119, 2000

[16] . Lin,Y., Cancer Letters, vol.124, pl.181, 1998

[17] . Begin, ME, et al., Prostaglandins, Leukotriennes, and Medicine, vol.19, p.177, Aug.1985; see also Begin, ME, Anticancer Research, vol.6, p291, 1986

[18] . Takeda, S., et al., Anticancer Research, vol.12, p.329, 1992

[19] . Vander Merwe, CF, et al., British J.Clin.Practice, vol.41, p.907, 1987

[20] . Begin, ME, et al., Prostaglandins, Leukotrienes & Medicine, vol.19, p.177, 1985

[21] . Brohult, A., et al., Acta.Obstet.Gynecol.Scand., vol.56, p.441, 1977

[22] . Brohult, A., et al., Acta.Obstet. Gynecol.Scand., vol.58, p.203, 1979

[23] . Brohult, A., et al., Acta. Chem.Scand., vol.24, p.730, 1970

[24] . Brohult, A., et al., Acta Obstet.Gynecol.Scand., vol.65, p.779, 1986; see also Acta.Obstet.Gynecol.Scand., vol.57, p.79, 1978

[25] . Riel, RR, J.Dairy Sci., vol.46, p.102, 1963

[26] . Knekt, P., et al., Br.J.Cancer, vol.73, p.687, 1996

[27] . Hirayama, T., in DIET AND HUMAN CARCINOGENESIS, Joosens, JV , p.191, Elsevier, NY

[28] . Sebedio, JL, et al., Biochimica et Biophysica Acta, vol.1345, p.5, 1997

[29] . Ip, C., et al., Nutrition & Cancer, vol.27, no.2, p.131, 1997

[30] . Ip, C., et al.; Cancer Research, vol.54, p.1212, 1994

[31] . Liew,C., et al., Carcinogenesis, vol.16, no.12, p.3037, 1995

[32] . Decker, EA, Nutrition Reviews, vol.53, no.3, p.49, Mar.1995

[33] . van den Berg,JJM, et al., Lipids, vol.30, no.7, p.599, 1995

[34] . Ip, C., et al., Carcinogenesis, vol.18, no.4, p.755, 1997

[35] . Ip, C., et al., Carcinogenesis, vol.17, no.5, p.1045, 1996

[36] . Belury, MA, et al., Lipids, vol.32, no.2, p.199, 1997

[37] . Shultz, TD, et al., Cancer Letters, vol.63, p.125, 1992; see also Visonneau, S., et al., J.Fed.Amer.Society Experimental Biology, vol.10, p.A182, 1996

[38] . Cook, ME, et al., Poultry Science, vol.72, p.1301, 1993; see also Miller, CC, et al., Biochem.Biophys.Res.Commun., vol.198, p.1107, 1994

[39] . Wong, MW, et al., Anticancer Research, vol.17, p.987, 1997

[40] . Houseknecht, KL, et al., Biochem. Biophys.Res.Commun., vol.244, p.678, 1998

[41] . Ip, C., et al., Nutrition & Cancer, vol.24, p.241, 1995

CHAPTER 19

★

MINERALS

"The war on cancer has been a qualified failure." John Bailar, MD,
PhD, former editor of the Journal of the National Cancer Institute

---

WHAT'S AHEAD?
Minerals are inorganic substances that provide structure and enzyme
activity in the human body.

↪ Since modern agriculture does not add trace
minerals back to the soil, our food is becoming
increasingly devoid of essential trace minerals.

↪ Selenium and magnesium play key roles in cancer prevention and
reversal.

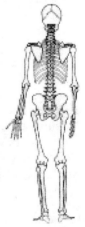

Minerals are the inorganic substances left over in ashes. Organic matter (based on carbon) can be burned. Minerals cannot be burned, although they will melt or vaporize at very high temperatures. Minerals in the human body work in many different arenas, from the structure provided by calcium in the bones and teeth, to the regulatory effect in enzymes provided by zinc, to the detoxifying effect from molybdenum and selenium. The body is a giant electrical battery, with minerals and water providing the conduction of electricity that keeps us healthy. While modern agriculture adds nitrogen (N), phosphorus (P), and potassium (K) to the soil, the remaining 60 minerals that are found in the human body are not added to the soil, thus are found in ever-diminishing amounts in our diet and bodies. This is not good. There are some crucial minerals involved in cancer prevention and reversal (such as selenium, zinc, chromium, magnesium). Iron is a unique mineral, since it is the rate-limiting mineral in new growth, from making babies, to growing your lawn, to spurring cancer growth. It is crucial that iron levels in your body and diet are ideal to recover from cancer and do not favor the growth of cancer.

> **MINERAL** (best form for absorption) suggested daily dosage
> Primary functions in human body, anti-cancer activities.

> **Calcium (glycinate, ascorbate) 100-500 mg**
> Electrolyte balance and cellular communication

Calcium is the most abundant mineral in the human body. While 99% of the body's calcium is bound up in the bones, the remaining 1% that is circulating is crucial for nerve and muscle function as well as regulating cell metabolism. There are calcium receptor sites on most cell membranes that help to control the flow of nutrients into and out of the cell as well as cell proliferation.

More than 5% of hospitalized cancer patients have elevated levels of calcium in the blood (hypercalcemia).[1] This is not because the patient is eating too much calcium, but caused by either a parathyroid hormone substance secreted by the tumor, or tumors cause the release of bone stores, or elevated calcium levels are caused by cell membranes not being able to maintain cell integrity. The calcium may get jettisoned when the cell has abnormal pH, perhaps from yeast infections.

Best food sources of calcium include dairy products, dark green leafy vegetables (like kale and spinach), and cooked bones (like in canned salmon. While the RDA of calcium is 800-1,200 milligrams daily, most Americans fall well short of this mark. Best supplemental sources of calcium are soluble forms of aspartate, citrate, lactate, orotate, etc. Calcium works with magnesium, sodium, potassium, and some ultra-trace minerals to regulate the "battery of life", or cell membrane potential that is crucial. Calcium also works with magnesium, phosphorus, protein, zinc, vitamin C, B-6, boron, and other nutrients to maintain proper mineralization of the skeleton, while dumping just the right amount of calcium into the bloodstream to keep the heart pumping merrily. Calcium metabolism is truly a delicate balancing act.

A low calcium intake increases the risk for colon cancer.[2] This effect may be due to calcium binding to bile acids in the colon to prevent carcinogenic by-products from forming, or due to the role calcium may play in regulating new cell growth. In human cancer patients, supplemental calcium increased the efficacy of radiation therapy to the bones and vulva.[3] Half of the patients with colon polyps (pre-cancerous growth) who were given supplements of calcium (1,250 mg as carbonate) had a significant decrease in cell proliferation. Calcium seems to tame the beast of hyperproliferative growth, like pre-cancerous growths.[4] Patients at high risk for developing colon cancer all showed a decrease in colon cell proliferation with calcium supplements.[5]

Magnesium (aspartate, glycinate)   150 mg
Essential for energy metabolism, low intake can spontaneously induce lymphoma

Magnesium is essential in at least 300 different enzyme reactions in the human body, including the pervasive conversion of ATP for energy. In animals, magnesium deficiency can spontaneously generate bone tumors and lymphomas.[6] Numerous studies show that a diet low in magnesium will increase the risk for various forms of cancer. Magnesium not only works with other electrolytes to maintain the sodium-potassium pump, but also has a central role in regulating DNA synthesis and the cell cycle.

The RDA for magnesium has been lowered from 400 milligrams daily to 350 mg, not because the evidence warranted this change but because few Americans came even close to consuming the RDA. The average American intake is 143-266 mg/day, which explains why low magnesium intake has been linked to an increase in the incidence of hypertension, heart disease, migraines, fatigue, immune suppression, fibromyalgia, glaucoma, and much more. Best food sources of magnesium are kelp, whole grains, nuts, and molasses. Magnesium aspartate is the best absorbed form of magnesium supplements.

Symptoms of magnesium deficiency include depression, excess sweating, fatigue, frequent infections, and high blood pressure, which are all common in cancer patients. Many drugs, including diuretics, and alcohol cause a loss of magnesium from the system.

Potassium (citrate)   300-500 mg
Essential ingredient for "electrolyte soup" that dictates healthy cell membrane

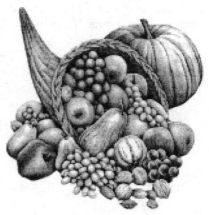

Potassium is the primary cation (positively charged ion) inside the human cell. Potassium is found primarily in plant foods, with the richest sources being avocado, banana, tomato, and potato. Meats and fish can provide a significant amount of potassium to the diet. Many studies show that a diet high in sodium (or salt) and low in potassium (found in plant food) increases the risk for heart disease and cancer, among other diseases.[7] Potassium is crucial for nerve and muscle function and the conversion of glucose into glycogen for storage. The first symptom of potassium deficiency is usually weakness and fatigue.

The FDA has set an upper limit of 99 mg allowed of potassium in tablet form due to the concerns that people with poorly functioning kidneys (less than 1% of the population) might suffer potassium overload. Meanwhile, 90% of the population do not get optimal amounts of potassium in the diet, especially in the right ratio with the other crucial electrolytes of sodium, calcium, and magnesium. The range of potassium intake that is recommended by the RDA board is 1.9 to 5.6 grams daily. Up to 3 grams daily can be lost in perspiration and through the use of diuretics, like anti-hypertensive medication, alcohol, and coffee. While many American health authorities have crusaded against the use of salt (sodium) at the table, actually a deficiency of potassium, magnesium, and calcium are much more likely to be at fault in hypertension, heart disease, and various forms of cancer.

Zinc (yeast bound, picolinate, or chelate)   10 mg
Potent immune stimulant, essential in over 200 enzyme reactions in the body, including immune cell production and cell replication.

Zinc is the most multi-talented mineral in the body, participating in everything from sexual development, to immunity, to maintenance of nerve tissue, to the zinc-dependent antioxidant enzyme SOD (superoxide dismutase). Apoptosis, or programmed cell death, which is missing in cancer cells, may be regulated by zinc.[8] The average American consumes about 10 milligrams of zinc daily, which is well shy of the 15 mg RDA. Best food sources of zinc include shell fish, organ meats, meat, fish, pumpkin seeds, ginger root, nuts, and seeds.

Zinc is a crucial mineral for optimal immune functioning. Low zinc status will lower T-cell counts, reduce thymic hormone levels, and reduce reactions to pathogens and cancer. Reduced zinc levels and cancer are both common in the elderly. Zinc supplements of only 20 mg/day improved immune functions via jump starting the thymus gland in institutionalized elderly subjects.[9] Loss of appetite is one of the first symptoms of zinc deficiency. Zinc supplements usually restore appetite, which is a common problem in cancer patients. A low intake of zinc increases the risk for cancers of the esophagus[10], lung[11], and prostate.[12] Cadmium from tobacco and pollution will readily replace zinc in the prostate and may lead to benign prostatic hypertrophy (enlarged prostate) and prostate cancer.[13]

SAFETY ISSUES. Supplements of zinc should be in the 20-60 mg/day range, since doses of 150 mg/day have been shown to trigger copper deficiency and depress the cardio-protective HDL-cholesterol.

Iron (yeast bound or chelate) 2-10 mg
   Essential for red blood cell synthesis (hematopoeisis) to properly oxygenate tissues, essential for energy metabolism and immune cell production

---

Iron has the narrowest "window of efficacy" of all nutrients and is the best nutritional example of "too much or too little will create a health problem". Iron is one of the most commonly deficient nutrients in America and around the world.[14] Yet consuming iron salts through enriched white flour without eating enough antioxidants can bring about a troublesome biochemical environment where the iron can create free radicals, damage the DNA, and cause heart disease or cancer.[15] Iron can be hoarded by infecting bacteria and cancer cells to further invade healthy tissue. I have seen many cancer patients who developed anemia while the cancer was winning the fight, yet had a sudden rise in serum ferritin iron stores when the cancer cells are being destroyed and releasing their iron content. Iron deficiency can lead to suppressed immune function.[16] Therefore, iron supplements must be provided:

◆ in conservative doses: 5-25 mg/day
◆ in the most bioavailable chelated form
◆ in conjunction with multiple antioxidants to protect against the potential free radical damage from iron.

   Iron is involved in:

✓ hemoglobin production for transporting oxygen to the cells
✓ myoglobin in the muscles
✓ oxidative burst as immune cells kill cancer cells
✓ one of the ways to induce cancer death through chemo drugs
✓ cytochromes for energy metabolism
✓ other iron-containing enzymes like NADH.

   Symptoms of deficiency include anemia, lethargy, behavioral problems, poor body temperature regulation, reduced immunity and others. Since the RDA for iron is 10-15 mg and most Americans do not consume this amount, the right form (chelated) of iron supplements may be extremely valuable for people who also get adequate antioxidants at the same time to prevent the metabolic wrecking-ball effect from iron as a free radical.

   SAFETY ISSUES. Many cancer patients are found to be anemic, which can precipitate the "knee jerk" response for recommending high doses of iron supplements, such as ferrous sulphate. This is a very bad idea. As mentioned above, iron supplements should be taken in conservative doses and in chelated versions, such as the heme form found in the blood. However, there is a prevailaing opinion among scientists that iron can be harmful and even carcinogenic.[17] Some scientists are using an iron-binding drug, Deferoxamine, to treat cancer patients[18], as if we haven't learned our lesson after 30 years of trying to "starve the cancer out of the patient" with anti-metabolites, such as leucovorin. If iron is such a bad guy, then why did researchers at the National Institutes of Health and Harvard find that the more iron in the person's serum, the lower the risk for heart disease (80% reduction in risk) and all-cause mortality (38% lower in men, 28% lower in women)?[19] Iron is an essential mineral for ALL OF LIFE, including humans and tumors. Unbound iron, which is caused by acidosis, is a serious issue that needs to be addressed by the health care practitioner.

Actually, iron is a rate-limiting growth nutrient for almost all forms of life, from a growing infant, to a tumor cell, to your lawn grass. The innate wisdom of the human body recognizes that iron can be a wrecking ball by generating free radicals and can also help the "enemy within" of any bacteria, yeast, or tumor cell to grow. That is why 99% of the iron in the human body is bound to hemoglobin or transferrin. It is UNBOUND iron that creates the problem for humans. And why does the iron become detached from its normal escort? The answer is: reduction in pH, or acidifying of the body tissues, probably from fungal metabolites. Yeast give off a host of organic acids that reduce the pH in the human body and create all sorts of problems, one of which is unbinding the iron. This effect is not unlike unhitching your prize stallion that normally does yoeman's work when attached to the plow or family wagon. But allowed to run amuck, the stallion (or iron) can do great damage. The key here is not to throw the baby out with the bathwater. We need adequate iron to extract energy from food (cytochrome system) and conduct aerobic metabolism (hemoglobin bringing oxygen to the cells). We also use iron as part of our immune system in killing invaders, such as cancer, with an oxidative burst. Any other strategy of supplementing iron can be counterproductive for the cancer patient.

Copper (chelate) 1 mg
    Involved in several important enzyme reactions, including cytochromes for energy and superoxide dismutase for free radical protection

---

Copper is important for the construction of tough connective tissues, which is how the body tries to envelop a tumor. Copper is crucial for energy metabolism via cytochrome c. Copper supplements have slowed tumor growth in animals.[20] Copper, via ceruloplasmin, helps to prevent the oxidation of fatty acids that can destroy DNA and cell membranes. The RDA of copper is 1.5-3 mg/day. Best sources of copper in the diet include organ meats, shellfish, and legumes.

Iodine (yeast bound, or kelp, or potassium iodide) 50-150 mcg
  Assists the thyroid gland in regulating basal metabolism, which is often low in cancer patients, is a selective toxin for disease-causing microorganisms in the gut

---

  Iodine is primarily involved in the thyroid hormone, thyroxin, which regulates basal metabolism throughout the body. Additionally, iodine seems to modify the effects of estrogen on breast tissue, thus reducing fibrocystic breast disease, which doubles the risk for developing breast cancer.[21] Low thyroid output is a fundamental insult in many women with breast cancer.[22]

  Seafood, especially kelp, provides the best sources of iodine. The fortification of salt with iodine (iodized salt) has been a classic example of public health measures that significantly reduced the incidence of goiter, or iodine deficiency expressed as clinical hypothyroidism. Yet, for various reasons, subclinical hypothyroidism is still rampant in the U.S. Iodine is also a selective toxin for microorganisms in the gut, helping to kill parasites and intestinal infections.

  NOTE. If basal temperature is below 97.8 F, then medical assistance may be needed in the form of prescription thyroxin supplements to bolster basal metabolism.

Manganese (yeast bound or chelate) 1-2 mg
  Essential mineral cofactor in various enzyme reactions, including an important antioxidant system of SOD (superoxide dismutase)

  Manganese-deficient animals develop low insulin output and problems with the connective tissue and processing of fats. Recommended intake is 2-5 milligrams daily for adults, with over half the female population consuming less than adequate amounts of manganese.[23] Best food sources of manganese are whole grains, nuts, and fruits grown on manganese-rich (properly fertilized) soil. There are at least 3 different minerals, including manganese, copper, and zinc, that play a role in variations of the critical antioxidant enzyme system SOD.

Chromium (yeast bound, picolinate, GTF niacinate) 200-600 mcg
  Essential mineral for proper energy metabolism, especially related to controlling blood sugar levels and preventing lean tissue wasting

---

  Chromium is at the center of the glucose tolerance factor (GTF) which works with insulin to allow glucose into body cells. Without adequate GTF in the body, insulin levels are raised, which can be disastrous. Glucose-dependent tissues, like the brain, lens of the eye, kidney, and lungs, suffer the most when blood sugar levels are abnormal. Without proper burning of glucose in the cells, the body resorts to the backup energy substrates of protein (which causes lean tissue wasting, a.k.a. cachexia) and fat (which elevates levels of fats in the blood for increased risk of heart disease). GTF is also critical for immune functions and may even play a role in regulating cell growth.[24] Deficiencies of chromium in humans typically lead to impaired glucose metabolism, elevated blood fats, and peripheral neuropathy (tingling numbness in extremities).

An estimated 90% of the American population do not consume the minimum recommended intake of 50 micrograms daily. Researchers at the United States Department of Agriculture have estimated that up to 25% of heart disease in America could be prevented merely by consuming adequate quantities of chromium. Human subjects who took 400 micrograms daily of chromium supplements lost more fat and gained more lean tissue than those who took 200 mcg.[25] Another study found that 600 mcg of chromium provided signficant drops in fasting blood glucose in diabetics.[26] Several studies have shown that chromium supplements lower fasting blood glucose levels in normal healthy individuals.[27] Remember, a crucial strategy in fighting cancer is to starve the cancer of its favorite fuel, which is sugar.

Chromium is concentrated in whole grains and beans grown on chromium-rich soil, which is rare since chromium is not typically used in fertilizer. Brewer's yeast, liver, black pepper and molasses are decent sources of chromium. Chromium is stripped out of most food refining processes, including the milling of wheat to white flour and cane sugar to refined 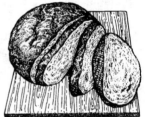 white sugar. 86% of Americans consume white bread rather than whole grain bread. The average American consumes 140 pounds per year of refined sugar, which increases the need for chromium while increasing the EXCRETION of chromium. The most bioavailable forms of chromium supplements are GTF, chromium picolinate, and chromium polynicotinate; the least bioavailable are the chromium salts like chromium chloride.

Selenium (yeast bound or selenomethionine) 200-600 mcg
Immune stimulant, detoxifying agent via glutathione peroxidase, may selectively control the growth of abnormal tissue

---

Selenium presents a fascinating story for the cancer patient. Until the 1960s, selenium was considered a toxic mineral by the FDA. In 1982, I developed a line of vitamin supplements made in the U.S. and shipped to Australia, which were rejected at their customs office because these supplements contained selenium, which was still considered toxic by the Australian FDA. An abundance of information beginning to appear in the 1960s showed that selenium may be one of our greatest allies in the war on cancer. Selenium is found in widely varying amounts in the diet, due to huge differences of selenium found in the soil. In places like South Dakota and Montana, there is so much selenium in the soil that animals grazing on the grass can develop selenium toxicity, or "blind staggers", which involves nerve and behavior problems. Some historians claim that General Custer's horses bolted on him in the Battle of Little Bighorn because the horses were suffering from selenium toxicity. In Finland, where the selenium-deficient soil leads to a high incidence of cancer and heart disease, wheat flour is enriched with selenium just like we add iron to our white flour.

Wheat germ, seafood, and Brazil nuts are the best sources of selenium. The RDA is 70 micrograms, while the average intake is just over 100 micrograms. When lining up maps showing selenium content in the soil with cancer incidence, there is a strong link between low selenium intake and higher cancer risk.[28] In a recent prospective double-blind human intervention study, supplements providing 200 mcg of selenium were able to reduce the incidence of various cancers by up to 60%.[29] Selenium is a potent immune stimulator.[30]

Selenium-deficient animals have more heart damage from the chemo drug, adriamycin.[31] Supplements of selenium and vitamin E in humans did not reduce the efficacy of the chemo drugs against ovarian and cervical cancer.[32] Animals with

CAN SELENIUM SUPPLEMENTS ALTER CANCER INCIDENCE?

REDUCTION IN CANCER INCIDENCE WITH 200 mcg/day SELENIUM

statistically significant P<0.05 results

cancer mort. 28/57
cancer incid. 77/119
lung cancer 17/31
prostate ca 13/35
colorectal ca 8/19

% less

STUDY DESIGN: 1312 patients 7 US clinics history basal/squamous ca, age 63 yr (18-80),randomized 1983-91, treated 4.5 yrs 200 mcg selenium (yeast), followup 6.4 yr., no diff.basal/squamous/melanoma incidence; Clark, JAMA, 276,1957,1996

implanted tumors were then treated with selenium and cis-platin (chemo drug) and showed a reduced toxicity to the drug with no change in anti-cancer activity.[33] Selenium supplements helped repair DNA damage from a carcinogen in animals.[34] Selenium was selectively toxic to human leukemia cells in culture.[35]

Garlic grown on selenium-enriched soil develops a unique anti-cancer activity. Selenium in a biological envelope, such as yeast-bound or selenomethionine, is the best absorbed and safest form of selenium.

SAFETY ISSUES. Selenium toxicity may begin as low as 1,000 mcg/day in some people, but toxicity is more common at about 65,000 micrograms (65 mg) for the average healthy adult.[36]

Molybdenum (yeast bound or chelate)   100-200 mcg
Essential mineral for detoxification pathways

Molybdenum functions as a mineral cofactor in hydroxylation enzyme reactions, such as uric acid and sulfite processing. When sulfites build up in the human system, cysteine metabolism is affected, which is crucial for detoxification. Most diets supply only around 50-100 micrograms daily of molybdenum and do not meet the safe and adequate levels of 75-250 mcg recommended by the Food and Nutrition Board. There is no RDA for molybdenum. Large-scale farming does not add molybdenum to the soil as part of broad spectrum fertilization, which further compounds the problems of common molybdenum deficiencies. It is found in vegetables that are grown on molybdenum-rich soil. Beans and organ meats are the best sources of molybdenum. This is an extremely non-toxic mineral, with animal studies showing that an intake of 100-5,000 milligrams per kilogram of diet is necessary to produce toxicity symptoms.[37]

Vanadium (vanadyl sulfate)   20-60 mcg
Crucial mineral for controlling blood glucose

Vanadium is not added back to the soil in agri-business, and hence may be missing from the American diet, which typically contains 10-60 micrograms daily of vanadium.[38] When non-insulin dependent diabetics were supplemented with 100 milligrams daily (100,000 micrograms) of vanadyl sulfate, blood glucose levels dropped by 14%.[39] Vanadium in the form of vanadyl sulfate has shown promise in helping to control rises in blood glucose in human diabetics.[40] Toxicity may begin at 13 milligrams (13,000 micrograms) of vanadium daily. Best food sources of vanadium include mushrooms, shellfish, dill, parsley, and black pepper.

PATIENT PROFILE: BEAT LUNG CANCER
E.M. was a 52 year old female with advanced lung cancer when she was admitted to our hospital. Her doctor back home had told her to "get her affairs in order." She began chemo and nutrition with excellent compliance in her diet. A year later, she was in complete remission. We planted a tree at our Celebrate Life Reunion in honor of her 5 year survival, the official definition of a cure by the American Cancer Society.

ENDNOTES

[1] . Heath, DA, Br., Med.J., vol.298, p.1468, 1989

[2] . Sorenson, AW, et al., Nutr.Cancer, vol.11, p.135, 1988

[3] . Iakovkeva, SS, Arkh.Patol., vol.42, p.93, 1980

[4] . Wargovich, MJ, J.Am.Coll.Nutr., vol.7, p.295, 1988

[5] . Buset, M., et al., Cancer Res., vol.46, p.5426, 1986

[6] . Seelig, MS, in ADJUVANT NUTRITION IN CANCER TREATMENT, p.284, Quillin, P (eds), Cancer Treatment Research Foundation, Arlington Heights, IL 1994

[7] . Jansson, B., Cancer Detect.Prevent., vol.14, p.563, 1991

[8] . Cousins, RJ, in PRESENT KNOWLEDGE IN NUTRITION, p.293, ILSI, Washington, 1996

[9] . Boukaiba, N, et al., Am.J.Clin.Nutr., vol.57, p.566, 1993

[10] . Barch, DH, J.Am.Coll.Nutr., vol.8, p.99, 1989

[11] . Allen, JI, et al., Am.J.Med., vol.79, p.209, 1985

[12] . Whelen, P., et al., Br.J.Urol., vol.55, p.525, 1983

[13] . Feustel, A., et al., Urol.Res., vol.12, p.253, 1984

[14] . Yip, R., et al., in PRESENT KNOWLEDGE IN NUTRITION, p.277, ILSI, Washington, 1996

[15] . Beard, J., in IRON DEFICIENCY ANEMIA, p.99, National Academy Press, 1993

[16] . Dallman, PR, Am.J.Clin.Nutr., vol.46, p.329, 1987

[17] . Reizenstein, P., Med.Oncol. & Tumor Pharmacother., vol.8, no.1, p.229, 1991

[18] . Donfrancesco, A, et al., Acta Haematol., vol.95, p.66, 1996

[19] . Corti, MC, et al., American J.Cardiology, vol.79, p.120, 1997

[20] . Sorenson, RJ, in TRACE SUBSTANCES IN ENVIRONMENTAL HEALTH XVI, U.Missouri 1982

[21] . Ghent, WR, et al., Can.J.Surg., vol.36,p.453, 1993

[22] . Callebout, E., in THE DEFINITIVE GUIDE TO CANCER, Diamond, J. (eds), p.116, Future Medicine, Tiburon, 1997

[23] . Keen, CL, et al., in PRESENT KNOWLEDGE IN NUTRITION, p.339, ILSI, Washington, 1996

[24] . Stoecker, BJ, in PRESENT KNOWLEDGE IN NUTRITION, p.347, ILSI, Washington, 1996

[25] . Evans, GW, et al., J.Inorganic Biochem., vol.49, p.177, 1993

[26] . Mossop, RT, Central African J.Med., vol.29, p.80, 1983

[27] . Anderson, RA, et al., Metabolism, vol.32, p.894, 1983

[28] . Schrauzer, GN, in VITAMINS, NUTRITION, AND CANCER, p.240, Karger, Basel, 1984

[29] . Clark, LC, et al., J.Amer.Med.Assoc., vol.276, p.1957, 1996

[30] . Kiremidjian-Schumacher, L., et al., Environmental Res., vol.42, p.277, 1987

[31] . Coudray, C., et al., Basic Res.Cardiol., vol.87, p.173, 1992

[32] . Sundstrom, H., et al., Carcinogenesis, vol.10, p.273, 1989

[33] . Ohkawa, K., et al., Br.J.Cancer, vol.58, p.38, 1988

[34] . Lawson, T., et al.,Chem.Biol.Interactions, vol.45, p.95, 1983

[35] . Milner, JA, et al., Cancer Research, vol.41, p.1652, 1981

[36] . Hathcock, JN, in MICRONUTRIENTS AND IMMUNE FUNCTIONS, vol.587, p.257, NY Acad.Sci., 1990

[37] . Nielsen, FH, in PRESENT KNOWLEDGE IN NUTRITION, p.359, ILSI, Washington, 1996

[38] . Harland, BF, et al., J.Am.Diet.Assoc., vol.94, p.891, 1994

[39] . Cohen, N., et al., J.Clin.Invest., vol.95, p.2501, 1995

[40] . Brichard, SM, et al., Trends Pharmacol.Sci., vol.16, p.265, 1995

CHAPTER 20

✲

ENZYMES

"Climb the mountains and get their good tidings. Nature's peace will flow into you as sunshine flows into trees. The winds will blow their own freshness into you, and the storms their energy, while cares will drop off like autumn leaves." John Muir, co-founder of national parks

---

WHAT'S AHEAD?

Enzymes are organic catalysts that either tear apart molecules or put them together. Life would be impossible without enzymes.

⤷ taking enzyme supplements with your meal can help to better digest and absorb the food

⤷ taking enzyme supplements (especially Wobenzym) in between meals can help to dissolve the coating around the cancer that makes it invisible to the immune system

---

Enzymes are organic catalysts that speed up the rate of a chemical reaction. In simple terms, enzymes in the body either "glue" stuff together (called conjugase) or tear stuff apart (called hydrolase). Without enzymes, life on earth could not exist. Enzymes wear out and are still a great source of mystery to leading researchers.

In the 1920s, scientists in Germany found that cancer patients seemed to lack a factor in the blood. They began injecting animal tumors with pineapple juice extract, which contains the proteolytic enzyme bromelain, and watched a measurable shrinkage or disappearance of many cancers in animals.

There are impressive studies showing that certain enzymes when taken orally as pills can reduce the toxicity of chemo and radiation, while extending the quality and quantity of life for most cancer patients. The German FDA has approved the use of injectable forms of enzymes, which are 100 times more potent than taking oral enzymes which must pass through the gut into the bloodstream. Enzymes taken in fairly large quantities on an empty stomach will be partially absorbed into the blood stream and may help fight the cancer. Enzymes taken with a meal will help digest the food in that meal, but probably will not be absorbed into the bloodstream to fight the cancer.

Enzymes (especially protease) 50,000 USP units or 200-1000 mg
Break up circulating immune complexes to improve efficiency of immune system, erode protective coating on tumor, break down toxic by-products of tumor metabolism that create weight loss and depression in cancer patients.

There are literally millions of enzymes produced by your body each second. Without hydrolase enzymes in your gut, the digestion of food could not occur. Our body makes digestive enzymes to break down large food particles into usable molecules:

-proteins are digested into amino acids by the action of proteases, including trypsin and chymotrypsin

-starches are digested into simple sugars by the action of amylase

-fats are digested into fatty acids and glycerol by the action of lipase.

Our ancestors ate a diet high in uncooked foods. Cooking food denatures enzymes, like changing the white on an egg from waxey to white when it is cooked. It makes no difference whether you cook the food over a fire, on the barbeque, in the microwave oven, or fry it on the stovetop...all forms of heat denature enzymes. All living tissue contains an abundance of hydrolase enzymes as part of the lysosomes, or "suicide bags", which are there to mop up cellular debris and destroy invading organisms. When our ancestors ate this diet high in uncooked food, they were receiving a regular infusion of "enzyme therapy" as a lucky by-product. These hydrolytic enzymes would help to digest the food, and about 10% of the unused enzymes would end up crossing through the intestinal wall into the blood stream.

It is clear that people who are undernourished without being malnourished live a longer and healthier life. Why this occurs is less obvious. Many good European studies support the use of digestive enzymes as a critical component of cancer treatment. Your mouth, stomach, and intestines will make a certain amount of enzymes to digest your food into smaller molecules for absorption through the intestinal wall into the bloodstream. Enzymes absorbed into the bloodstream help to break up immune complexes, expose tumors to immune attack, and assist in cell differentiation. People who eat less food may live longer because they are able to absorb a certain percentage of their unused digestive enzymes, which then have many therapeutic benefits. Indeed, as far back as 1934, an

Austrian researcher, Dr. E. Freund, found that cancer patients do not have the "solubilizing" tumor-destroying enzymes in their blood that normal healthy people have.

The vast majority of cancer patients are older people, who have demonstrated a reduced output of digestive enzymes. Raw foods, which are high in hydrolytic enzymes, may sometimes help cancer patients.

There are 30 years of good research from Europe showing that enzyme therapy may help cancer patients. Digestive enzymes can:

♦ reduce tumor growth and metastasis in experimental animals.[1]
♦ prevent radon-induced lung cancer in miners.[2]
♦ improve 5 year survival in breast cancer patients. Stage I at 91%, stage II at 75%, and stage III at 50%.[3]
♦ bromelain (enzyme from pineapple) inhibited leukemic cell growth and induced human leukemia cells in culture to revert back to normal (cytodifferentiation).[4]
♦ reduce the complications of cancer, such as cachexia (weight loss), pain in joints, and depression.
♦ reduced the secondary infections that result from certain chemo and radiation methods, especially bleomycin-induced pneumotoxicity.[5]

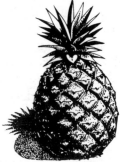

Proteolytic enzymes (proteases), such as bromelain from pineapple, seem to dissolve the "stealth" coating that keeps tumors invisible from the cancer patient's "radar". Proteases also break up "circulating immune complexes", which makes the immune system more efficient against cancer. Proteases have recently been found to be part of the body's complex regulation and communication system, possibly helping to induce apoptosis (suicide) in cancer cells.[6] Best food sources of these proteolytic enzymes are pineapple, papaya, mango, and kiwi.

Wobenzym is a unique clinically-tested product from Germany with a proprietary blend of various plant and animal-derived digestive enzymes, coupled with rutin (a bioflavonoid) all packaged in an enterically coated pill to survive the acid bath of the stomach and move into the intestines for absorption.

Serrapeptase (technically Serrato Peptidase) is a proteolytic enzyme produced by bacteria in the gut of silkworms. Serrapeptase has been studied and used extensively in Europe and Asia for over a quarter century, and seems to reduce swelling and digest unnecessary fibrin in the body. In one study, 70 women with

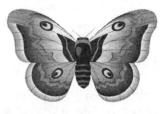

fibrocystic breast disease were randomly divided into either treatment with serrapeptase or placebo group. The serrapeptase group had a greater reduction in breast swelling and pain than the placebo group.[7]

Enzymes are measured in USP (United States Pharmacopeia) comparison to pancreatic extract. One of the functions of the pancreas is to make digestive enzymes. A 4x label on your enzymes means "4 times the potency of pancreatin USP". Therefore, 500 mg of 4X pancreatin is equal in digestive capacity to 2,000 mg of pancreatin USP. 50,000 USP units is a good target for any given meal or in between meal dosage.

Enzymes taken with a meal will help to digest the food, but will not be absorbed into the bloodstream to help fight the cancer. About 10% of enzymes taken on an empty stomach will be absorbed into the bloodstream to help fight the cancer. Enzymes are one of the more fragile molecules in nature, easily denatured by temperatures above 108 F.

PATIENT PROFILE: J.L. was a 54 year old school teacher who was diagnosed with advanced breast cancer. She underwent a bilateral mastectomy, followed by adjuvant chemo. She later had reconstructive surgery to create a very shapely figure, which was important to her. She changed her diet markedly, discarding the abundance of sweets that used to be her staples. She began taking a wide assortment of nutrition supplements. She also realized that the world did not need her as "director of the universe". She reached a peaceful settlement with her teenage daughter, who demanded too much of B.J. B.J. now spends lots of time walking the beaches near her home on the Atlantic Ocean. B.J. not only is disease-free, but says that cancer is the best thing that ever happened to her in rearranging her priorities in life.

ENDNOTES

[1]. Ransberger, K, et al., Medizinische Enzymforschungsgesellschaft, International Cancer Congress, Houston 1970

[2]. Miraslav, H., et al., Advances in Antimicrobial and Antineoplastic Chemotherapy, proceedings from 7th international congress of chemotherapy, Urban & Schwarzenberg, Munchen, 1972

[3]. Rokitansky, O., Dr. Med., no.1, vol.80, p.16ff, Austria

[4]. Maurer, HR, et al., Planta Medica, vol.54, no.5, p.377, 1988

[5]. Schedler, M., et al., 15th International Cancer Congress, Hamburg, Germany, Aug.1990

[6]. Mynott, TL, et al., J. Immunology, vol.163, no.5, p.2568, Sept.1, 1999

[7]. Kee, WH, Singapore Med.J., vol.30, no.1, p.48, 1989

Chapter 21

✴

VITAMINS

✴

"The optimum treatment of the cancer patient requires a concerted multi-disciplinary approach employing the full resources of surgery, radiotherapy, chemotherapy, immunotherapy and supportive care. The last named has received the least attention, although it might well possess great potential for therapeutic advance."[1]

Linus Pauling, PhD, Nobel Laureate, 1974

WHAT'S AHEAD?

Many vitamins are essential in the human diet, but are missing in the typical American diet. Vitamins in therapeutic levels are an essential part of a full-spectrum attack on cancer.

↳ some vitamins, such as vitamin E succinate and K, may help to destroy tumor cells directly

↳ some vitamins, such as C, can become a selective toxin against tumor cells

↳ some vitamins, such as B-6 and E, improve immune functions to help the body recognize and destroy cancer cells

---

A (palmitate) 2000-20,000 iu
    Down-regulates cancer at genetic level, immune stimulant, improves cell differentiation process, helps with cell-to-cell communication.

Along with iron, vitamin A is one of the most common micronutrient deficiencies in the world. Around the world, an estimated 500,000 people each year go permanently blind because of clinical vitamin A deficiency. Vitamin A was the first micronutrient to be recognized for its role in preventing cancer. Vitamin A is one of the most multi-talented of all substances in human nutrition and plays a key role in preventing and reversing cancer. While vitamin A and beta-carotene are considered interchangeable, more recent evidence shows that these two nutrients have some overlapping functions and some distinctly different functions. A drug analog of vitamin A (all trans retinoic acid) has become a near cure all for acute promyelocytic leukemia, with one study showing a 96% cure rate.[2] Some companies use an emulsified vitamin A so that it stays in the blood stream longer, which may be important for extremely high doses of A (>100,000 iu/day) in cancer patients.

All of the known functions of vitamin A relate either directly or indirectly to the cancer patient:

♦ **Cell division**. Billions of times each day, cells divide in the precarious process of cell division, i.e. proliferation or hyperplasia. Without vitamin A, this fragile process can easily turn into cancer, or neoplasia. Vitamin A is crucial for cancer prevention.[3] Vitamin A deficiency may be one of the primary insults leading to lung cancer.[4] There are probably binding sites on the human DNA for vitamin A. Researchers found that one of the most common cancers in Third World countries, cervical cancer, was linked to Human Papilloma Virus, which was then linked to shutting off the cancer-protective gene, called p53, which was then linked to a low intake of vitamin A. Essentially, vitamin A keeps the p53 active and protecting our DNA against cancer, even from viral attack.

♦ **Cell-to-cell communication**, a.k.a. gap junction. Cells communicate via a "telegraph" system of ions floating in and out of cell membrane pores. This intercellular communication helps to maintain cooperation and coordination of cell functions. Without vitamin A, the "telegraph" system becomes distorted, and cancer can arise.

♦ **Maintenance of epithelial tissue**, or skin. The vast majority of cancers, including lung, breast, colon, and prostate, all arise from the epithelial tissue and are called carcinomas. Other categories of cancers include: leukemia (cancer of the bone marrow that produces red & white cells), lymphoma (cancer of the lymph cells and glands), and sarcomas (cancers of the structural tissue).[5] When the body is deprived of vitamin A, skin (epithelial) cancer is more likely to result. Giving therapeutic doses of vitamin A has been shown to slow down and reverse some forms of cancer.

◆ **Immune stimulant**. Vitamin A deficiency brings changes in the mucosal membranes, changes in lymphocyte sub-populations, and altered T- and B-cell functions.[6] There are many studies linking vitamin A supplements to the curing of measles.[7] Vitamin A supplements brought a 19% reduction in respiratory infections in children.[8] HIV-positive pregnant women with the lowest quartile of serum vitamin A had a 400% increase in the risk of transmitting their HIV virus to their unborn infant.[9]

◆ **Anti-cancer activity**. Vitamin A supplements as sole therapy in patients with unresectable (cannot be surgically removed) lung cancer measurably improved immune functions and tumor response.[10] Vitamin A, and not beta-carotene, improved lymphocyte levels and reduced complications after surgery in lung cancer patients.[11] In patients treated for bladder cancer, the incidence of recurrence was 180% higher in patients who consumed the lowest quartile of vitamin A in the diet.[12] High doses of vitamin A (200,000 iu/week) were able to reduce damaged and potentially cancerous mouth cells by 96%.[13] Vitamin A and its synthetic analogues have been shown to improve cancer treatment in oral leukoplakia, laryngeal papillomatosis, superficial bladder carcinoma, cervical dysplasia, bronchial metaplasia, and preleukemia.[14] Vitamin A supplements of 300,000 iu per day were provided in a placebo-controlled trial with 307 patients with stage I non-small-cell lung cancer. 37% of the treated group experienced a recurrence, while 48% of the non-treated group had a recurrence, thus bringing a 25% reduction in tumor recurrence, when used as the sole therapy.[15]

SAFETY ISSUES. While vitamins, in general, are much safer than drugs, it is important to discuss vitamin A toxicity, which is by far the most common cause of vitamin toxicity. Up to 1 million iu of vitamin A per day has been given for 5 years without side effects in European cancer clinics.[16] One study found that women taking as little as 10,000 iu/day during pregnancy had a slightly elevated risk for having a child with birth defects (teratogenicity).[17] Another study from the National Institutes of Health found no increase in birth defects in women taking 25,000 iu/day of vitamin A. An FDA biochemist, John Hathcock, PhD, states that toxicity with vitamin A at these low levels mainly involves people with confounding medical conditions, including compromised liver function.[18] Cancer clinics in Europe often administer up to 2.5 million iu/day of vitamin A in emulsified form for several months under medical supervision. While these doses are not recommended without medical supervision, it shows the relative safety of vitamin A in the general population. Giving at least 300,000 iu per day of retinol palmitate in 138 lung cancer patients for at least 12 months created self-terminating unremarkable symptoms in less than 10% of these patients and only caused interruption of treatment in 3% due to symptoms that were potentially related to vitamin A excess. Upset stomach (dyspepsia), headache, nosebleeds, and mild hair loss were the most common and self-limiting symptoms.

Since primitive meat-eating populations would usually eat the liver of the animal first, which is the most concentrated source of pre-formed vitamin A, descendants of carnivorous people probably have a much greater tolerance and need for higher doses of A. By increasing the intake of vitamin E, many people will be able to avoid toxicity from high doses of vitamin A, since it is the lipid peroxide products from A that can cause damage to the liver. Vitamin E prevents lipid peroxidation. **PREGNANT WOMEN SHOULD NOT USE HIGH DOSES OF VITAMIN A.**

Beta-carotene 15 mg (=25,000 iu) as mixed natural carotenoids
Immune stimulant, helps with cell-to-cell communication

It is easy to appreciate the beauty of carotenoids on a crisp, fall day with the autumn foliage at its peak. Carotenoids are usually pigmented substances produced by plants to assist in photosynthesis and to protect the plant from the damaging effects of the sun's radiation. Of the 800 or so carotenoids that have been isolated, the most famous are beta-carotene, alpha-carotene, lutein, zeaxanthin, lycopene, and beta-cryptoxanthin. Most carotenoids are pigmented molecules that are red, yellow, or orange in color. A few carotenoids, such as phytoene and phytofluene, are colorless.

Over 200 epidemiological studies[19] show that a diet rich in fruit and vegetables will lower the risk for a variety of cancers. Of the 15% of annual lung cancer patients who are not smokers, which totals over 22,000 deaths per year, fruits and vegetables can provide major protection against lung cancer.[20]

Beta-carotene and other carotenoids have been thoroughly reviewed regarding their role in cancer and it has been found: "...carotenoids exert an important influence in modulating the actions of carcinogens."[21] Beta-carotene has been shown to play a major role in the "telegraph"-like communication between cells that prevents or reverses abnormal growths. This "gap junction communication" is one of many reasons why beta-carotene protects us from cancer.[22] Beta-carotene selectively inhibited the growth of human squamous cancer cells in culture.[23] Beta-carotene and canthaxanthin provided significant protection in animals against the cancer-causing effects of radiation.[24]

Carotenoids may partially compensate for the "sins" of our unhealthy lifestyles. In one study, researchers from the National Cancer Institute and Harvard tracked over 47,000 healthy individuals and found that lycopenes, even from pizza sauce, were protective against prostate cancer.[25] Other studies have found that beta-carotene supplements can reverse the pre-cancerous condition (oral leukoplakia) brought about by chewing betel nut,[26] which is a Third World version of chewing tobacco.

Beta-carotene affects the cancer process in a variety of ways:

♦ alters the adenylate cyclase activity in melanoma cells in culture, which affects cell differentiation and, thus, whether a cell will turn cancerous or not[27]

♦ potent anti-oxidant,[28] which spares immune cells in the microscopic "war on cancer" and protects the healthy prostaglandins

♦ provides a certain level of tumor immunity in mice inoculated with cancer cells[29]

♦ protects the DNA against the damaging effects of carcinogens[30]

♦ according to studies by Food and Drug Administration researchers, beta-carotene protects against the cancer causing effects of a choline deficient diet in animals

♦ once cancer has been initiated, either chemically or physically, beta-carotene inhibits the next step in the cancer process of neoplastic transformation[31]

♦ there is a synergistic benefit of using vitamin A with carotenoids in patients who have been first treated with chemo, radiation, and surgery for common malignancies[32]

♦ beta-carotene and vitamin A together provided a significant improvement in outcome in animals treated with radiation for induced cancers[33]

♦ carotenoids (from Spirulina and Dunaliella algae) plus vitamin E and canthaxanthin were injected in animal tumors, with the result being complete regression, as mediated by an increase in Tumor Necrosis Factor (TNF) in macrophages in the tumor region[34]

♦ in 20 patients with mouth cancer who were given high doses of radiation and chemo, beta-carotene provided significant protection against mouth sores (oral mucositis) induced by medical therapy, although there was no significant difference in survival rates[35]

♦ in animals, beta-carotene provided cancer protection against a carcinogenic virus, which would normally damage the DNA[36]

Betatene is a special, mixed carotenoid extract from Dunaliella algae that has been shown in scientific studies to potently inhibit the development of breast tumors in animals.[37] Betatene consists of a rich mixture of various carotenoids, primarily naturally-occurring betacarotene, along with smaller amounts of lycopene, alpha-carotene, zeaxanthin, cryptoxanthin, and lutein.

BETA-CAROTENE CAUSES LUNG CANCER?

SAFETY ISSUES. There is virtually no toxicity to beta-carotene at any dosage, other than the mild pigmentation (carotenemia) that occurs in the skin region.[38] With our primitive analytical tools, scientists isolated the most likely champion of the carotenoids, beta-carotene, and conducted several human intervention trials funded by the National Cancer Institute to examine whether beta-carotene would reduce the incidence of lung cancer in heavy smokers. It didn't.[39] And in two studies, the beta-carotene supplemented groups had slightly elevated incidences of lung cancer. The press loved this huge controversy and made sure that everyone knew about it. Unfortunately, only a small portion of the story was told.

Issues not covered by the press included:

-Those individuals who had the highest SERUM beta-carotene at the start of these two studies had a lower incidence of lung cancer. Beta-carotene ABSORBED does indeed reduce the risk of suicidal lifestyles, such as smoking.

- Prominent researchers in nutrition and cancer have published papers showing that antioxidants, like beta-carotene, can become pro-oxidants in the wrong biochemical environment, such as the combat zone of free radicals generated by heavy tobacco use.[40] Nowhere in Nature do we find a food with just beta-carotene. All foods contain a rich and dazzling array of anti-oxidants.

-After 35 years of heavy smoking, the damage is done. The damaging effects of tobacco cannot be neutralized by one "magic bullet" pill of synthetic beta-carotene, with coal tar-based food dyes added to ensure a homogenous color in the beta-carotene capsules.

-It is the synergism of multiple carotenoids that protects people. If beta-carotene truly provoked lung cancer, then what about the 200 studies showing that a diet rich in fruit and vegetables (best sources of beta-carotene) significantly lowers the incidence of cancer?

-At the International Conference on Nutrition and Cancer, sponsored by the University of California at Irvine, held in July 1997, there were several watershed presentations showing that one nutrient alone may be ineffective or counterproductive for cancer patients, while a host of compatible nutrients in the proper ratio can be extremely effective at slowing or reversing cancer.

D-3 (cholecalciferol) 200-2000 iu
Helps to squelch cancer at genetic level, reducing the production of gene fragments (episomes) by working with calcium receptors

---

As the fledgling science of nutrition grows in knowledge and analytical tools, we keep discovering more nutrients and more functions of the nutrients that we thought we already understood. Such is true for vitamin D, which actually is not a real vitamin in the sense of needing it in the diet.[41] We can manufacture vitamin D in the body by the action of sunlight on the skin converting cholesterol to D.

As a simple metaphor, think of most human cells containing a "switch" that can activate cancer, called the oncogene. Vitamin D puts a protective plate over that oncogene "switch" to prevent cancer from starting or spreading.

Nature always seems to provide. In areas of the world where sunshine is unpredictable at best, indigenous people had traditional diets that were rich in fish liver, which is the most concentrated food source of vitamin D. Cloudy regions of the world have had notoriously higher rates of tuberculosis; cancers of the breast[42], ovaries[43], colon[44], and prostate; hypertension and osteoporosis[45]; multiple sclerosis; and other health problems.

IS SUN EXPOSURE GOOD FOR US?

♥excess sun exposure (free radicals) on fair skin with excess PUFA diet (vulnerable to free radicals) with AOX deficient diet= cataracts, basal & squamous carcin, mac.deg.

♦Lowest incidence of melanoma found in outdoor constr.workers.
Sunnier climates have 50% reduction in risk for most other cancers.
Sun exposure lowers incidence of depression, auto-immune diseases.
Sunlight (UVB) generates 10,000 iu/day vit.D semi-naked adult.
RDA vit.D=400 iu
Most older Americans deficient in vitamin D
Vitamin D effective against infections, cancer, heart disease, osteoporosis, depression, auto-immune diseases.
40,000 iu (1000 mcg=1 mg) toxic
Vieth, R., Am.J.Clin.Nutr., vol.69, no.5, p.842,May 1999; Am.J.Clin.Nutr.,vol.77, p.204,Jan.2003

If sunshine is the "medicine" in these diseases, then vitamin D and melatonin are the most likely by-products of sunlight exposure. Vitamin D has demonstrated the ability to enhance the immune system to fight off tuberculosis.[46] Our primitive ancestors consumed or produced about 5 times more vitamin D than we get, because they ate whole foods, ate lots of fish, and lived outside in the sun. Most Americans and nearly all women receive far below the RDA (200-400 iu) for vitamin D.[47] One international unit (1 iu) of vitamin D-3 (a measurement of biological activity) is equal to 0.025 micrograms in weight.

Ergosterol is a plant steroid that is converted commercially to vitamin D-2 and used to fortify milk, a move that has virtually eliminated the deficiency syndrome of rickets in cloudy regions of the world. Vitamin D-3, cholecalciferol, is the natural vitamin produced in the skin by the action of sunlight. Once activated in the kidneys and liver, the steroid version of vitamin D-3 is: 1 alpha 25 dihydroxy cholecalciferol (1,25 D-3), which works with the hormones of parathyroid and calcitonin to regulate calcium metabolism, absorption, transport, and more.

So, how does all this information relate to the cancer process?-- probably by regulating calcium transport into and out of the cell, which has been shown to be crucial in the cell differentiation process.[48]

- In animals fed a high fat diet, which normally would produce a higher incidence of colon cancer, supplements of calcium and vitamin D blocked this carcinogenic effect of the diet.[49]
- Vitamin D inhibits the growth of breast cancer in culture, and also seems to subdue human breast cancer.[50]
- Cells from human prostate cancer were put into a "...permanent nonproliferative state.", or shut down the cancer process, by the addition of vitamin D.[51]
- Human cancer cells have been shown to have receptor sites, or stereo-specific "parking spaces" for vitamin D.[52]

Vitamin D prevents the formation of gene fragments, or episomes, that may be the beginning of the cancer process. Bone cells that generate new blood and immune cells (hematopoietic cells) have receptors for 1,25 D-3, and activated macrophages from the immune system can synthesize 1,25 D-3.[53] Vitamin D induces differentiation to suppress cell growth in numerous tumor lines tested.[54] In tumor-bearing mice, vitamin D-3 supplements inhibited the immune suppression from the tumor secretion (granulocyte/macrophage colony stimulating factor, GM-CSF), while also reducing tumor growth and metastasis.[55] Due to the success of vitamin D at down-regulating various forms of cancer, many drug companies are researching patentable vitamin D analogs to treat cancer. But nothing works like Mother Nature's original.

SAFETY ISSUES. Nature has checkpoints in place to control the possibility of vitamin D toxicity in the body. People who are native to sunny climates have darker skin, which is full of melanin to reduce the production of vitamin D in the skin, while also protecting against the damaging effects of ultraviolet light. Dark-skinned people are also more vulnerable to rickets (vitamin D deficiency) when moving to cloudy climates. Also, African-American men have a much higher incidence of prostate cancer, perhaps due to variations in vitamin D metabolism.

In order for dietary intake of vitamin D to become toxic, there needs to be activation of vitamin D in the kidney and liver, which are other safeguards in the body. Nonetheless, young children are potentially vulnerable to vitamin D toxicity, which may begin as low as 1,800 iu/day for extended periods of time.[56] Symptoms of toxicity include hypercalcemia, hypercalciuria, anorexia, nausea, vomiting, thirst, polyuria, muscular weakness, joint pains, and disorientation.[57] On a summer's day, a sunbather at the beach will produce about 10,000 iu of vitamin D before the body says "that's enough" and shuts off the production mechanism for D. Good research published in the *American Journal of Clinical Nutrition* shows that vitamin D toxicity for most adults begins at 40,000 iu per day.[58] Since there are 40 iu per microgram, this means that toxicity is at 1000 micrograms=1 milligram of D.

> # E (succinate, and/or mixed natural tocopherols) 200-1000 iu
> Natural E stimulates immune functions and works as an antioxidant. E succinate may be selectively toxic to tumor cells.

More than a few physicians have assumed that since vitamin E is an antioxidant, and chemo and radiation work by generating pro-oxidants to kill cancer cells, therefore vitamin E will reduce the efficacy of medical therapy in cancer patients. Nothing could be further from the truth. Vitamin E is a valuable ally for both the cancer patient and the oncologist.

My college professors in the 1970s would facetiously chuckle at the "health nuts" who popped vitamin E capsules, claiming that "vitamin E was a vitamin in search of a disease." In one study, healthy students were deprived of vitamin E in the diet for up to 2 years with no blatant vitamin deficiency syndrome, such as is found with vitamin C and scurvy, or vitamin D and rickets. Deficiencies of vitamin E cause an increase in lipid peroxidation (pro-oxidants) that decrease energy production (due to mitochondrial membrane damage), increase mutation of DNA, and alter the normal transport mechanisms in the cell membrane.[59] Hemolytic anemia (premature bursting of red blood cells) has been found in infants who are fed a diet high in polyunsaturated fats (which generate lipid peroxides) and iron (which can be a pro-oxidant). Malabsorption syndromes, such as biliary cirrhosis (blockage of the liver duct to the gallbladder), can generate blatant vitamin E deficiency in humans.[60]

Actually, clinical deficiencies of vitamin E probably take decades to turn into full blown cataracts, Alzheimer's, heart disease, arthritis, or cancer. While 1 milligram of vitamin E (alpha tocopheryl acetate) equals 1 international unit (iu), other versions (racemates) of E are not as potent, and hence have less iu per mg.

Most substances in life are either fat soluble (can be dissolved in alcohol) or water soluble, with a few magical substances, like lecithin, able to work in either universe. Vitamin E is the most critical of all fat soluble antioxidants. Imagine that little "fires", or pro-oxidants, break out all over the human body all of the time. The primary "fire extinguisher" that can put out fires in the fat soluble portion of the body, including the vulnerable cell membrane,

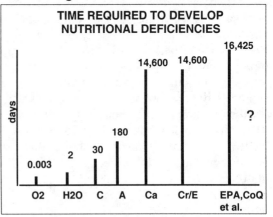

TIME REQUIRED TO DEVELOP NUTRITIONAL DEFICIENCIES

days

16,425
14,600 14,600
180
30
2
0.003
?

O2   H2O   C   A   Ca   Cr/E   EPA,CoQ et al.

is vitamin E.[61] Because of this fundamental role in cell biology, vitamin E helps to:

- protect the beneficial prostaglandins
- stimulate immune function
- protect healthy cells against toxins and radiation, while making cancer cells more vulnerable to medical therapy
- a special form of vitamin E (succinate) is selectively toxic to cancer cells.

Vitamin E actually refers to a family of 8 related compounds, the tocopherols and tocotrienols. Tocopherols got their name from "pherein", meaning to carry, and "tocos", meaning birth, because vitamin E from wheat germ was found to be essential for fertility. True natural vitamin E is a mixture of alpha, beta, delta, and gamma tocopherols plus some tocotrienols, which are more concentrated in rice bran and palm oil. Vitamin E may help the cancer patient in numerous ways:

NUTRITIONAL SYNERGISM. Zinc deficiency in animals further compounds a vitamin E deficiency, meaning that zinc must be present to properly utilize vitamin E.[62] Also, vitamin E protects the body against the potentially damaging effects of iron and rusting fish oil. Human volunteers given high doses of fish oil experienced an immune abnormality (mitogenic responsiveness of peripheral blood mononuclear cells to concanavalin A), which was reversed with supplements of vitamin E.[63]

IMMUNE REGULATOR. Vitamin E plays a powerful role as an immune regulator.[64] When 32 healthy elderly adults were given supplements of 800 iu daily of vitamin E, there were measurable improvements in immune functions.[65] Following 28 days of supplements of vitamins E, C, and A researchers found that 30 elderly institutionalized patients had substantial improvements in immune functions (absolute T-cells, T4 subsets, T4:T8 ratio, and lymphocyte proliferation).[66] E seems to work by protecting immune factors from immediate destruction in their suicidal plunge at cancer cells. E also works by bolstering the activity of the thymus and spleen organs to stimulate lymphocyte proliferation. In burned animals, vitamin E supplements offered substantial protection in the intestinal mucosa to prevent bacterial translocation (gut bacteria migrating into the blood to cause septicemia).[67]

PROTECTION FROM TOXINS. Vitamin E protected animals from the cancer-causing effects of alcohol on the esophagus[68] and a carcinogen on the colon.[69] Vitamin E and selenium protected animals against the potent carcinogenic effects of DMBA from tobacco.[70] Vitamin E protected the damaged liver of rats from developing fatty liver and collagen content.[71] Vitamin E protects us against the greatest toxin and essential nutrient of them all--oxygen, as shown in exercised animals.[72] By sparing fats in the blood from becoming lipid peroxides, vitamin E supplements were very effective at preventing heart disease.[73] Vitamin E prevents the formation of one of the more common carcinogenic agents in humans--nitrosamines--which are formed by the combination of nitrates in the diet and amino acids in the stomach. Vitamin E prevents damage to the skin from ultraviolet radiation.[74] According to researchers from Bulgaria, vitamin E protects us against the harmful effects of too many iron-generating free radicals and damage to our detoxification system, cytochrome P-450. Much of the damage caused by iron in the human body is due to:

1) wrong form of iron, we need chelated iron, not iron salts as we get in fortified white flour

2) not enough antioxidants to prevent this oxidizing metal from "rusting" in the cell and creating harm.

3) lowering of pH, or acidosis, which causes iron to become unbound from its protective shells of hemoglobin and transferrin

REVERSE PRE-CANCEROUS CONDITION. Vitamin E supplements (200-400 mg/d for 3 months) reversed fibrocystic breast disease (a major risk for breast cancer) in 22 out of 26 women.[75] Other women have found reversal of fibrocystic breast disease through elimination of caffeine, chocolate, and colas, which contain methylxanthines.

PROSTAGLANDINS. We can generate very healthy prostaglandins, if we have the right dietary precursors in our blood, which come from:

- enough fish oil (EPA) or flax oil (ALA) and borage oil (GLA)
- healthy levels of blood sugar (60-100 mg%)
- optimal amounts of vitamin E[76]

Because of this beneficial impact on prostaglandins, vitamin E helps to inhibit platelet adhesion[77], which helps to slow down the spreading of cancer. And yet, as shown below, vitamin E does not influence blood clotting, or prothrombin time, which is good news for people worried about proper clotting during and after surgery.

SLOWS AND REVERSES CANCER. In human studies, low intake of vitamin E increases the risk for cancer of various body sites.[78] Patients with head and neck cancers are more likely to have a recurrence if they have low blood levels of vitamins E, A, and beta-carotene.[79] Vitamin E injected into animal mouth tumors was able to significantly reduce or completely eliminate tumors.[80] In patients with colorectal cancer, vitamin E, C, and A supplements were able to reduce the growth of abnormal cells in the colon, indicating a possible slowing of the cancer process.[81] In human epidemiology studies, people with the highest intake of E (still very low compared to ideal intake) had a 40% reduction in the risk for colon cancer.[82] In animals, vitamin E supplements prevent lung tumors from developing.[83]

VITAMIN E SUCCINATE AND CANCER. When vitamin E is esterified (combined) with succinic acid, a new molecule is formed with surprising ability to selectively shut down cancer growth, but not harm healthy tissue,[84] slowing the growth of brain (glioma and neuroblastoma) and melanoma cells in culture.[85] E succinate is able to reduce the genetic expression of c-myc oncogenes in cultured cancer cells.[86] E succinate inhibits virally-induced tumors in culture.[87] E succinate has been studied as a potent regulator of cell proliferation.[88]

IMPROVES MEDICAL THERAPY OF CANCER. Vitamin E helps generally toxic medical therapies to distinguish between healthy and cancerous cells. The best proposed mechanism for this action is the anaerobic state of many tumors. Vitamin E apparently is not well absorbed, or needed, by tumors, since they are anaerobic (without oxygen). An antioxidant is of little interest to an oxygen-independent cell. Because of this function of vitamin E, chemotherapy and radiation can be made much more selectively toxic to the cancer cells, while protecting the patient from host damage.

It has long been known that a vitamin E deficiency, common in cancer patients, will accentuate the cardiotoxic effects of adriamycin.[89] The worse the vitamin E deficiency in animals, the greater the heart damage from adriamycin.[90] Patients undergoing chemo, radiation, and bone marrow transplant for cancer treatment had markedly depressed levels of serum antioxidants, including vitamin E.[91] Given the fact that both chemo and radiation can induce cancer, which reduces the chances for survival, it is noteworthy that vitamin E protects animals against a potent carcinogen, DMBA.[92] Vitamin E supplements prevented the glucose-raising effects of a chemo drug, doxorubicin.[93] Since cancer is a sugar-feeder, preventing this glucose-raising effect may be another valuable contribution from vitamin E in patients receiving chemo. Meanwhile, vitamin E improves the tumor kill rate of doxorubicin.[94] Vitamin E modifies the carcinogenic effect of daunomycin (chemo drug) in animals.[95]

Human prostate cancer cells were killed at a higher rate when adriamycin (chemo drug) was combined with vitamin E at concentrations that can easily be obtained from supplementation.[96] Vitamin E supplements (1,600 iu/day) taken one week prior to adriamycin therapy protected 69% of patients from hair loss, which is nearly universal in adriamycin-treated patients.[97] Vitamin E helped to repair kidney damage caused by adriamycin in animals.[98] Vitamin E and selenium supplements in animals helped to reduce the heart toxicity from adriamycin.[99] Selenium and vitamin E supplements were given to 41 women undergoing cytotoxic therapy for ovarian and cervical cancers, with a resulting drop in the toxicity-related rise in creatine kinase.[100] Vitamin E, A, and prenylamine reduced the toxicity of adriamycin on the hearts of animals studied.[101]

In animals with implanted tumors, those pretreated with vitamin E had a much greater tumor kill from radiation therapy.[102] Radiation therapists know that the ability to kill cancer with radiation diminishes as the tumor becomes more anaerobic or hypoxic. Vitamin E seems to sensitize tumors, making them more vulnerable to radiation therapy. In cultured human cancer cells, vitamin E increased the damaging effects of radiation on tumor cells.[103] Brain cancer cells were easier to kill once pretreated with vitamin E succinate.[104] Tumor kill in animals receiving radiation therapy was greatly increased by pretreatment with vitamin E.[105] Vitamin E supplements reduced the breakage of red blood cells in animals given radiation therapy.[106] Vitamin E supplements improved the wound recovery in animals given preoperative radiation.[107]

Vitamin E combined with vitamin K, leucovorin (anti-metabolite cancer drug), and 5FU (fluorouracil) significantly enhanced the cell growth inhibition curves for 5FU.[108] One of the more troublesome side effects of chemotherapy is peripheral neuropathy, or a tingling numbness in the extremities. Low vitamin E status is likely to blame for peripheral neuropathy.[109]

Oral mucositis, or sores in the mouth, is a common problem arising from the use of many chemotherapy drugs. These mouth sores are so painful that cancer patients stop eating, creating malnutrition, which really deteriorates the general health picture. Vitamin E topically applied healed 67% of cancer patients in a double-blind trial at M.D. Anderson Hospital in Houston.[110] To use this therapy, puncture the end of a soft gelatin vitamin E capsule and spread the vitamin E oil over the mouth sore. Do this several times each day.

Can't get enough in food

Vitamin E supplements have even been endorsed by the National Cancer Institute[111], American Heart Association, and the United States Department of Agriculture, because in order to consume 400 international units of vitamin E, you would have to eat either:

-2 quarts of corn oil, or

-5 pounds of wheat germ, or

-8 cups of almonds, or

-28 cups of peanuts

SAFETY ISSUES. Taking many times the RDA of vitamin E had some researchers worried about toxicity, so they fed 900 iu (90 times the RDA) daily to healthy college students for 12 weeks with no changes in liver, kidney, thyroid, **blood clotting,** or immunoglobulin levels.[112] These results are valuable, because vitamin E inhibits the platelet aggregation that can cause stroke, heart disease, or cancer metastasis; yet it does not alter blood clotting activity. Therefore, pre-surgical patients do not need to reduce vitamin E intake for fear of not clotting during and after surgery. According to a review of the world's literature on vitamin E toxicity, there are virtually no side effects at dosages under 3,200 iu/day.[113] For a review of other issues regarding risks with vitamin E, see chapter 15 on Supplements.

K (menadione)   50-200 mcg
Selectively toxic to tumor cells. In combination with vitamin C forms anti-cancer compound.

When vitamin K was first researched in 1929, it was labelled the "Klotting" factor by the Dutch scientist Henrik Dam. Since then, much has been learned about this fascinating molecule. There are three primary variations of vitamin K, all with certain levels of activity in the body.

♦ K-1, or phylloquinone, is produced in higher plants such as spinach, broccoli, Brussels sprouts, and kale.

♦ K-2, or menaquinone, is produced by bacterial fermentation, which means that we manufacture varying amounts of vitamin K in a healthy human gut. Fermented foods such as cheeses and soy foods also carry some K.

♦ K-3, or menadione, is the synthetically-derived version of vitamin K, called Synkavite in drug form.

Although mother's milk will quickly begin generating vitamin K in the infant's gut, physicians have developed a standard hospital protocol of giving injections of Synkavite to all newborns. About 1/3 of all patients with chronic gastrointestinal problems have clinical vitamin K deficiency.[114]

There are several handsome lessons to be learned as we review vitamin K in :

♦ **Metavitamin functions**. Many nutrients develop unique functions when given at anything beyond survival doses. Niacin, vitamin A, vitamin C, fish oil, and others all reflect the fact that low dose of a nutrient will give you basic survival functions, while higher doses give us "above-vitamin" or meta-vitamin functions. In this case, vitamin K is basically a clotting factor that helps to activate prothrombin, so that we do not bleed to death when cutting open the skin envelope.[115] In higher doses, vitamin K becomes a potent anti-cancer agent that is non-toxic to healthy cells.[116]

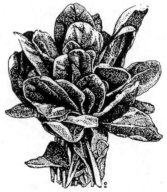

♦ **Synergism yields two main benefits**:
1) significant increase in healing capacity; 2) the need for lower

doses. Researchers found that combining vitamins C and K-3 against cultured human breast cancer cells allowed for inhibition of the cancer growth at doses 90-98% less than was required if only one of these vitamins was used against the cancer.[117]

♦ **Look beyond the obvious**. Coumarin (a.k.a. dicumarol, warfarin) is an anti-coagulant drug that holds promise in cancer treatment by shutting down cancer cell metabolism and helping to slow metastasis. Vitamin K has a primary function of inducing coagulation. The obvious deduction is that vitamin K (a coagulant) would neutralize the benefits of coumarin (anti-coagulant). In real life, Vitamin K-3 does not neutralize the effects of coumarin[118] but actually improves the anti-cancer effects of coumarin.[119] While K-1 reverses the effects of coumarin, K-3 does not reverse the effects of coumarin due to the slight difference in chemical structure in which K-3 cannot participate in the gamma carboxylation of prothrombin.

♦ **Similar is not the same as identical, in chemical structures**. Oftentimes, drug companies find a substance that has therapeutic action, such as vitamin A or indole-3-carbinol from broccoli, and will try to create a slightly different molecule, so that it can be patented. These slight differences nearly always translate into high toxicity from these newly-formed molecules. For instance, the difference between a man and woman rests primarily in the difference between the hormones testosterone and estrogen, which are nearly identical molecules except for one OH group. Over 40 years ago, Professor J.S. Mitchell of England showed that patients receiving K-3 had measurable shrinkage of tumors. Later, the drug doxorubicin was introduced as an anti-cancer drug. K-3, doxorubicin, and coumarin all share related chemical structures as "naphthoquinone" molecules. Yet, of all these compounds, K-3 has been shown by Chlebowski and colleagues at the University of California Los Angeles to have 70 times (7,000%!!!) more anti-cancer activity than coumarin and 25 times more cancer-killing capacity than vitamin K-1.

Vitamin K-3 works against cancer both by directly antagonizing cell replication in cancer cells[120] and also by inhibiting metastasis. K-3 also works as a potentiator of radiation therapy. In one study, patients with mouth cancer who were pre-treated with injections of K-3 prior to radiation therapy doubled their odds (20% vs. 39%) for 5-year survival and disease-free status.[121] Animals with implanted tumors had greatly improved anti-cancer effects from all chemotherapy drugs tested, when vitamins K and C were given in combination.[122] In cultured leukemia cells, vitamins K and E added to the chemotherapy drugs 5FU (fluorouracil) and leucovorin provided a 300% improvement in growth inhibition when compared to 5FU by itself.[123] Animals given methotrexate and K-3 had improvements in cancer reversal, with no increase in toxicity to the host tissue.[124] In one case study, a patient with recurrent and drug-refractory bone cancer metastasized to the lungs was put on a regimen of hydrazine sulfate and vitamin K-3 injections, with a resulting weight gain and complete regression of her cancer.[125] In 13 cancer patients, some with demonstrated drug-resistant tumors, menadiol (vitamin K analog, a.k.a. K-4) was given at up to 3200 mg per meter squared per week along with various chemo drugs, with no increase in host toxicity, but some improvements in tumor responses.[126]

SAFETY ISSUES. There is no known toxicity associated with the plant-derived version, K-1.[127] The toxicity of menadione (K-3) is very low, with animals having no adverse side effects after being fed 1,000 times the daily requirement.[128] The typical dietary intake of K-1 in America is somewhere between 100-500 micrograms daily, with little understanding of the role played by the production of K-2 in the healthy human gut.

A special note on coumarin. Many cancer patients on coumarin are directed by their physician to avoid foods high in vitamin K-1, including kale, spinach, broccoli, and other anti-cancer greens. Actually, much more important is to have a PREDICTABLE intake of vitamin K-1. The doctor will take blood samples and conduct a Pro test (prothrombin test, time required for the blood to clot) and prescribe coumarin based on this test. It is much more essential to have a PREDICTABLE amount of vitamin K-1 in the diet than to avoid it, which will allow for the safest and most effective use of anti-coagulant drugs.

C 200-10,000 mg (from ascorbic acid and/or buffered sources like sodium ascorbate or calcium ascorbate)
Immune stimulant, antioxidant, helps envelop cancer, shuts down cancer growth

---

If vitamin A is the mother of all anti-cancer vitamins, then vitamin C is the grandmother of all. The problem started millions of years ago, when primates lost the liver enzyme necessary to convert sugar into vitamin C.[129] Of the millions of animals, reptiles, amphibians, insects, and other things that walk, crawl, fly, and swim--humans are among the few creatures on earth that do not make our own vitamin C. Our primitive ancestors were able to consume 300-500 milligrams daily of vitamin C, which definitely prevents scurvy. Throughout the golden ages of world exploration by ship, thousands of people died--sometimes up to half of the crew--due to scurvy. Highly perishable fresh fruits and vegetables are the richest sources of vitamin C and were unavailable on ship voyages longer than a few weeks. Around 1750, the English physician, James Lind, found that limes could prevent and reverse scurvy (does that make limes a prescription drug?).

"Time lags" are a known phenomenon that separate a discovery from the actual implementation of a breakthrough. It was another 50 years after Dr. Lind's research before limes were required to be carried aboard ships, thus costing the world thousands of unnecessary deaths in this delay. Are we doing the same thing by delaying aggressive nutrition support for millions of cancer patients?

Vitamin C is one of the more versatile vitamins in human nutrition. Its functions include:

♦ protector against free radicals
♦ maintainer of tough connective tissue (collagen and elastin), which is the "glue" that keeps our body together
♦ producer of adrenaline for energy
♦ producer of serotonin for thought and calmness
♦ stimulater of various immune components to protect against infections and cancer
♦ converter of cholesterol into bile for its elimination in the bowels
♦ maintainer of fat stores in the adipose tissue to prevent heart disease
♦ regulator of bone formation
♦ detoxifier to better tolerate pollutants
♦ reducer of allergic reactions by preventing histamine release
♦ regulator of insulin to better control blood sugar levels

HOW MUCH???

Part of the controversy surrounding vitamin C is the extreme range of dosages that can be consumed in humans or produced in animals:

⇒ 10 milligrams daily will prevent blatant scurvy in most healthy adults
⇒ 60 mg is the Recommended Dietary Allowance
⇒ 200-300 mg would be consumed by people who are following the NCI suggestion of 5 servings of fruit and vegetables daily
⇒ 300 mg of supplemental vitamin C was shown to increase quantity of life by 6 years in men
⇒ 1000 mg is required in many hospitalized patients, just to maintain adequate serum ascorbate levels
⇒ 10,000 to 20,000 mg is often taken by many people using C to curtail some illness, such as cancer, AIDS, viral infections, and injury recovery
⇒ 100,000 mg/day has been given intravenously with no side effects
⇒ 20,000 mg is produced daily by many animals, such as goats and dogs, on a per weight basis using a 154 pound reference man; internal production goes up further when the animal is exposed to stress, infections, or toxins

---

Although Linus Pauling, PhD, was not the first scientist to suggest that vitamin C might help cancer patients, he was definitely the most vocal and decorated of the lot. With two unshared Nobel prizes and three Presidential citations, you would think that the scientific community would be more open to Dr. Pauling's comments. Though Pauling was considered to be one of the two greatest scientists of the 20th century, along with Albert Einstein, the 1970s found Pauling to be an academic nomad for his innovative views on vitamin C.

However, as time marched on, data continued to gather to support Pauling's viewpoint. By 1982, the National Academy of Sciences was willing to admit that vitamin C might prevent cancer.[130] And by 1990, the National Institutes of Health hosted a conference on "Vitamin C and Cancer", which showed that Pauling was truly on to something.[131] While Pauling's strident critics claimed that he was trying to cure cancer with vitamin C, in fact Pauling only suggested high doses of C in concert with medical therapies would augment cancer outcome,

Pauling later went on to explain the reasons that vitamin C may improve outcome in cancer treatment, including the increased need for C in cancer patients, the ability of C to prevent cancer breaking down connective tissue for metastasis, the ability of C to help "wall off" or encapsulate the tumor, the role of C in immune attack on cancer, and the role of C in hormonal balance.[132] One of the highlights of my career was having Dr. Pauling eat supper at my house in 1992, spry and alert at 91 years of age.

Vitamin C can help cancer patients in several critical categories:

1) Prevention. Cancer patients have already demonstrated a genetic vulnerability to cancer and to toxins. Cancer patients will likely be exposed to even more potent carcinogens in medical therapy. Therefore, the need to prevent secondary and iatrogenic tumors is great. In a study encompassing 16 groups in 7 countries covering 25 years, higher vitamin C intake was strongly related to lowering cancer incidence.[133] Another study examined the cancer-protective effect of vitamin C and found that 33 of 46 epidemiological studies showed it helped, while none showed any increase in cancer with higher vitamin C intake.[134] Vitamin C protects humans against a whole assortment of toxic chemicals[135] while accelerating wound recovery[136] and stabilizing iron compounds (ferritin) in the blood.[137] Vitamin C reduced the incidence and severity of kidney tumors in animals exposed to the hormones estradiol or diethylstilbestrol.[138] Through a wide variety of mechanisms, vitamin C is a potent inhibitor of cancer.[139]

2) Augmenting medical therapy. C may be able to enhance the toxicity of chemo and radiation against the cancer cells, while protecting the patient from possible harm. C was able to enhance the effectiveness of a drug (misonidazole) that improves outcome in radiation treatment of cancer.[140] C improved the tumor-stopping abilities of a wide range of medical therapies against brain cancer (neuroblastoma) cells in culture.[141] Animals given the chemo drugs vincristine (from the periwinkle plant) and vinblastine were given supplements of vitamin C, with an increase in the excretion of these very toxic drugs.[142] Animals given adriamycin (a common chemotherapy drug) along with vitamin C had a significant prolongation of life and reduction in the expected heart damage (cardiotoxicity) from this drug.[143] Given the widespread use of adriamycin and its known lethal toxicity on the heart[144], it should be standard procedure to give high doses of antioxidants prior to administration of adriamycin.

Animals with implanted tumors were injected with high doses of C one hour prior to whole-body radiation therapy, all scaled to mimic the effects in a human cancer patient. Vitamin C did not affect the tumor-killing capacity of the radiation, but did provide substantial protection to the animals.[145] 50 previously untreated cancer patients were randomly divided into 2 groups, with group #1 receiving radiation therapy only and group #2 receiving radiation plus 5 grams daily of C. After 1 month, 87% of the vitamin C group had achieved a complete response (disappearance of all tumors) compared to 55% in the control group.[146]

3) Slowing or reversing cancer. High doses of C are preferentially toxic to tumor cells, while not harming healthy tissue. One of the explanations why C kills cancer but not healthy cells lies in the fact that C generates large amounts of hydrogen peroxide, H2O2, a potent free radical, which is neutralized in healthy cells by catalase.[147] Cancer cells do not have catalase to protect them. Animals exposed to a carcinogen and then vitamin C had their basal cell cancers examined under electron microscope. The cancer cells exposed to C showed a disintegration of cell structure, cell membrane disruption, increased collagen synthesis, and general reduction in the number and size of tumors.[148] The researcher concluded: "...vitamin C exerts its antineoplastic effects by increasing cytolytic and autophagic activity, cell membrane disruption, and increased collagen synthesis, and thus, inhibits cancer cell metabolism and proliferation."

C may be the ultimate selective toxin against cancer that researchers have been searching for.[149] Recent studies have found that vitamin C is absorbed well by tumor tissue. This study led to the "assumption" that cancer patients should not take vitamin C because it might reduce the effectiveness of chemo and radiation. Actually, no study has ever found that to be true. Vitamin C selectively kills cancer cells while protecting healthy tissue from the damaging effects of chemo and radiation. Vitamin C is absorbed by tumor cells because C is so similar in structure to glucose (sugar). Yet large amounts of a single antioxidant in an anaerobic environment, such as a tumor, have been shown to become a pro-oxidant, just like chemo, except the vitamin C only destroys cancer cells. Antioxidants in a team effort in an aerobic cell, such as healthy tissue, work in harmony to protect that cell against oxidation, like chemo and radiation.

Vitamin C was toxic to melanoma cells but not to healthy cells in culture.[150] When researchers took leukemia cells from 28 patients and cultured them with vitamin C, 25% of the cultures were inhibited by at least 79%.[151] In animals with implanted tumors, vitamin C and B-12 together provided for significant tumor regression and 50% survival of the treated group, while all of the animals not receiving C and B-12 died by the 19th day.[152] C and B-12 seemed to form a cobalt-ascorbate compound that selectively shut down tumor growth. When vitamin C and K were combined with cancer cells in culture, the dosage required to slow and kill cancer cells dropped to only 2% compared to the dosage required by either of these vitamins alone.[153] Vitamin C or essential fatty acids were able to inhibit the growth of melanoma in culture, yet when combined, their anti-cancer activity was much stronger.[154]

In both case studies and clinical trials in the scientific literature, C helps many cancer patients and hurts no one. Show me a drug that has the same risk-to-benefit-to-cost ratio. In one case report, a 70 year old man had been treated for kidney cancer, and then experienced a metastatic recurrence. He refused further medical therapy and started on 30 grams daily of intravenous vitamin C. Six weeks later, his chest X-rays showed that he was disease free.[155] A 42-year-old man with reticulum cell sarcoma was treated on two different occasions with high-dose intravenous vitamin C as sole therapy, and each time resulted in a complete remission with 17 years of followup.[156]

Pauling and Cameron found that 10,000 mg (10 grams) daily of vitamin C brought a 22% survival rate in end-stage untreatable cancer patients after 1 year on C, compared to a 0.4% survival in patients without C.[157] Charles Moertel, MD, of the Mayo Clinic allegedly followed the Pauling protocol and found no benefit with vitamin C.[158] Actually, even though Moertel did not follow Pauling's protocol, none of the untreatable, drug-refractory colon cancer patients in Moertel's study died while on vitamin C for 3 months.

Finnish oncologists used high doses of nutrients (including 2-5 grams of C) along with chemo and radiation for lung cancer patients. Normally, lung cancer is a "poor prognostic" malignancy with a 1% expected survival at 30 months, under normal treatment. In this study, however, 8 of 18 patients (44%) who were given vitamin C and other nutrients were still alive 6 years after diagnosis.[159]

Oncologists at West Virginia Medical School randomized 65 patients with transitional cell carcinoma of the bladder into either the "one-per-day" vitamin supplement providing the RDA, or into a group which received the RDA supplement plus 40,000 iu of vitamin A, 100 mg of B-6, 2000 mg of vitamin C, 400 iu of vitamin E, and 90 mg of zinc. After 10 months, tumor recurrence was 80% in the control group (RDA supplement) and 40% in the experimental "megavitamin" group. Five-year projected tumor recurrence was 91% for controls and 41% for "megavitamin" patients. Essentially, high-dose nutrients, including vitamin C, cut tumor recurrence in half.[160]

In a non-randomized clinical trial, Drs. Hoffer and Pauling instructed patients to follow a reasonable cancer diet (unprocessed food low in fat, dairy, and sugar), coupled with therapeutic doses of vitamins (including 12 grams of C) and minerals.[161] All 129 patients in this study received concomitant oncology care. The control group of 31 patients who did not receive nutrition support lived an average of less than 6 months. The group of 98 cancer patients who received the diet and supplement program lived an average of 6 years.

4) Higher need. There is an elevated need for this nutrient during disease recovery. In one study, 15 patients with melanoma and colon cancer who were receiving immunotherapy (interleukin 2 and lymphokine-activated killer cells) showed blood levels of vitamin C indicative of scurvy.[162] In 20 adult hospitalized patients on Total Parenteral Nutrition (TPN), the mean daily vitamin C needs were 975 mg, which is over 16 times the RDA, with the range being 350-2250 mg.[163] Of the 139 lung cancer patients studied, most tested deficient or scorbutic (clinical vitamin C deficiency).[164] Another study of cancer patients found that 46% tested scorbutic, while 76% were below acceptable levels for serum ascorbate.[165]

SAFETY ISSUES. Vitamin C is extremely safe, even in high doses. In one review of the literature regarding safety of vitamin C, 8 different double-blind placebo-controlled trials giving up to 10,000 mg daily of C for years produced no side effects.[166] In some sensitive individuals, doses of as little as 1,000 mg produce gastrointestinal upset, including diarrhea. Allegations that vitamin C mega-doses would produce oxalate kidney stones or cause B-12 deficiency have never been seen in millions of humans taking mega-doses of C for years. Up to 100,000 mg of C has been safely administered IV. As doses of oral C increase, the percentage that is absorbed goes down. Some experts claim that 10-20 grams of C per day is the upper threshold of what humans can tolerate and efficiently absorb. Use VitaChek C paper strips (316-682-3100) to monitor the vitamin C in urine. Maintaining maximum vitamin C in the urine can be helpful. Meanwhile, mineral-bound ascorbate provides a more prolonged and sustained blood level of serum ascorbate.

B-1 (thiamine mononitrate) 2-20 mg
Improves aerobic metabolism

When the British first learned to mill wheat and remove the outer bran and inner germ, they called the remaining cadaver of a food substance "the Queen's white flour". Bringing this technology around the world, the Dutch showed the South Pacific people of Java how to refine their rice, leaving only white rice behind and disposing of the bran and germ. Many of these people developed a condition of weakness and inability to function, called beri-beri, or literally translated: "I cannot. I cannot." Thiamin was one of the first vitamins to be studied and isolated in the early 20th century.

The importance of thiamin lies in its critical role in energy metabolism and the need for energy in every cell of the body. Thiamin becomes incorporated into a critical enzyme (thiamin pyrophosphate) for production of ATP energy. Low intake of thiamin was associated with an increase in the risk for prostate cancer.[167] Although thiamin is added back to enriched white flour, it is not added back to pastry flour (as in doughnuts) and is often deficient in the elderly[168] and those who regularly consume alcohol.[169] Best food sources of thiamin include brewers yeast, peas, wheat germ, peanuts, whole grains, beans, and liver.

B-2 (riboflavin)   2-20 mg
   Improves aerobic metabolism

Again, like thiamin above, riboflavin is mainly concerned with generating ATP energy from foodstuffs through the enzyme FAD (flavin adenine dinucleotide). However, riboflavin is also essential for the generation of a critical protective enzyme, glutathione peroxidase, which mops up free radicals. With optimal amounts of riboflavin in the body, there is less damage to cell membranes, DNA, and immune factors. Low intake of riboflavin is associated with an increased risk for cancer of prostate and esophagus. Although riboflavin is added back to enriched white flour, many elderly[170] and poor people are low in riboflavin intake.[171] Alcohol interferes with the absorption and metabolism of riboflavin. Best food sources of riboflavin include brewer's yeast, kidney, liver, broccoli, wheat germ, milk, and almonds.

B-3 (inositol hexanicotinate)   100-1500 mg
   Improves aerobic metabolism and tumor-killing capacity of medical therapy, also may work like an enzyme to dissolve protective coating surrounding tumor

---

Like the energy vitamins mentioned above, niacin generates ATP energy via the enzyme NAD (nicotinamide adenine dinucleotide) and also has other duties that impact the cancer patient. Niacin supplements in animals were able to reduce the cardiotoxicity of adriamycin, while not interfering with its tumor-killing capacity.[172] Niacin combined with aspirin in 106 bladder cancer patients receiving surgery and radiation therapy provided for a substantial improvement in 5-year survival (72% vs. 27%) over the control group.[173]

Tumors can hide from radiation therapy as hypoxic (low oxygen) lumps. Niacin seems to make radiation therapy more effective at killing these hypoxic cancer cells.[174] Loading radiation patients with 500 mg to 6000 mg of niacin has been shown to be safe and is one of the most effective agents known to eliminate acute hypoxia in solid malignancies.[175] There is also intriguing evidence that high doses of niacin can act like enzymes, which means:

⇒ changing the coating of the tumor to make it more vulnerable to the immune system and to medical intervention.

⇒ breaking up inefficient clumps of immune cells, or circulating immune complexes

⇒ altering Tumor Necrosis Factor (TNF) that can lead to depression, weight loss, and pain.

B-5 (D-calcium pantothenate)   10-40 mg
Improves stress response

Pantothenic acid is named for "pantos", which is Greek for "found everywhere".   Indeed, all plants and animals require or make pantothenic acid as part of a crucial energy enzyme, acetyl coenzyme A, which is vital for generating ATP energy and a chemical for stress response.   Injections of pantothenic acid improved wound healing in rabbits.[176]   Based on the fact that the average American diet provides about 6 mg of pantothenic acid daily, the recommended intake (no formal RDA) is 4-7 mg. Deficiencies of pantothenic acid will generate symptoms of paresthesia (burning, prickling, tingling of extremities), headache, fatigue, insomnia, and GI distress.   Pantothenic acid works closely with carnitine and CoQ to maximize the efficiency of burning dietary fats.   Supplements of pantothenic acid can help in the stress response, proper balancing of adrenal hormones, energy production, and manufacturing of red blood cells.   Best food sources of pantothenic acid are royal bee jelly, liver, kidney, egg yolk, and broccoli.

B-6 total of 50 mg; 2-3 mg from pyridoxal 5 pyrophosphate, and 10-40 mg from pyridoxine HCl
Improves immune functions and may reduce toxicity from radiation therapy

---

B-6 occurs in three natural forms: pyridoxine, pyridoxal, and pyridoxamine. B-6 works chiefly in an enzyme, pyridoxal-5-phosphate, which shifts amine groups from molecule to molecule.   At least 100 different enzyme systems in humans involving protein metabolism, catabolism, anabolism, or enzyme production all require B-6.   B-6 is essential for:

- regulating proper blood glucose levels
- production of niacin from tryptophan
- lipid metabolism and carnitine synthesis
- making nucleic acids (RNA and DNA)
- immune cell production
- regulation of hormones.

Among its many functions, B-6 is required for producing thymidine, without which cells are more likely to develop cancerous mutations.[177] In a group of 12 non-medicated, newly diagnosed cancer patients who had been smokers, all showed indications (based on coenzyme stimulation) of B-6 deficiency.[178] A low intake of B-6 increases tumor susceptibility and tumor size.[179]

In huge surveys conducted by the United States Department of Agriculture, 80% of Americans did not consume the RDA of 2 mg daily of B-6. There are many aspects of the typical American lifestyle that will exacerbate a marginal deficiency of B-6: many drugs, common food dyes, alcohol, and a high protein intake. Deficiency symptoms will reflect the functions of B-6, which means that almost anything can go wrong.

In one study, 25 mg (1250% of RDA) provided measurable improvements in immune functions in healthy adults. B-6 supplements (50-500 mg) have been shown to cure up to 97% of Carpal Tunnel Syndrome, a painful condition of the wrist and hands. B-6 is very helpful in preventing and reversing neuropathy, or a tingling numbness in the hands and feet, which is common in chemo patients and also preventing the "tanning" of blood proteins, a.k.a. glycosylation or glycation, which occurs when too much sugar is regularly found in the bloodstream.[180]

Above-normal intake of B-6 offers many possible benefits to the cancer patient, including immune stimulation[181], blood sugar control, protection from radiation damage, and inhibition of growth in melanoma.

Early studies in animals indicated that depriving them of B-6 might slow down tumor growth and increase survival time.[182] More recent studies find the opposite to be true. Animals supplemented with B-6 and then injected with a deadly strain of cancer, melanoma, showed an enhanced resistance to the disease.[183] B-6 inhibits melanoma in vivo.[184] B-6 supplements of 25 mg/day in 33 bladder cancer patients provided for marked reduction in tumor recurrence compared to the control group.[185] More recently, oncologists randomized 65 patients with transitional cell carcinoma of the bladder into either the "one-per-day" vitamin supplement providing the RDA, or into a group which received the RDA supplement plus 40,000 iu of vitamin A, 100 mg of B-6, 2000 mg of vitamin C, 400 iu of vitamin E, and 90 mg of zinc. High-dose nutrients, including B-6, cut tumor recurrence in half.[186] B-6 supplements of 300 mg/day throughout 8 weeks of radiation therapy in patients with endometrial cancer provided a 15% improvement in survival at 5 years.[187]

SAFETY ISSUES. Less than 500 mg/day appears to be safe for most adults.[188] P-5-P appears to be the more readily available and active form of B-6, yet most people can convert pyridoxine into active P-5-P.

B-12 (cyanocobalamin)   500 mcg-3000 mcg
Assists in proper cell growth, i.e. making of new immune factors and proper division of other cells. Combines with vitamin C to create selective anti-cancer compound

---

In 1926, Minot and Murphy were awarded the Nobel prize for showing that feeding large quantities of liver could cure the dreaded disease, pernicious anemia, or B-12 deficiency. As people mature beyond age 40, the likelihood of developing pernicious anemia goes up substantially as the gut loses its efficiency at binding with this gigantic molecule and escorting it across the intestinal mucosa. The RDA of 2 micrograms (mcg) can easily be obtained in a typical "meat and potatoes" diet in America, since the best sources are liver, meat, fish, chicken, clams, and egg yolk. However, absorbing the nutrient is another challenge. When this "intrinsic factor" in the gut is missing, large amounts in the diet can somewhat overwhelm the mucosal barrier in the gut and allow some absorption into the bloodstream, which is what happened when liver was used to cure pernicious anemia.

Since B-12 is a methyl donor, it is involved in all new cell growth, which makes it rather important in processes like red blood cell and immune cell formation, energy metabolism, and nerve function. There is a huge body of data now pointing to B-12 and folacin as primary nutrients that can interrupt the production of homocysteine, which is a major risk factor in heart disease.

For the cancer patient, B-12 supplements may bolster host defense mechanisms, plus it can combine with vitamin C to form a unique cobalt ascorbate complex that is selectively toxic to tumor cells.[189]

Folic acid   100-800 mcg
Assists in proper cell growth, is an immune stimulant, helps to check abnormal DNA production

---

Folic acid (a.k.a. folate, folacin) presents a unique challenge in cancer treatment. On one side of the fence stand the oncologists who have used the chemotherapy drug methotrexate for decades as an antagonist to the B vitamin, folic acid, to slow cancer growth, with leucovorin (folinic acid) as the rescue agent to summon the patient back from near death, or "the vital frontier". On the other side stand nutritionists who understand the pivotal role that folic acid plays in HEALTHY cell growth. The efficacy of methotrexate, now being used to treat some cases of rheumatoid arthritis, is not affected by patients taking supplements of folic acid.[190]

Without optimal amounts of folic acid in the cell, growth is erratic and prone to errors, such as birth defects and cancer. Low folate status during pregnancy will generate common birth defects, including spina bifida. Humans with low B-12 and folate status present a clinical picture that looks like leukemia.[191] The importance of folate in new cell growth is highlighted in the fact that it is the only nutrient whose requirement doubles during pregnancy.

Folic acid may be the most common vitamin deficiency in the world, since more people are choosing animal foods (poor source of folic acid) over plant foods.[192] The name, folic acid, comes from the Latin term "folium", meaning foliage, since dark green leafy vegetables are a rich source of folic acid. Other good sources of folic acid include brewer's yeast, legumes, asparagus, oranges, cabbage, root vegetables, and whole grains. Since folic acid is essential for all new cell growth, disturbances in folic acid metabolism are far-reaching, including heart disease (due to more homocysteine in the blood), birth defects, immune suppression, cancer, premature senility, and a long list of other conditions. Without adequate folate in the diet, cell growth is like a drunk driver heading down the highway--more likely to do some harm than not.

Since folic acid and B-12 work together in methyl donor reactions, a deficiency of one can be masked by an excess of the other. Hence, the FDA has stipulated that non-prescription supplements cannot contain more than 800 micrograms of folic acid. Experts have estimated that up to 20% of all senility in older adults is merely a long-term deficiency of folic acid and vitamin B-12. The RDA of folate is 200 mcg for adults and 400 mcg for pregnant women, although the Center for Disease Control has recommended that 800 mcg of folic acid would prevent most cases of spina bifida. Without adequate folic acid in the body, there is a buildup of homocysteine in the blood, which probably generates 10% or more of the 1 million cases of heart disease each year in the U.S.

Cancer is not an "on-off" switch. There are varying shades of gray in between the black and white of normal cells and full-blown metastatic malignancies. In cervical cancer, there is a rating system where a stage I dysplasia shows abnormal cell growth, while stage IV is life-threatening cancer. In one study, 40% of women with stage I and II cervical dysplasia showed clear signs of folic acid deficiency.[193] In a double-blind placebo-controlled trial, 10 milligrams daily of folate (50 times the RDA) reversed cervical dysplasia in the majority of women tested.[194] Low folate intake increases the risk for colorectal cancer.[195] Human cells in a culture of low folate show immune suppression (impaired delayed hypersensitivity).[196]   Folate deficiency is common throughout the world and America, especially among the elderly and adolescent females.[197]   Alcohol and many drugs interfere with the absorption and metabolism of folate. Average intake of folate in the U.S. is about 240 mcg, which is one half to one fourth of what a good diet will contribute.

Biotin   10-50 mcg
     Improves energy metabolism for glucose and fats, is involved in pH maintenance through carbon dioxide binding, and helps regulate cell growth

---

     Biotin is a B vitamin that is incorporated into 4 different carboxylase enzymes, which makes it essential for processing fats, sugar, and various amino acids. Biotin is also involved in the production of glucokinase, an enzyme in the liver that is essential for burning glucose. Biotin supplements have been helpful at improving glucose tolerance in insulin-dependent diabetics (Type 1, using 16 milligrams/day) and non-insulin-dependent diabetics (Type 2, using 9 mg/day).[198]   Biotin supplements have been able to improve peripheral neuropathy (tingling numbness) in diabetics. Peripheral neuropathy is common in patients after extensive chemotherapy.
     Richest food sources of biotin are brewer's yeast, liver, soy, rice, peanut butter, and oats. Biotin is also produced in the intestines through bacterial fermentation, which complicates the understanding of what an optimal intake might be. A healthy gut environment of adequate fiber, fluid, and probiotics probably improves the production of biotin in the gut. Recommended intake of biotin is 30-300 mcg per day.

PATIENT PROFILE: CONQUERED BREAST CANCER
D.S. was a 61 year old female diagnosed with Stage III breast cancer. Underwent radical mastectomy (1 breast) with 4 of 22 nodes found to have cancer. Two subsequent rounds of chemotherapy produced severe side effects--patient passed out within 5 minutes of beginning chemo. Told by oncologist that without chemo, D.S. had a 5% chance of survival. Discontinued chemotherapy anyway. Two years later went to different physician who detected possible disease in the remaining breast. Surgeon performed lumpectomy and there was no cancer in this tissue, as per the pathologist report. D.S. then began nutrition therapy as sole therapy. Three months later, she was found to have enlarged lymph nodes with possible recurrent breast cancer.   Three months later these nodes disappeared. Last time I saw her was 3 years later and she was still in complete remission.   She is very pleased with the healing power of nutrition.

ENDNOTES

[1] . Cameron, E, and Pauling, L., Chem.Biol.Interactions, vol.9, p.272, 1974

[2] . Huang, ME, Am.J.Hematol., vol.28, p.124, 1988

[3] . Watson, R., et al., Nutr.Res., vol.5, p.663, 1985

[4] . Zhang, XM, et al., Virchows Archiv.B Cell.Pathol., vol.61, p.375, 1992

[5] . Friedberg, EC, CANCER QUESTIONS, p.32, Freeman & Co, NY, 1992

[6] . Semba, RD, Clin. Infect.Dis., vol.19, p.489, 1994

[7] . Rumore, MM, Clin.Pharm., vol.12, p.506, 1993

[8] . Pinnock, CB, et al., Aust.Paediatr.J., vol.22, p.95, 1986

[9] . Nutrition Reviews, vol.52, p.281, 1994

[10] . Micksche, M., et al., Onkologie, vol.1, p.57, 1978

[11] . Vagner, VP, et al., Klin.Med., vol.69, p.55, 1991

[12] . Michalek, AM, et al., Nutrition and Cancer, vol.9, p.143, 1987

[13] . Stich, HF, Am.J.Clin.Nutr., vol.53, p.298S, 1991

[14] . Lippman, SM, et al., J.Am.Coll.Nutr., vol.7, p.269, 1988

[15] . Pastorino, U., et al., J. Clin.Oncol., vol.11, p.1216, 1993

[16] . Hruban, Z, Am.J.Pathol., vol.76, p.451, 1974

[17] . Rothman, KJ, et al., N.Engl.J.Med., vol.333, p.1369, 1995

[18] . Hathcock, JN, et al., Am.J.Clin.Nutr., vol.52, p.183, 1990

[19] . Block, G., et al., Nutr.Cancer, vol.18, p.1, 1992

[20] . Mayne, ST, et al., J. Nat.Cancer Inst., vol.86, p.33, 1994

[21] . Krinsky, NI, Amer.J.Clin.Nutr., vol.53, p.238S, 1991

[22] . Zhang, L., et al., Carcinogenesis, vol.12, p.2109, 1991

[23] . Schwartz, JL, Biochem.Biophys Res.Comm., vol.169, p.941, 1990

[24] . Mathews-Roth, MM, et al., Photochem Photobiol., vol.42, p.35, 1985

[25] . Giovannucci, E., et al., J.Nat.Cancer Inst., vol.87, p.1767, 1995

[26] . Garewal, HS, et al., Archives Otolaryngol Head Neck Surg., vol.121, p.141, Feb.1995

[27] . Hazuka, MB, et al., J. Amer.Coll.Nutrition, vol.9, p.143, 1990

[28] . Burton, GW, J.Nutrition, vol.119, p.109, 1989

[29] . Tomita, Y., et al., J.Nat.Cancer Inst., vol.78, p.679, 1987

[30] . Santamaria, L., et al., Modulation and Mediation of Cancer by Vitamins, p.81, Karger, Basel, 1983

[31] . Bertram, JS, et al., Nutrients and Cancer Prevention, Prasad, KN (eds), p.99, Humana , 1990

[32] . Santamaria, L., et al., Nutrients and Cancer Prevention, p.299, Prasad, KN (eds), Humana , 1990

[33] . Seifter, E., et al., J.Nat.Cancer Inst., vol.71, p.409, 1983

[34] . Shklar, G., et al., Eur.J.Cancer Clin.Oncol., vol.24, p.839, 1988

[35] . Mills, EED, British J.Cancer, vol.57, p.416, 1988

[36] . Seifter, E., et al., J.Nat.Cancer Inst., vol.68, p.835, 1982

[37] . Nagasawa, H., et al., Anticancer Res., vol.9, p.71, 1989

[38] . Meyers, DG, et al., Archives Internal Med., vol.156, p.925, 1996

[39] . Alpha tocopherol beta-carotene cancer , New England J of Medicine, vol.330, p.1029, 1994

[40] . Schwartz, JL, Journal of Nutrition, vol.126, 4 suppl, p.1221S, 1996

[41] . Norman, AW, in PRESENT KNOWLEDGE IN NUTRITION, p.120, Ziegler, EE (eds), ILSI, Washington 1996

[42] . Gorham, ED, et al., Intern.J.Epidemiol. vol.20, p.1145, Dec.1991

[43] . Lefkowitz, ES, et al., Intern.J.Epidemiol., vol.23, p.1133, Dec.1994

[44] . Garland, CF, et al., Lancet, p.1176, Nov.18, 1989

[45] . Barger-Lux, MJ, J. Nutr., vol.124, p.1406S, Aug.1994

[46] . Crowle, AJ, et al., Infection and Immunity, vol.55, p.2945, Dec.1987

[47] . Newmark, HL, Adv.Exp.Med.Biol., vol.364, p.109, 1994

[48] . Lancet, p.1122, May 16, 1987

[49] . Pence, B., et al., Proc Amer.Assoc. Cancer, vol.28, p.154, 1987

[50] . Colston, KW, et al., Lancet, p.188, Jan.28, 1989

[51] . Peehl, DM, et al., J. Endocrinol. Invest., vol.17, p.3,, 1994

[52] . Eisman, JA, et al., Modulation and Mediation of Cancer by Vitamins, p.282, Karger, Basel, 1983

[53] . Kizaki, M., et al., Vitamins and Cancer Prevention, p.91, Wiley-Liss, NY, 1991

[54] . DeLuca, HF, Nutrients and Cancer Prevention, p.271, Humana Press, NY, 1990

[55] . Rita, M., et al., Cancer Immunol. Immunother., vol.41, p.37, 1995

[56] . Food and Nutrition Board, National Research Council, Recommended Dietary Allowances, National Academy Press, p.97, Washington, DC, 1989

[57] . Buist, RA, Intern.Clin.Nutr.Rev., vol.4, p.159, 1984

[58] . Vieth, R., Am.J.Clin.Nutr., vol.69, no.5, p.842, May 1999; see also Vieth, R., Am.J.Clin.Nutr., vol.77, p.204, Jan.2003

[59] . Sokol, RJ, in PRESENT KNOWLEDGE IN NUTRITION, p, 132, Ziegler, ILSI, Wash DC, 1996

[60] . Munoz, SJ, et al., Hepatology, vol.9, p.525, 1989

[61] . Niki, E. et al., Amer.J.Clin.Nutr., vol.53, p.201S, 1991

[62] . Bunk, MJ, et al., Proc.Soc.Exp.Biol.Med., voo.190, p.379, 1989

[63] . Kramer, TR, et al., Am.J.Clin.Nutr., vol.54, p.896, 1991

[64] . Nutrition Reviews, vol.45, p.27, Jan.1987

[65] . Meydani, SN, et al., Am.J.Clin.Nutr., vol.52, p.557, 1990

[66] . Penn, ND, et al., Age Ageing, vol.20, p.169, 1991

[67] . Kuroiwa, K, et al., J.Parenteral Enteral Nutr., vol.15, p.22, 1991

[68] . Odeleye, OE, et al., Nutr.Cancer, vol.17, p.223, 1992

[69] . Cook, MG, et al., Cancer Research, vol.40, p.1329, 1980

[70] . Horvath, PM, et al., Anticancer Research, vol.43, p.5335, Nov.1983

[71] . Sclafani, L, et al., J.Parenteral Enteral Nutr., vol.10, p.184, 1986

[72] . Packer, L., Med.Biol., vol.62, p.105, 1984

[73] . Rimm, EB, et al., New Engl J.Med., vol.328, p.1450, 1993

[74] . Record, IR, et al., Nutr.Cancer, vol.16, p.219, 1991

[75] . J.Amer Med.Assoc, vol.244, p.1077, 1980

[76] . Panganamala, RV, et al., Annals NY Acad Sci, vol.393, p.376, 1982

[77] . Jandak, J., et al., Blood, vol.73, p.141, Jan.1989

[78] . Knekt, P., et al., Am.J.Clin.Nutr., vol.53, p.283S, 1991

[79] . deVries, N., et al., Eur.Arch.Otorhinolaryngol, vol.247, p.368, 1990

[80] . Shklar, G., et al., J.Nat.Cancer Inst., vol.78, p.987, 1987

[81] . Paganelli, GM, et al., J.Nat.Cancer Inst., vol.84, p.47, 1992

[82] . Longnecker, MP, et al., J.Nat.Cancer Inst., vol.84, p.430, 1992

[83] . Yano., T., et al., Cancer Letters, vol.87, p.205, 1994

[84] . Prasad, KN, et al., J. Amer.Coll.Nutr., vol.11, p.487, 1992

[85] . Rama, BN, et al., Proc.Soc.Exper.Biol. Med., vol.174, p.302, 1983

[86] . Cohrs, RJ, et al., Int.J.Devl.Neuroscience., vol.9, p.187, 1991

[87] . Kline, K., et al., Nutr.Cancer, vol.14, p.27, 1990

[88] . Prasad, KN, et al., NUTRIENTS AND CANCER PREVENTION, Prasad, KN (eds), p.39, Humana Press, 1990

[89] . Singal, PK, et al., Mol.Cell.Biochem., vol.84, p.163, 1988

[90] . Singal, PK, et al., Molecular Cellular Biochem., vol.84, p.163, 1988

[91] . Clemens, MR, et al., Am.J.Clin.Nutr., vol.51, p.216, 1990

[92] . Shklar, G., et al., J.Oral Pathol.Med., vol.19, p.60, 1990

[93] . Geetha, A., et al., J.Biosci., vol.14, p.243, 1989

[94] . Geetha, A., et al., Current Science, vol.64, p.318, Mar.1993

[95] . Wang, YM, et al., Molecular Inter Nutr.Cancer, p.369, , Arnott, MS, (eds), Raven Press, NY, 1982

[96] . Ripoll, EAP, et al., J.Urol., vol.136, p.529, 1986

[97] . Wood, L, N.Engl.J.Med., vol.312, p.1060, 1985

[98] . Washio, M., et al., Nephron, vol.68, p.347, 1994

[99] . VanVleet, JF, et al., Cancer Treat.Rep., vol.64, p.315, 1980

[100] . Sundstrom, H., et al., Carcinogenesis, vol.10, p.273, 1989

[101] . Milei, J., et al., Am.Heart J., vol.111, p.95, 1986

[102] . Kagerud, A., et al., vol.20, p.1, 1981

[103] . Prasad, KN, et al., Proc.Soc.Exper.Biol.Med., vol.161, p.570, 1979

[104] . Sarria, A., et al., Proc.Soc.Exper.Biol.Med., vol.175, p.88, 1984

[105] . Kagerud, A., et al., Anticancer Research, vol.1, p.35, 1981

[106] . Hoffer, A., et al., Radiation Research, vol.61, p.439, 1975

[107] . Taren, DL, et al., J.Vit.Nutr.Res., vol.57, p.133, 1987

[108] . Waxman, S., et al., Eur.J.Cancer Clin.Oncol., vol.18, p.685, 1982

[109] . Traber, MG, et al., N.Engl.J.Med., vol.317, p.262, 1987

[110]. Wadleigh, RG, et al., Amer.J.Med,vol.92, p.481, May 1992

[111]. J.Nat.Cancer Inst., vol.84, p.997, July 1992

[112]. Kitagawa, M., et al., J. Nutr.Sci. Vitaminology, vol.35, p.133, 1989

[113]. Hathcock, JN, NY Acad Sciences, vol.587, p.257, 1990

[114]. Nutrition Reviews, vol.44, p.10, Jan.1986

[115]. Suttie, JW, in PRESENT KNOWLEDGE IN NUTRITION, p.137, Ziegler, EE (eds), ILSI, Washington, 1996

[116]. Chlebowski, RT, et al., Cancer Treatment Reviews, vol.12, p.49, 1985

[117]. Noto, V., et al., Cancer, vol.63, p.901, 1989

[118]. Dam,H., in Harris, VITAMINS AND HORMONES, p.329, vol.18, Academic Press, NY, 1960

[119]. Chlebowski, RT, et al., Proc.Am.Assoc.Cancer Res., vol.24, p.653, 1983

[120]. Nutter, LM, et al., Biochem.Pharmacol., vol.41, p.1283, 1991

[121]. Krishanamurthi, S., et al., Radiology, vol.99, p.409, 1971

[122]. Taper, HS, et al., Int.J.Cancer, vol.40, p.575, 1987

[123]. Waxman, S., et al., Eur.J.Cancer Clin.Oncol., vol.18, p.685, 1982

[124]. Gold, J., Cancer Treatment Reports, vol.70, p.1433, Dec.1986

[125]. Gold, J., Proc.Amer Assoc Cancer Researchers, vol.28, p.230, Mar.1987

[126]. Nagourney, R., et al., Proc.Amer.Assoc.Clin.Oncol., vol.6, p.35, Mar.1987

[127]. National Research Council, VITAMIN TOLERANCE OF ANIMALS, National Academy Press, Washington, DC 1987

[128]. Suttie, IBID

[129]. Levine, M., et al., in PRESENT KNOWLEDGE IN NUTRITION, p.146, ILSI, Washington, 1996

[130]. National Academy of Sciences, DIET NUTRITION AND CANCER, National Academy Press, Washington, 1982

[131]. Block, G., Annals Intern.Med., vol.114, p.909, 1991

[132]. Cameron, E., Pauling, L., Cancer Research, vol. 39, p.663, Mar.1979

[133]. Ocke, MC, et al., Int.J.Cancer, vol.61, p.480, 1995

[134]. Block, G., Am.J.Clin.Nutr., vol.53, p.270S, 1991

[135]. Tannenbaum, SR, et al., Am.J.Clin.Nutr., vol.53, p.247S, 1991

[136]. Ringsdorf, WM, et al., Oral Surg, p.231, Mar.1982

[137]. Nutrition Reviews, vol.45, p.217, July 1987

[138]. Liehr, JG, Am.J.Clin.Nutr., vol.54, p.1256S, 1991

[139]. Bright-See, E., et al., Modulation and Meditation of Cancer by Vitamins, p.95, Karger, Basel., 1983

[140]. Josephy, PD, et al., Nature, vol.271, p.370, Jan.1978

[141]. Prasad, KN, et al., Proc.Natl.Acad.Sci., vol.76, p.829, Feb.1979

[142]. Sethi, VS, et al., in Modulation and Mediation of Cancer by Vitamins, p.270, Karger, Basel, 1983

[143]. Fujita, K., et al., Cancer Research, vol.42, p.309, Jan.1982

[144]. Minow, RA, et al., Cancer Chemother.Rep., vol.3, p.195, 1975

[145]. Okunieff, P., Am.J.Clin.Nutr., vol.54, p.1281S, 1991

[146]. Hanck, AB, Prog.Clin.Biol.Res., vol.259, p.307, 1988

[147]. Koch, CJ, et al., J.Cell.Physiol., vol.94, p.299, 1978

[148]. Lupulescu, A., Exp.Toxic.Pathol. vol.44, p.3, 1992

[149]. Riordan, NH, et al., Medical Hypotheses, vol.44, p.207, 1995

[150]. Bram, S., et al., Nature, vol.284, p.629, Apr.1980

[151]. Park, CH, et al., Cancer Research, vol.40, p.1062, Apr.1980

[152]. Poydock, ME, Am.J.Clin.Nutr., vol.54, p.1261S, 1991

[153]. Noto, V., et al., Cancer, vol.63, p.901, 1989

[154]. Gardiner, N, et al., Pros.Leuk., vol.34, p.119, 1988

[155]. Riordan, HD, et al., J. Orthomolecular Med., vol.5, p.5, 1990

[156]. Campbell, Al, Oncology, vol.48, p.495, 1991

[157]. Cameron, E., Pauling, L., Proc.Natl.Acad.Sci., vol.75, p.4538, Sept.1978

[158]. Moertel, CG, et al., N.Engl.J.Med., vol.312, p.137, 1985

[159]. Jaakkola, K., et al., Treatment with antioxidant and other nutrients in combination with chemotherapy and irradiation in patients with small-cell lung cancer, Anticancer Res 12,599-606, 1992

[160]. Lamm, DL, et al., Megadose vitamin in bladder cancer: a double-blind clinical trial, J Urol, 151:21-26, 1994

[161]. Hoffer, A, Pauling, L, Hardin Jones biostatistical analysis of mortality data of cancer patients, J Orthomolecular Med, 5:3:143-154, 1990

[162]. Marcus, SL, et al., Am.J.Clin.Nutr., vol.54, p.1292S., 1991
[163]. Abrahamian, V., et al., Ascorbic acid requirements in hospital patients, JPEN, 7, 5, 465-8, 1983
[164]. Anthony, HM, et al., Vitamin C status of lung cancer patients, Brit J Ca, 46, 354-9, 1982
[165]. Cheraskin, E., Scurvy in cancer patients?, J Altern Med, 18-23, Feb.1986
[166]. Bendich, A., in BEYOND DEFICIENCIES, NY Acad.Sci., vol.669, p.300, 1992
[167]. Kaul, L., et al., Nutr.Cancer, vol.9, p.123, 1987
[168]. Bowman, BB, et al., Am.J.Clin.Nutr., vol.35, p.1142, 1982
[169]. Rindi, G., in PRESENT KNOWLEDGE IN NUTRITION, p.163, ILSI, Washington, 1996
[170]. Elsborg, L., Int.J.Vitamin Res., vol.53, p.321, 1983
[171]. Lopez, R., et al., Am.J.Clin.Nutr., vol.33, p.1283, 1980
[172]. Schmitt-Graff, A., et al, Pathol.Res.Pract., vol.181, p.168, 1986
[173]. Popov, AI, Med.Radiol. Mosk., vol.32, p.42, 1987
[174]. Kjellen, E., et al., Radiother.Oncol., vol.22, p.81, 1991
[175]. Horsman, MR, Radiotherapy Oncology, vol.22, p.79, 1991
[176]. Aprahamian, M., et al., Am.J.Clin.Nutr., vol.41, p.578, 1985
[177]. Prior, F., Med.Hypotheses, vol.16, p.421, 1985
[178]. Chrisley, BM, et al., Nutr.Res., vol.6, p.1023, 1986
[179]. Ha, C., et al., J.Nutr., vol.114, p.938, 1984
[180]. Solomon, LR, et al., Diabetes, vol.38, p.881, 1989
[181]. Gridley, DS, et al., Nutrition Research, vol.8, p.201, 1988
[182]. Tryfiates, GP, et al., Anticancer Research, vol.1, p.263, 1981
[183]. DiSorbo, DM, et al., Nutrition and Cancer, vol.5, p.10, 1983
[184]. DiSorbo, DM, et al., Nutrition and Cancer, vol.7, p.43, 1985
[185]. Byar, D., et al., Urolog7, vol.10, p.556, Dec.1977
[186]. Lamm, DL, et al., Megadose vitamin in bladder cancer: a double-blind clinical trial, J Urol, 151:21-26, 1994
[187]. Ladner, HA, et al., Nutrition, Growth, & Cancer, p.273, Alan Liss, Inc., 1988
[188]. Cohen, M., et al., Toxicology Letters, vol.34, p.129, 1986
[189]. Poydock, ME, Am.J.Clin.Nutr., vol.54, p.1261S, 1991
[190]. Leeb, BF, et al., Clin.Exper.Rheumat., vol.13, p.459, 1995
[191]. Dokal, IS, et all, Br.Med.J., vol.300, p.1263, 1990
[192]. Bailey, LB, FOLATE IN HEALTH AND DISEASE, Marcel Dekker, NY 1995
[193]. Fekete, PS, et al., Acta. Cytologica, vol.31, p.697, 1987
[194]. Butterworth, CE, et al., Am.J.Clin.Nutr., vol.35, p.73, 1982
[195]. Freudenheim, J., Int.J.Epidemiol., vol.20, p.368, 1991
[196]. Levy, JA, BASIC AND CLINICAL IMMUNOLOGY, p.297, Lange, Los Altos, 1982
[197]. Werbach, M., NUTRITIONAL INFLUENCES ON ILLNESS, p.625, Third Line , Tarzana, 1996
[198]. Koutsikos, D., et al., Biomed.Pharmacother., vol.44, p.511, 1990

CHAPTER 22

FOOD EXTRACTS

✭

"If people let the government decide what foods they eat and what medicines they take, their bodies will soon be in as a sorry state as the souls who live under tyranny."   *- Thomas Jefferson*

WHAT'S AHEAD?
While whole foods are the foundation of this nutrition program, some ingredients in foods are so valuable as cancer fighters that they merit inclusion as concentrated supplements to:

↳ stimulate immune functions
↳ regulate the body's cell division
↳ escort any excess estrogen from the body
↳ detoxify the body

Cruciferous (as diindolylmethane DIM) 50-200 mg
Detoxifying agent, helps to neutralize the damaging effects of estrogen, may selectively slow the cancer process

---

It was the cabbage family that was first highlighted in this new and exciting field of phytochemicals. Although the father of modern medicine, Hippocrates, taught us 2,400 years ago "Let food be your medicine and medicine be your food", modern medicine has only recently begun to accept the importance of this ancient truth. For instance, researchers in the Cold War era of 1950 fed two different groups of animals either beets or cabbage and then exposed them to radiation. The animals fed cabbage had much less hemorrhaging and death from radiation. But since no one in those days could conceive of a radio-protective effect of a food, the scientists concluded that "something in beets makes radioactive exposure more lethal."[1] Actually, "something" in cabbage makes radiation much less damaging to healthy tissue.

Cruciferous vegetables include cabbage, broccoli, Brussels sprouts, cauliflower, and others. Among the phytochemicals in cruciferous vegetables that have been researched, sulforaphane is one of the more promising as a cancer fighter. It was Professor Lee Wattenburg of Minnesota who found that cabbage extract has the ability to prevent the initiation and promotion of cancer cells.[2] The various fractions in cruciferous plants, including indole-3-carbinol, isothiocyanates, glucosinolates, dithiolethiones, and phenols, are able to:[3]

♦ Prevent chemicals from being converted into cancer-causing compounds
♦ Induce liver detoxification systems, such as glutathione S-transferase and P-450, to help rid the body of poisons
♦ Scavenge free radicals, thus working as an antioxidant
♦ Prevent tumor promoters from reaching their cell targets, such as blocking the binding of estrogen to estrogen-dependent tumors

---

Maitake D-fraction (10-60 mg)
  Adaptogen, immune stimulant

Mushrooms, or fungi, have long been valued for their contributions as foods and medicines for humans. Penicillin was first discovered as bread mold, or fungi, and found to inhibit bacterial growth. Mushrooms usually grow as mold on rotten tree stumps or in manure. Of the various mushrooms that have been tested for their medicinal value, including lentinan, Shiitake, and PSK, Maitake (Grifola frondosa) has shown the most consistent anti-cancer effects from oral intake. The other mushrooms may have active ingredients that are effective when injected, but not when orally consumed.

Maitake literally means "dancing mushroom" since Japanese people who discovered these basketball-sized mushrooms growing on tree stumps would "dance with joy" at the prospects of the taste and health-giving properties. In the 1980s, Japanese firms began cultivating Maitake mushrooms on sawdust and intensely investigating the therapeutic value of this mushroom. An isolated fraction, D-fraction with active constituents of 1,6 and 1,3 beta-glucans, has been found to be the most potent and best-absorbed from the diet.

Maitake may help cancer patients via:

♦ Immune stimulation, capable of doubling the activity of Natural Killer cells in animals. D-fraction was able to increase interleukin-1 production from macrophages and potentiate delayed type hypersensitivity response, which is indicative of tumor growth suppression[4]
♦ Adaptogen that lowers hypertension[5], lowers excess blood sugar levels, protects the liver, and has anti-viral activity[6]
♦ Inhibition of metastasis of cancer by 81% in one animal study[7]
♦ Augmenting the anti-cancer activity of drugs like Mitomycin. In a comparison study between Maitake D-fraction and Mitomycin C,

Maitake provided superior tumor growth inhibition of 80% vs. 45% for the drug. Yet when both were given together, but at half the dosage for each, tumor inhibition was 98%

♦ Reducing toxic side effects from chemotherapy while augmenting tumor kill of the drug. There was a 90% drop in the incidence of appetite loss, vomiting, nausea, hair loss, and leukopenia (deficiency of immune cells) in human cancer patients treated with Maitake D-fraction while undergoing chemotherapy

---

Garlic (Kyolic) 500-2000 mg
Immune stimulant[8], detoxifying agent, antioxidant[9], powerful antifungal compound[10], protects[11] and rebuilds the liver[12], controls blood sugar levels, reduces the toxic effect of chemotherapy and radiation[13] on healthy cells, increases energy

---

First mentioned as a medicine about 6,000 years ago, garlic has been a major player in human medicines throughout the world. In the tomb of the Egyptian king, Tutankhamen, were found gold ornaments and garlic bulbs. Slaves who built the Great Pyramids relied heavily on the energizing power of garlic for their work. Hippocrates, father of modern medicine, used garlic to heal infections and to reduce pain. Although garlic has been a medical staple of many societies for over 4,000 years, only in the past few decades when over 2,000 scientific studies have proven its healing value, has garlic received the respect and attention that it deserves.

Garlic grown on selenium-rich soil, such as found in Kyolic, may be directly toxic to tumor cells.[14] Garlic may be able to impact the cancer process[15] by inhibiting:

♦ carcinogen formation in the body (i.e. nitrosamines)
♦ the transformation of normal cells to pre-cancerous cells[16]
♦ the promotion of pre-cancerous cells to cancer[17]
♦ spreading (metastasis) of cancer cells to the surface of blood vessels
♦ formation of blood vessels in tumor mass, i.e. anti-angiogenesis

The debate continues regarding the active ingredients in garlic, but they may include amino acids (like the branched chain amino acids of leucine and isoleucine), S-allyl cysteine, allicin, and organically-bound selenium. In a double-blind trial in humans with high serum cholesterol, aged deodorized garlic with no allicin content was able to lower serum cholesterol by 7%.[18] While garlic in general, as either aged, fresh, cooked, or in supplement form, is a healthy addition to anyone's nutrition program, aged garlic extracts were effective at protecting animals from liver damage.[19] An extensive review of the literature on garlic and its influence on the cancer process shows the impressive and multiple ways that garlic can help the cancer patient.[20] In a Chinese study, people who ate more garlic had a 60% reduction in the risk for stomach cancer.[21]

Aged garlic was effective at preventing the initiation and promotion phase of esophageal cancer in animals.[22] In one animal study, garlic was more effective against bladder cancer than the drug of choice in human bladder cancer, BCG (bacillus Calmette-Guerin).[23] Garlic grown on selenium-rich soil was more effective than selenium supplements at inhibiting carcinogen-induced tumors in animals.[24] A study published in the *Journal of the National Medical Association* referred to garlic as "...a potent, non-specific biologic response modifier."[25] Garlic protects against the DNA-damaging potential of DMBA[26] and the liver carcinogen, aflatoxin.[27] It stimulates immune functions by activating macrophages and spleen cells[28] as well as enhancing Natural Killer cell activity.[29]

Lycopene 3-9 mg
     Potent antioxidant and immune stimulant

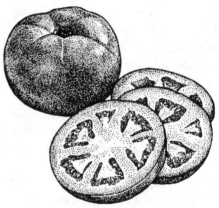

Lycopene is one of the most potent antioxidants yet tested, having double the protective capacity of beta-carotene.[30] Lycopene is the reddish pigment from the carotenoid family. Tomatoes are the richest source of lycopenes, with watermelon and red grapefruit containing appreciable amounts of lycopenes.[31] 100 grams of raw tomatoes, or about 1 cup, contains about 3 milligrams of lycopene. Lycopene has made headlines around the world, and cheers in many college dorms, in December of 1995 when a scientific study published in the *Journal of the National Cancer Institute* found that men who ate more PIZZA experienced less prostate cancer.[32] Pizza is obviously not a "nutrient dense" healthy food with all the fat, difficult-to-digest cheese, and white flour. Yet lycopene from tomatoes is such a potent antioxidant, immune stimulant, and regulator of cancer gene expression that a little tomato sauce on the pizza could neutralize the otherwise unhealthy meal of pizza and offer significant protection against the second most common cancer in American men.

As little as one serving per week of tomatoes could reduce esophageal cancer risk by 40% and other sites by 50%.[33]. In another study, blood samples from 25,000 people were frozen for 15 years. Of the people in this study who developed cancer, those with the highest levels of lycopenes had the lowest incidence of pancreatic cancer.[34]

Bovine cartilage 2-9 gm
 Immune stimulant, anti-mitotic agent (shuts down cell division in abnormal cells), anti-angiogenesis (shuts down production of blood vessels from tumors), adaptogen

---

 Bovine tracheal cartilage (BTC) is one of the more crucial and expensive of all nutrition factors to help the cancer patient, so we will spend more than a little time discussing this ingredient. Imagine these headlines: "Major drug company finds new treatment for cancer, arthritis, shingles, and many other infectious disorders". The story would be featured on TV and newspapers around the world. The stock value of that company would skyrocket. But what if that same substance was a humble little unpatentable food extract? Would the enthusiasm be as great? Bovine cartilage may be in that category.

 Good luck never hurt anyone's career. In 1954, John Prudden, MD (Harvard), PhD (Columbia), noticed an article from the reknowned Columbia-Presbyterian researchers, Drs. Meyer, Regan, and Lattes, on how topical cartilage could neutralize the disastrous effect that cortisone had on inhibiting wound recovery. This tip on the therapeutic value of cartilage had come from a mysterious "Dr. Martin" from Montreal, who has never since been located.

 The next lucky event for Prudden came when a 70-year-old woman came to him with advanced breast cancer that was literally eating away her chest cavity, in stage IV fungating breast cancer. Prudden tried the topical bovine cartilage along with injecting bovine cartilage solutions into obvious tumor areas with the hopes that it might help to heal these awful, ulcerated wounds. Surprisingly, the woman returned to Dr. Prudden with the wounds healed AND the cancer gone. It has been said that "chance favors the prepared mind".

 Over the course of 40 years, Prudden has been involved in $7 million of research to better understand BTC. Prudden received a patent on cartilage in 1962 for its anti-inflammatory properties when topically applied to arthritic regions of the body. Prudden was an affable man and dog lover who saved one of his dogs from mastocytoma (a terminal cancer) using BTC, before passing away in 1998.

 Prudden found that the wind pipe of cows was considered offal, among the waste products of the butchering process. Given the world's hunger for beef, this seemed to be a bountiful supply of inexpensive raw material. Prudden developed the complex process for removing the fat from the cartilage, then drying, and powdering it. He named his original product Catrix, short for Cicatrix, which means "healed wound".

Cartilage resembles fetal mesenchyme, which is the source for developing muscle, bones, tendons, ligaments, skin, fat, and bone marrow. It probably is this unique origin that gives rise to the many therapeutic benefits of cartilage. Initially, there was some interest in using only young (less than 6 month old) cows for BTC. Prudden believed that this is an unnecessary effort and an unproven theory.

Anti-angiogenesis? Lane's theory that shark cartilage may shut down the making of blood vessels from tumors (anti-angiogenesis) has some foundation. In 1976, Dr. Robert Langer of MIT and Dr. Judah Folkman of Harvard published work showing that something in cartilage can shut down angiogenesis in cultured tumors.[35] Later studies by this same group showed that rabbits with corneal cancers had measurable benefits from cartilage topically applied in slowing the growth of tumors.[36] In 1983, Langer and colleague Anne Lee found that something in shark cartilage could slow the growth of tumors through anti-angiogenesis.[37]

Langer pursued this line of research, finding that tumors could not grow larger than 1-2 centimeters (1/2 to 1 inch) without vascularization to support further growth.[38] Dr. Patricia D'Amore of Harvard endorsed the concept that if you shut down angiogenesis, then you shut down tumor growth.[39] Folkman's team then found that when a cell switches from normal growth (hyperplasia) to rapid and uncontrolled tumor growth (neoplasia), then the angiogenesis process gears up dramatically.[40] Other Harvard researchers found that something in cartilage definitely shuts down angiogenesis, which is essential for tumor growth.[41] Japanese researchers reported on this anti-angiogenic agent found in shark cartilage.[42] More Harvard researchers reported on the strong link between angiogenesis and tumor progression.[43] Folkman further explained the importance of anti-angiogenesis in cancer, yet added that perhaps genetic regulation is more important than some dietary protein.[44]

In discussions with pathologists and Dr. Prudden, there seems to be a difference between the blood vessels that extend cork screw-like from a tumor and the blood vessels that extend "tree

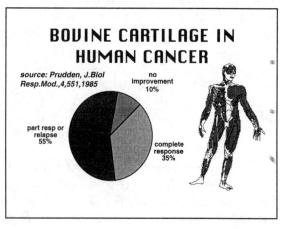

BOVINE CARTILAGE IN HUMAN CANCER

source: Prudden, J.Biol Resp.Mod.,4,551,1985

no improvement 10%

part resp or relapse 55%

complete response 35%

root-like" from healthy tissue. If there is an anti-angiogenesis factor in cartilage, then it cannot inhibit the making of normal healthy blood vessels. How does a baby shark grow into a large adult shark if shark cartilage shuts down the making of ALL blood vessels?

Prudden believed that BTC is effective because it is a biodirector, or "normalizer". There are parallels of these "homeostatic regulators" in the botanical medicine field called adaptogens, such as ginseng or astragalus, which will raise your blood pressure if it is too low or lower it if it is too high. Think about the enigma of cartilage:

⇒ topically applied, it **accelerates** healthy growth for wounds, but **slows** abnormal cancer growth

⇒ taken internally, it **increases** various immune factors, including B-cells (from the bone), macrophages (literally: "big eaters"), and cytotoxic T-cells (important in the "war on cancer"); YET it also **slows** down auto-immune attacks involved in allergies, arthritis, and lupus

⇒ taken internally, it slows the wasting disease, cachexia, caused by cancer and AIDS

⇒ taken internally, it **slows** the division in abnormal cells (anti-mitotic), but **allows** healthy cells to divide

⇒ taken internally, it **reduces** inflammation, such as in arthritis

Prudden pioneered the use of BTC for its

• wound healing properties, which culminated in textbook acceptance[45]
• anti-inflammatory agent in arthritis[46]
• anti-cancer activity.[47]

Prudden's peer-reviewed article showed a 90% response rate in 31 human cancer patients followed for 15 years. Of the 31 total patients, 35%, or 11 of these terminal patients were **cured** using 9 grams daily of oral bovine tracheal cartilage as sole therapy, while 55% or 17 showed some benefit then relapsed, and 10% or 3 showed no improvement. Prudden used BTC in over 1,000 cancer patients, with good follow-up on 100 patients. His latest research paper has been submitted for peer review before being published in a journal.

Dr. Brian Durie has found equally impressive results using BTC to halt cancer growth in vitro.[48] Prudden's other research shows that BTC probably works by turbo-charging the immune system.[49] For his noteworthy persistence and brilliance in spearheading BTC research, Prudden received the coveted "Linus Pauling Scientist of the Year" award at the Third International Symposium on Adjuvant Nutrition in Cancer Treatment in Tampa, in September of 1995.

Of all the impressive healing agents in Nature's "pharmacy", none is more safe, cost-effective, versatile, and promising than BTC.

Nucleic acids (nucleotides from brewer's yeast): DNA 500-1500 mg and RNA 500-1500 mg

Immune stimulants, help to regulate genetic expression and discourage the excessive production of Tumor Necrosis Factor, which can lead to tissue wasting

---

At the very core of our cells are the "blueprints" of DNA that allow that cell to make another exact copy. RNA has various forms that basically are the "servants" of DNA, clamping on the DNA to read the base pair sequence, then going out into the cell to construct proteins, enzymes, or whatever the cell needs based on the DNA blueprints. Obviously, this is a very crucial pathway for human health. When DNA goes awry, cancer can result. Somehow the DNA in the healthy host tissue can become corrupted and start creating cells that lack normal regulation properties, have no plan, and reproduce without any restraint.

We make our own DNA and RNA (also called nucleic acids) in our cells from amino acids in the purine and pyrimidine pathways. We also eat some DNA/RNA in metabolically active foods including brewer's yeast, liver, seeds (especially the germ), organ meats, and bee pollen. The debate has never been over the value of DNA/RNA, but rather "can we absorb these nutrients into the bloodstream intact?" To answer that question, we need to step back and look at other examples of:

♦ fatty acids that are dissected with bile salts and enzymes in the GI tract and then reassembled in the bloodstream
♦ the known passage of large proteins through the intestinal wall to cause food allergies in the bloodstream
♦ the use of glandular therapy (such as natural dessicated thyroid) to treat the target gland with a large protein molecule that should be destroyed in the acid bath of the gut.
♦ how infants receive their immunity from the immunoglobulins in mother's millk.

Either these molecules have special "windows" in the gut or these molecules are torn apart in the gut and then reassembled on the other side of the intestinal mucosa in the bloodstream. Supplements of RNA/DNA have shown benefits in both immunity and wound recovery, when taken orally in both human and animal studies.

Animals fed a nucleotide-deficient diet had impaired immune functions which were corrected when fed uracil (a DNA precursor).[50] In protein depletion, RNA supplements may be essential in order to return immune functions to normal.[51] Several human trials have studied an enteral formula, Impact, which uses RNA, arginine, and fish oil to provide substantial improvement in immune factors.[52] RNA seems to improve wound recovery after surgery.[53] RNA supplements provide a boost to memory in the elderly.[54] RNA supplements were able to help regenerate the damaged livers of rats.[55] Early indications were that RNA may be able to help cancer patients.[56] Of course, a patentable drug (Poly A/Poly U) was developed to continue these studies, with very encouraging results.[57] RNA supplements seem to encourage Natural Killer cells to attack cancer and bacteria.[58]

In personal discussions with Arsinur Bircaglu, MD, an oncologist from Turkey, she showed very intriguing human clinical data that large amounts of RNA and DNA taken orally could shut down the tissue wasting process (cachexia) that is so common in cancer and AIDS. Precursors to make more nucleic acids seem to dampen down the cytokines (Tumor Necrosis Factor) that trigger the downward spiral of cancer cachexia.

Probiotics (billions of live Lactobacillus acidophilus, Bifidobacterium bifidum, Saccharomyces boulardi)
Reduced production of carcinogens in the gut, maintenance of gut integrity and immune functions

---

It was the Nobel Laureate from Russia, Dr. Eli Metchnikoff, who told us at the turn of the century: "Death begins in the colon." Metchnikoff isolated the bacteria in yogurt, Lactobacillus, that ferments milk sugar, and he spent much of his illustrious career shedding light on the function of bacteria in the gut.

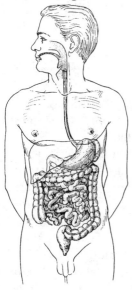

In order to better appreciate the importance of probiotics for cancer patients, we need to rewind the video cassette recorder to Louis Pasteur's deathbed confession in 1895: "I have been wrong. The germ is nothing. The terrain is everything." Pasteur was the famous French chemist who developed pasteurization, or the killing of bacteria with heat. Pasteur spent much of his life trying to figure out how to kill all the bacteria in the universe. Didn't work. By "terrain", Pasteur was referring to the land that bacteria grow in--your body. We now find that some bacteria are helpful, such as those that manufacture biotin and vitamin K in the gut. Many bacteria are relatively harmless, unless we have compromised immune functions. Many bacterial infections are called "opportunistic" because they only happen when the bacteria seize the opportunity while the host is weakened. Many bacteria in the gut can produce carcinogens and estrogens, to further a cancer process.[59] To finally give long overdue respect to an important area of human nutrition, the classical textbook MODERN NUTRITION IN HEALTH AND DISEASE now contains a chapter on probiotics or intestinal microflora.[60]

Oncologists have toiled for three decades trying to isolate cancer patients from all external bacteria, since death from infections is so common in cancer patients, especially those treated with chemotherapy. Oncologists working in bone marrow transplant (BMT) units will isolate cancer patients from family members and tell the patient to avoid fruits and vegetables, hoping to prevent an infection in the immune-compromised patient. Some BMT units even autoclave the food to try to reduce exposure to bacteria. Meanwhile, we have more bacteria in our gut than all the cells in our body. There is an ongoing struggle in your gut between bifidobacteria (good guys) and putrefactive bacteria (bad guys). The typical American diet (too much fat, sugar, and beef and not enough whole grains, fruits, and vegetables) will often create a very lethal mixture of bacteria in the gut. One pound of fecal matter contains over 50 billion bacteria.

What happens in too many cancer patients is that the infection comes from the inside, called bacterial translocation, not from the outside.[61] Only one of three factors needs to be present for disease-causing bacteria from the intestines to slide through the intestinal wall and create a life-threatening infection in the blood (sepsis):

⇒ Disruption of the ecological balance of the normal intestinal microflora, resulting in overgrowth of certain harmful bacteria
⇒ Impairment of host immune functions
⇒ Physical disruption of the gut mucosal barrier

Over 40% of our immune system is clustered around the gastro-intestinal tract. Lymph nodes sit on the intestinal wall like international border guards, keeping dangerous bacteria inside the gut from migrating into the bloodstream. Bacteria in the human gut can decompose undigestible plant matter into butyric acid, a potent anti-cancer agent.

Probiotics include a wide assortment of favorable bacteria, including Lactobacillus acidophilus from yogurt. When comparing the dietary habits of 1,000 women with and 1,000 women without breast cancer, yogurt was found to be the most protective of all foods analyzed.[62] Yogurt also helped to prevent the normal intestinal side effects caused by radiation therapy in women undergoing radiation for ovarian and cervical cancer.[63] There are soil-based organisms found in Natur-Earth (Nature's Biotics 800-622-8986) that are equally intriguing as means of rectifying an imbalanced collection of bacteria in the human gut. Since dairy products are the most allergy-producing food in the world and can produce mucous in many individuals, it is unwise to recommend widespread use of yogurt for all cancer patients, though probiotic supplements can be of benefit.

Think of probiotics as "biological controls" within the gut. We have a septic tank inside of us. Our colon holds more than enough bacteria and fungi to kill us, yet when the gut flora is in balance, these deadly bacteria pass through us without doing any harm. Compare the balance of organisms in our gut with a healthy balanced organic garden. The birds and frogs (probiotics) eat the insects (unfriendly bacteria) and leave the vegetables (food in our gut) for us to digest and absorb.

Researchers in Russia gave gunshot-wounded animals either antibiotics, or probiotics, or no treatment (control) and found that probiotics were more effective than antibiotics at preventing surgical infection.[64] Bacterial translocation was dramatically reduced in animals who were given surgery on the gut, then probiotics.[65] Antibiotics can kill off the friendly bacteria in the gut, leaving the distinct possibility of bacterial translocation of the nasty bacteria into the bloodstream. In an animal study, the probiotic Saccharomyces boulardii was able to reduce the incidence of bacterial translocation from antibiotics.[66] Bone marrow transplantation operations often trigger a "graft versus host" disease, which means the patient who received the new immune cells is having an allergic response because this is not the patient's own DNA. German oncologists found that giving yogurt to patients undergoing allogeneic bone marrow transplantation (getting immune cells from someone else versus getting your own—autologous) dramatically reduced the bacterial translocation of enteric bacteria.[67]

Rather than discouraging the intake of friendly bacteria, as oncologists now do, it would be much wiser to encourage the cancer patient to develop a healthy gut microflora through the use of fermented foods, like yogurt, and supplements with probiotics.

Bee pollen 600 mg
Rich in amino acids, B-vitamins, and bioflavonoids; historically used as an energizer, blood builder, and immune stimulant

---

Bee pollen is a rich and well-balanced collection of B-vitamins, vitamin C, RNA and DNA, amino acids, polyunsaturated fats, enzymes, trace minerals, bioflavonoids, and an assortment of other unidentified nutrition factors.

Bee pollen has been used throughout history as a superfood to restore energy and recuperative powers to the ailing individual.[68] Bee pollen improves allergies in many individuals, and hence may have a regulating effect on the immune system by helping to dampen unnecessary autoimmune attacks, which saves immune warriors for the real cancer battle. There is no toxicity to bee pollen. Other bee products with extraordinary healing properties include royal bee jelly and propolis, which is the antibiotic compound used by bees to disinfect their hives before occupation. Some people use propolis as a substitute for antibiotics in non-life threatening infections.

Lecithin (phosphatidylcholine) 1-3 grams
　　Helps to detoxify the liver, regulates cell growth, contributes choline for many other functions in the body, becomes part of healthy cell membranes for proper nutrient intake and toxin removal

---

　　Lecithin is an incredible substance with great potential to help the cancer patient. Most substances in life are either fat soluble, such as butter, or water soluble, such as vitamin C. Lecithin is on a very short list of substances that can dissolve both fat and water soluble substances at the same time, also known as an emulsifier. Lecithin is used widely in the food industry to prevent separation of ingredients in cookies, etc. The richest sources of lecithin are soybeans and egg yolks. For a little experiment, next time you finish with blending some eggs for scrambling, add water to the container and use an electric blender to see the "soap bubbles" rise from the leftover lecithin-rich egg yolks.

　　Lecithin is a molecule that is similar in structure to triglycerides found in soy oil and beef, except that one of the fatty acids has been replaced by phosphatidylcholine. This simple exchange gives lecithin unique properties, including:

⇒ lowering of serum cholesterol and reduction of platelet aggregation in humans[69]

⇒ reversing the skin disease psoriasis[70]

⇒ improving the course of Alzheimer's disease[71]

⇒ reducing the tremors in tardive dyskinesia[72]

　　Lecithin seems to work in the cell membrane to enhance "cell membrane dynamics", works in the nervous tissue (sphingomyelin), and contributes a key B-vitamin, choline. Choline works with folate, methionine, and B-12 as methyl donors, which are responsible for all new cell growth.

　　Choline is one of the few nutrients tested in which merely a deficiency (without any other compounding factor, such as toxins or aging) is enough to spontaneously generate liver cancer in animals.[73] In animal and human studies, choline deficiency leads to fatty liver and compromised liver functions.[74] Lecithin is a major protective nutrient for the liver, helping to regenerate healthy liver tissue and excrete toxins. Protecting the liver, with substances like lecithin and milk thistle, is crucial for cancer patients.

> **Genistein (from non-genetically modified organism soy) 6 mg**
> Helps to selectively slow down cancer growth

When scientists reviewed the world's cancer incidences, they found some strange disparities. Japanese men had 1/5 the incidence of prostate cancer and Japanese women had 1/5 the incidence of breast cancer when compared to Americans. The reasons could be many, including a lower fat diet, more exercise, less beef, less obesity, and more vegetables and seaweed. But researchers settled in on soybean products, including tofu and tempeh, as the primary protector against cancer. It has now been well established that regular consumption of soy products may lower the incidence of many forms of cancer.[75] While there is a rich collection of isoflavones, protease inhibitors, and lectins in soybeans, researchers have focused on genistein as perhaps the cancer-protective bioflavonoid in soy.

Genistein may be able to:

♦ selectively kill cancer cells
♦ reduce the tumor growth capacity of sex hormones in both men and women
♦ induce programmed cell death (apoptosis) in cancer
♦ inhibit metastasis
♦ inhibit angiogenesis[76] (making of blood vessels from tumors)
♦ induce differentiation, to help regulate proper cell growth.[77]

Genistein is one of the few agents on planet earth that may be able to revert a cancer cell back to a normal healthy cell, in a process called prodifferentiation.[78] Scientists have worked diligently to better understand the anti-cancer effects of protease inhibitors in soy.[79] Dr. Ann Kennedy spent 20 years at Harvard, and is now working at the University of Pennsylvania, researching the extraordinary ability of the Bowman Birk Inhibitor (a protease inhibitor found in soy) to prevent and reverse cancer while also reducing the toxic effects of chemo and radiation on animals.[80]

Soy and breast cancer. Based on the fact that soy contains weak phytoestrogens that can induce infertility in zoo animals kept on a high soy diet, some experts have cautioned against the use of soy in estrogen/progesterone-positive breast cancer. Tamoxifen is an estrogen binder drug that is given to women with estrogen-positive breast cancer. Tamoxifen has a similar chemical structure to genistein, yet genistein does not have any of the toxic side effects of Tamoxifen. Once again, Nature comes up with another brilliantly helpful molecule in genistein, which inhibits both breast and prostate cancer.[81] Genistein actually slows the growth of breast cancer cells in culture.[82] The macrobiotic diet uses large amounts of soy to help slow the growth of many cancers, including breast cancer. A fermented and concentrated soy product, Haelen 851, has been used successfully to reverse breast cancer. For more on this subject, refer to the explanation of ginseng, which also contains phytoestrogens.

PATIENT PROFILE: REVERSING STAGE 4 STOMACH CANCER
B.C. was a 46 year old male diagnosed with stage 4 stomach cancer that had spread to 40% of his liver. His doctor gave him 6 months to 2 years to live. B.C.'s wife put him on the nutrition program in this book for a month at which point he then took chemo. He tolerated the chemo much better than the doctors had anticipated, probably because B.C. was taking many nutrition supplements which the doctor told him not to do. Three months later, the stomach cancer was gone and liver showed 3 remaining spots. Added herbal teas to their regimen which reduced the abdominal bloating. CAT scans 5 months later showed only 1 small spot remaining on the liver. Doctor was ecstatic. B.C. credits his wife's nutrition research with saving his life.

ENDNOTES

[1]. Lourau, G., et al., Experientia, vol.6, p.25, 1950
[2]. Wattenburg, LW, Cancer Res. (suppl), vol.52, p. 2085S, 1992
[3]. Kensler, TW, et al., p.154-196, in FOOD CHEMICALS AND CANCER PREVENTION, vol.1, American Chemical Society, Wash DC, 1994
[4]. Hishida, I., et al., Chem.Pharm.Bull., vol.36, p.1819, 1988
[5]. Adachi, K., et al., Chem.Pharm.Bull., vol.36, p.1000, 1988
[6]. Nanba, H., J. Orthomolecular Med., vol.12, p.43, 1997
[7]. Nanba, H., Cancer Prevention, NYAS, p.243, Sept.1995
[8]. Lau, BHS, et al., Molecular Biotherapeutics, vol.3, p.103, June 1991
[9]. Imai, J., et al., Planta Medica, p.417, 1994
[10]. Tadi, PP, et al., International Clinical Nutrition Reviews, vol.10, p.423, 1990
[11]. Nakagawa, S., et al., Phytotherapy, Research, vol.1,p.1, 1988
[12]. Horie, T., et al., Planta Medica, vol.55, p.506, 1989
[13]. Lau, BHS, International Clinical Nutrition Reviews, vol.9, p.27, 1989
[14]. Ip, C., et al., Nutr.Cancer, vol.17, p.279, 1992
[15]. Dausch, JG, et al., Preventive Medicine, vol.19, p.346, 1990
[16]. Wargovich, MJ, et al., Cancer Letters, vol.64, p.39, 1992
[17]. Belman, S, Carcinogenesis, vol.4, p.1063, 1983
[18]. Steiner, M., et al., Amer.J.Clin.Nutr., vol.64, p.866, 1996
[19]. Nakagawa, S., et al., Phytotherapy Res., vol.1, p.1, 1988
[20]. Dausch, JG, et al., Preventive Med., vol.19, p.346, 1990
[21]. You, WC, et al., J. Nat.Cancer Inst., vol.81, p.162, 1989
[22]. Wargovich, MJ, et al., Cancer Letters, vol.64, p.39, 1992
[23]. Marsh, CL, et al., J. Urology, vol.137, p.359, Feb.1987
[24]. Ip, C., et al., Nutrition and Cancer, vol.17, no.3, p.279, 1992
[25]. Abdullah, TH, et al., J.Nat.Med.Assoc., vol.80, p.439, 1988
[26]. Amagase, H., et al., Carcinogenesis, vol.14, p.1627, 1993
[27]. Yamasaki, T., et al., Cancer Letters, vol.59, p.89, 1991
[28]. Hirao, Y., et al., Phytotherapy Research, vol.1, p.161, 1987

[29]. Abdullah, TH et al., Onkologie, vol.21, p.53, 1989

[30]. DiMascio, P., et al., Arch.Biochem.Biophysics, vol.274, p.532, 1989

[31]. Mangels, AR, et al., J.Am.Diet.Assoc., vol.93, p.284, 1993

[32]. Giovannucci, E., et al., J.Nat.Can.Inst., vol.87, p.1767, 1995

[33]. Franceschi, S., et al., Int.J.Cancer, vol.59, p.181, 1994

[34]. Comstock, GW, et al., Amer.J.Clin.Nutr., vol.53, p.260S, 1991

[35]. Langer, R. et al., Science, p.70, July 1976

[36]. Langer, R. et al., Proceedings National Academy of Sciences, vol.77, no.7, p.4331, July 1980

[37]. Lee, A., et al., Science, vol.221, p.1185, Sept.1983

[38]. Folkman, J, et al., Science, vol.235, p.442, Jan.1987

[39]. D'Amore, PA, Seminars in Thrombosis & Hemostasis, vol.14, p.73, 1988

[40]. Folkman, J., et al., Nature, vol.339, p.58, May 1989

[41]. Moses, MA, et al., Science, vol.248, p.1408, June 1990

[42]. Oikawa, T., et al., Cancer Letters, vol.51, p.181, 1990

[43]. Weidner, N., et al., New England Journal of Medicine, vol.324, p.1, Jan.1991

[44]. Folkman, J., Journal Clinical Oncology, vol.12, p.441, Mar.1994

[45]. Madden, JW, in SABISTON'S TEXTBOOK OF SURGERY, p.268, WB Saunders, Philadelphia, 1972

[46]. Prudden, JF, et al., Seminars in Arthritis and Rheumatism, vol.3, p.287, Summer 1974

[47]. Prudden, JF, Journal of Biological Response Modifiers, vol.4, p.551, 1985

[48]. Durie, BGM, et al., Journal of Biological Response Modifiers, vol.4, p.590, 1985

[49]. Rosen, J, et al., Journal of Biological Response Modifiers, vol.7, p.498, 1988

[50]. Kinsella, J., et al., Crit.Care Med., vol.18, p.S94, 1990

[51]. Pizzini, RP, et al., Surgical Infection Society abstract, p.50, 1989

[52]. Cerra, FB, Am.J.Surg., vol.161, p.230, 1991; see also Cerra, FB, et al., Nutrition, vol.6, p.88, 1990; see also Lieberman, M., et al., Nutrition, vol.6, p.88, 1990

[53]. Aarons, S., et al., J.Surg.Onc., vol.23, p.21, 1983

[54]. Cameron, DE, et al., Am.J.Psychiatry, vol.120, p.320, 1963

[55]. Newman, EA, et al., Amer.J.Physiol., vol.164, p.251, 1951

[56]. Pilch, YH, Am.J.Surg., vol.132, p.631, 1976

[57]. Michelson, AM, et al., Proc.Soc.Exper.Biol. Med., vol.179, p.1, 1985

[58]. Wiltrout, RH, et al., J.Biol.Resp.Mod., vol.4, p.512, 1985

[59]. Tomomatsu, H., Food Technology, p.61, Oct.1994

[60]. Goldin, BR, et al., MODERN NUTRITION, Shils, ME (eds), p.569, Lea & Febiger, Phila, 1994

[61]. Deitch, EA, Archives Surgery, vol.125, p.403, Mar.1990

[62]. Le, MG, et al., J.Nat.Cancer Inst., vol.77, p.633, Sept.1986

[63]. Salminen, E., et al., Clin.Radiol., vol.39, p.435, 1988

[64]. Nikitenko, VI, J.Wound Care, vol.13, no.9, p.363, Oct. 2004

[65]. Seehofer, D., J.Surg.Res., vol.117, no.2, p.262, Apr.2004

[66]. Herek, O, Surg. Today, vol.34, no.3, p.256, 2004

[67]. Gerbitz, A, Blood, vol.103, no.11, p.4365, Jun 1, 2004

[68]. Page, LR, HEALTHY HEALING, p.76, Healthy Healing Publ, 1996

[69]. Brook, JG, et al., Biochem.Med.Metab.Biol.,vol. 35, p.31, 1986

[70]. Gross, P, et al., NY State J.Med., vol.50, p.2683, 1950

[71]. Little, A., et al., J.Neurology, Neurosurgery & Psychiatry, vol.48, p.736, 1985

[72]. Jackson, IV, et al., Am.J.Psychiatry, vol.136, p.11, Nov.1979

[73]. Yokoyama, S, et al., Cancer Res., vol.45, p.2834, 1985

[74]. Zeisel, SH, et al., Fed Amer Soc Exper Biol., vol.5, p.2093, 1991

[75]. Messina, M., et al., J.Nat.Cancer Inst., vol.83, p.541, 1991

[76]. Fostis, T., et al., Proc. Natl. Acad.Sci., vol.90, p.2690, 1993

[77]. Boik, J., CANCER & NATURAL MEDICINE, p.184, Oregon Medical, Princeton, MN 1995

[78]. Watanabe, T., et al., Exp.Cell Res., vol.183, p.335, 1989

[79]. Hocman, G., Int.J.Biochem., vol.24, p.1365, 1992

[80]. Kennedy, AR, in ADJUVANT NUTRITION IN CANCER TREATMENT, p.129, Quillin, P. (eds), Cancer Treatment Research Foundation, Arlington Heights, IL 1994

[81]. Adlercreutz, H., et al., Lancet, vol.342, p.1209, Nov.1993

[82]. Peterson, G., et al., Biochem.Biophy.Res.Commun., vol.179, p.661, 1991

CHAPTER 23

ACCESSORY FACTORS

*

"The bad news is that half of what we have taught you is wrong. The worse news is that we can't tell you which half is wrong."
spoken at a medical school graduation

WHAT'S AHEAD?
Accessory factors are nutritional compounds that are not yet considered essential, yet may hold the key to optimal health by:
↳ improving energy metabolism
↳ providing full-spectrum antioxidant protection
↳ bolstering detoxification pathways

While there are around 50 nutrients that are considered essential in the diet of humans, there are literally thousands of other "accessory factors" found in various foods. There is increasing evidence that we may need these substances in our diet in order to maintain optimal health. These accessory factors may someday be considered "conditionally essential" nutrients, which means that during some phases of life (i.e. very young, older, sick), these nutrients would become essential in the diet. Cancer patients often have a compromised system that is unable to manufacture optimal amounts of these nutrients in the body. The difference between "surviving" and "thriving to beat cancer" may rest in the intake of these accessory factors.

Coenzyme Q-10, 100-300 mg
Improves aerobic metabolism, immune stimulant, membrane stabilizer, improves prostaglandin metabolism.

CoQ is found in the energy transport system of mammals, specifically the mitochondrial membrane. Dr. Peter Mitchell was awarded the Nobel prize for his work in 1975 on CoQ. CoQ is nearly a wonder drug in reversing cardiomyopathy.[1] CoQ is either manufactured in the human body from the amino acid tyrosine and mevalonate or consumed in the diet, with heart and liver tissue being particularly rich in CoQ-10 for humans. Hence, CoQ, along with carnitine, EPA, and other nutrition factors, are considered "conditionally essential nutrients", since we may not be able to manufacture enough of these nutrients at certain phases of the life cycle. Niacin is an essential vitamin that also is produced within the body (endogenous source) and consumed in the diet (exogenous sources). CoQ is also called ubiquinone, since various forms of this molecule are found everywhere (as in ubiquitous). CoQ may help cancer patients by:

◊ correcting CoQ deficiency states[2], since we don't eat liver or heart and lose the capacity to make CoQ within as we age

◊ radical scavenger (antioxidant) that works with vitamin E in the fat-soluble portions of the body and cells[3]

◊ stabilizing cell membranes through interaction with phospholipids[4]

◊ correction of mitochondrial "leak" of electrons during oxidative respiration, which improves aerobic production of ATP[5]

◊ improving prostaglandin metabolism[6]

◊ stabilizing calcium-dependent channels on cell membrane receptor sites[7]

CoQ may enhance immune functions.[8] CoQ reduces the damage to the heart (probably by sparing mitochondrial membranes) from the chemotherapy drug adriamycin.[9] Long-term users of adriamycin risk cardiac arrest, unless given adequate CoQ, vitamin E, niacin, and other nutrients to reduce the damage to the heart. Using 300 mg daily of CoQ as sole therapy, 6 of 32 breast cancer patients (19%) experienced partial tumor regression, while one woman took 390 mg daily and gained complete remission.[10] Given the fact that CoQ probably becomes an essential nutrient as we age and become ill, there are good reasons to include CoQ in your nutrition supplement program. CoQ is best absorbed in the presence of fats in your digestive tract, especially lecithin, fish, shark, and borage oils.

Lipoic acid 30-100 mg

Alpha lipoic acid (a.k.a. thioctic acid) is involved in energy metabolism, but also works as a potent antioxidant, regulator of blood sugar metabolism, chelator (remover) of heavy metals, improves memory, discourages the growth of cancer, and prevents glycation (sugar binding to cell membranes) that can change the flexibility of cell membranes and blood vessels.

Lipoic acid works with pyruvate and acetyl CoA in a critical point in energy metabolism.[11] Partly because of this pivotal job in generating ATP, lipoic acid becomes an incredibly multi-talented nutrient. Though lipoic acid is not considered an essential nutrient yet, as humans age we produce less and less of lipoic acid internally.[12] Because of its unique size and chemical structure, lipoic acid works as an antioxidant that can penetrate both fat-soluble (like vitamin E) and water-soluble (like vitamin C) portions of the body.[13] This gives lipoic acid access to virtually the entire body, whereas most antioxidants only protect isolated areas of the body.

Lipoic acid prevents "glycation" or glycosylation, which means the binding of sugar molecules to important proteins in the bloodstream, cell membrane, nerve tissue, etc. Glycation is a disastrous "tanning" that occurs, not unlike turning soft cow skin into hard leather in the tanning process. These new proteins that are bound to sugars do not have the same abilities as before the glycation process. Supplements of lipoic acid have been found to reverse the peripheral neuropathy from diabetes in as little as 3 weeks.[14] Lipoic acid improves blood flow to the nerves, which then improves nerve conduction.[15] Many cancer patients suffer peripheral neuropathy as a by-product of the damaging effects of chemotherapy. Lipoic acid may prevent and reverse this destruction of nerve tissue. Because of its role in aerobic metabolism, lipoic acid supplements in animals provided an increase in the amount of oxygen reaching the heart by 72% and the liver by 128%. Since cancer is an anaerobic growth, enhancing aerobic metabolism in a cancer patient is like shining daylight on a vampire.

Lipoic acid increases the available levels of other antioxidants in the body, like vitamin E[16] and glutathione.[17] While there are many antioxidants found in a healthy diet and produced in the body (like uric acid), lipoic acid is the only antioxidant that meets the "wish list" of Dr. Lester Packer of the University of California at Berkeley. That "perfect" antioxidant should:
⇒ neutralize free radicals
⇒ be rapidly absorbed and quickly utilized by the body cells
⇒ be able to enhance the action of other antioxidants
⇒ be concentrated both inside and outside cells and cell membranes
⇒ promote normal gene expression
⇒ chelate metal ions, or drag toxic minerals out of the body.[18]

Because of its role as an antioxidant and the critical need for immune cells to be protected from their own cellular poisons, lipoic acid has been shown to improve antibody response in immunosuppressed animals.[19]

Lipoic acid also works to improve the efficiency of insulin by allowing blood glucose into the cells. Animal studies showed that supplements of lipoic acid increased insulin sensitivity by 30-50% and reduced plasma insulin and free fatty acids by 15-17%.[20]

SAFETY ISSUES. In over 30 years of extensive use and testing in European clinical trials, there have been no serious side effects reported from the use of lipoic acid.

L-glutathione (reduced) 100-300 mg
   Stimulator of immune system, detoxification, re~ division and prostaglandin metabolism.

Glutathione is one of the most widely distributed and important antioxidants in all of nature, yet there has been some confusion regarding its use in cancer patients and its absorption. So keep your thinking cap on as we review this nutrient.

Glutathione is a tripeptide, meaning a molecule formed from three amino acids: glutamine, cysteine, and glycine. Some clinicians have chosen to use N-acetyl-cysteine as a means of augmenting the production of glutathione in the body. Glutathione, also abbreviated GSH, is one of the most widely-distributed antioxidants in plants and animals, and is the chief thiol (sulfur-bearing) molecule in most cells. Glutathione plays a central role in the enzyme system glutathione peroxidase, which is crucial for cell metabolism, cell regulation, detoxification, DNA synthesis and repair, immune function, prostaglandin metabolism, and regulation of cell proliferation through apoptosis (programmed cell death).[21] GSH is particularly helpful in protecting the liver from damage upon exposure to toxins.[22] GSH levels are decreased in most disease states, infertility, aging, toxic burden, and other unfavorable health conditions.[23] Lower levels of blood GSH are associated with more illness, higher blood pressure, higher percent body fat, and reduced general health status.[24] Cancer patients have less GSH in their blood than healthy people.[25] So far, no controversy.

glutamine+cysteine+glycine=glutathione

Help cancer patients? Some oncologists have reasoned that GSH provides one of the main protective mechanisms for cancer cells to develop resistance to chemotherapy.[26] Thus, efforts have been made to develop drugs that deplete the cancer patient of GSH. However, supplements of glutathione in patients being treated for ovarian cancer with the drug cisplatin had an improvement in outcome and reduced kidney toxicity from the cisplatin.[27] In another study of 55 patients with stomach cancer, GSH prevented the neurotoxicity usually associated with cisplatin and did not reduce the anti-neoplastic activity of the drug.[28] In animals exposed to a potent carcinogen (DMBA), GSH provided significant reduction in the size and incidence of tumors.[29] Animals exposed to DMBA and given GSH, vitamin C, E, and betacarotene had substantial reduction in the number and size of cancers.[30]

In animals with chemically-induced (aflatoxin) liver cancer (an extremely poor prognostic cancer), 100% died within 20 months, while 81% of the animals with liver cancer that were treated with GSH were disease-free 4 months later.[31] Eight patients with advanced refractory (resistant to medical therapy) liver cancer were given 5 grams daily of oral GSH, with most surviving longer than expected and one being cured.[32] Glutathione in the diet has been shown to protect the intestinal wall of animals from the insult of chemical carcinogens.[33] In cultured cancer cells, GSH was able to induce apoptosis (programmed cell death), which may be one of the ways that GSH can assist cancer patients.[34]

Can you absorb GSH in the gut? In one study, 7 healthy human subjects were given increasingly higher oral supplements of GSH up to 3 grams daily with blood levels showing no significant increase in glutathione, cysteine, or glutamate.[35] However, many other studies with humans and animals[36] have found GSH well absorbed into the bloodstream. Best sources of GSH are dark green leafy vegetables, fresh fruit, and lightly cooked fish, poultry, and beef. Processing reduces the GSH levels of foods.

Trimethylglycine 10-500 mg (aka betaine)
Detoxifier, protects liver, lowers homocysteine, and energizer.

Trimethylglycine, or TMG, is the oxidative product of choline. If the body is made up of "bricks", then methylation is the laying of each individual bricks. TMG is heavily involved in methylation throughout the body, which means that TMG:

➢ lowers the cardiotoxic levels of homocysteine[37]
➢ protects the liver from alcohol ingestion[38]
➢ in animal studies, protects the liver from carcinogens[39]
➢ reverses non-alcoholic steatosis (fatty infiltration and deterioration of the liver)[40]

L-carnitine 100-300 mg
Involved in energy metabolism of fats, thus preventing fatty buildup in heart and liver and encouraging the complete combustion of fats for energy. Cancer cells cannot use fat for energy.

Think of carnitine as the "shoveller throwing fresh coals into the furnace" of the cell's mitochondria. Carnitine was first isolated from meat extracts in 1905, hence the "carnitine", refers to animal sources. Indeed, there is virtually no carnitine in plant foods, with red meats having the highest carnitine content.[41] The typical American diet provides from 5-100 mg/day of carnitine. Humans can manufacture carnitine in the liver and kidney from the precursors (raw materials to make) of lysine and methionine, and the cofactors of vitamin C, niacin, B-6, and iron. A deficiency of any of these precursors may lead to a carnitine deficiency, which involves buildup of fats in the blood, liver, and muscles and may lead to symptoms of weakness. Since infants require carnitine in their diet and other individuals have been found to have clinical carnitine deficiencies, some nutritionists have lobbied to have carnitine included as an essential nutrient, not unlike niacin.[42]

Carnitine may help the cancer patient by:
◊   protecting the liver from fatty buildup[43]
◊   improving energy and endurance[44]
◊   protecting the heart against the damaging effects of adriamycin.[45]
◊   In cultured cells, carnitine supplements provided for bolstering of immune functions (polymorphonuclear chemotaxis) and reduced the ability of fats to lower immune functions.[46]

Carnitine is probably essential in the diet for people who are very young, or sick, stressed, older, burdened with toxins, etc.

> **Tocotrienols 20-40 mg**
> Antioxidant, immune stimulant, regulates fatty acid metabolism.

I hiked up to the top of Mount San Gorgonio in southern California in 1984. The view was spectacular. However, when I pulled out my binoculars, I could see much more detail. And when I borrowed a pair of high-powered binoculars from a friend, the details of the surrounding landscape became even more defined and clear. The same thing is happening in the field of nutrition. As our analytical equipment becomes more sophisticated, our ability to see subsets of molecules that work together becomes more impressive. The star nutrient of today may become a supporting actress tomorrow. Such may be the case for vitamin E (tocopherols) and its kissing cousin, tocotrienols.

While some nutritionists campaign against the use of palm oil, since it has a higher content of saturated fats than soy or corn oil, the data actually show that palm oil may LOWER the risk for heart disease, since it is rich in tocotrienols, which are potent antioxidants that protect the blood vessel walls.[47] Palm oil is the second largest volume of vegetable oil produced in the world.

Tocotrienols are very similar in structure to tocopherols, which is vitamin E. Palm oil and rice bran are the richest sources of tocotrienols. Tocotrienols have only 30% the vitamin E activity when compared to D-alpha-tocopherol, the "gold standard" of vitamin E.[48] Yet tocotrienols have demonstrated a greater anti-cancer activity than vitamin E.[49] Tocotrienols were able to delay onset of cancer in animals, while mixed carotenes from palm oil were able to regress these same cancers.[50] In vitro and in vivo, dietary palm oil (richest source of tocotrienols) was able to exhibit a "dose dependent" anti-tumor activity against several carcinogenic compounds.[51] Just as some researchers now feel that bioflavonoids are more important in human nutrition than the vitamin C that was discovered first, there are some very bright scientists who feel that the primary role of vitamin E is to help manufacture and protect tocotrienols, which may have the ultimate antioxidant and immune-stimulating activity in the human body.

Quercetin 100-400 mg
     Bioflavonoid with unique immune stimulating and anti-neoplastic activity.

While a review paper from 1983 estimated that about 500 varieties of bioflavonoids existed in nature[52], more current estimates go as high as 20,000 different bioflavonoid compounds. Bioflavonoids are basically accessory factors used by plants to assist in photosynthesis and reduce the damaging effects from the sun. Best sources of bioflavonoids are citrus, berries, onions, parsley, legumes, green tea, and bee pollen. The average Western diet contains somewhere between 150 mg/day[53] and 1,000 mg/day[54] of bioflavonoids, with about 25 mg/day of quercetin. Best source of quercetin is the white rind in citrus fruits. Of all the nutrition factors discussed in this book, only a few, including quercetin, have shown the potential to revert a cancerous cell back to a normal healthy cell, called prodifferentiation.[55]

Quercetin has many talents that may help the cancer patient:[56]

◊ Induces apoptosis, or programmed cell death in otherwise "immortal" cancer cells
◊ Inhibits inflammation, by reducing histamine release
◊ Inhibits tumor cell proliferation
◊ Competes with estrogen for binding sites, thus defusing the damaging effects of estrogen
◊ Helps to inhibit drug resistance in tumor cells[57]
◊ Potent antioxidant
◊ May inhibit angiogenesis (making of blood vessels from the tumor)
◊ Inhibits capillary fragility, which protects connective tissue against breakdown by tumors
◊ Has anti-viral activity
◊ Reduces the "stickiness" of cells, or aggregation, thus slowing cancer metastasis

◊ Reduces the toxicity and carcinogenic capacity of substances in the body[58] YET at the same time may enhance the tumor-killing capacity of cisplatin[59]

◊ Helps to eliminate toxic metals through chelation[60]

◊ Increases the anti-neoplastic activity of hyperthermia (heat therapy) on cancer cells

◊ May revert cancer cells back to normal cells (prodifferentiation), possibly by repairing the defective energy mechanism in the cancer cells[61]

Quercetin was considered a possible carcinogen based upon the Ames in vitro test in 1977, since it caused mutagenic changes to cells. Yet, new studies show that quercetin is not a carcinogen, but may be one of the most potent anticarcinogens in nature.[62]

Another area of debate surrounding quercetin is bioavailability. One study gave a 4 gram oral dose once of quercetin to 6 healthy volunteers, then measured for quercetin in the blood. No quercetin could be found in the blood or urine, and 53% of the dose ended up in the stools, giving suspicions that quercetin is not well absorbed from the diet.[63] However, since then, many studies giving oral doses of quercetin to animals and humans have found major therapeutic benefits, indicating that it is somehow absorbed into the bloodstream, according to world-reknowned experts in the field, Elliott Middleton, MD, and Chithan Kandaswami, PhD. Quercetin may travel through the bloodstream as a similar structure molecule (called an analog), making it difficult to detect in bioavailability studies.

In animals fed 5% of their diet as quercetin, there was a 50% reduction in the incidence of tumors after exposure to carcinogens, while animals fed 2% quercetin had a 25% reduction in tumor incidence.[64] Quercetin has been shown to inhibit estrogen-dependent tumors by occupying the critical estrogen receptor sites on the tumor cell membranes.[65] Quercetin, at relatively low concentration, has been shown to inhibit the proliferation of squamous cancer cells.[66] Quercetin and other bioflavonoids have shown the ability to inhibit metastasis in cultured cells.[67] Quercetin significantly increased the tumor kill rate of hyperthermia (heat therapy) in cultured cancer cells.[68] Head and neck squamous cancers in humans are resistant to most medical therapies and have a high rate of tumor recurrence. Quercetin was selectively toxic in both in vitro and in vivo head and neck cancers in a dose-dependent fashion.[69]

One problem for cancer patients can be inflammation, or swelling of tissue. This is a crucial "tightrope walk", in which you want a certain amount of alarm in the immune system, which creates dumping of free radicals and swelling; yet you don't want too much of this, or it creates weakness, pain, discomfort, and tissue wasting. Rigdon Lentz, MD is a pioneering oncologist who has developed and patented a device for filtering the factors in the blood of cancer patients (Tumor Necrosis Factor inhibitors) that prevent the immune system from attacking the tumor. Dr. Lentz finds that he must provide a gradual attack on the tumor, or else swelling and tumor lysis (bursting of cancer cells) can actually kill the cancer patient with toxic by-products. Quercetin can help reduce swelling by helping to produce anti-inflammatory prostaglandins.[70] Quercetin inhibits the release of histamine from mast cells, thus reducing allergic reactions.[71] Quercetin also helps to stabilize cell membranes, decrease lipid peroxidation, and inhibit the breakdown of connective tissue (collagen) by hyaluronidase (one of the ways that cancer spreads).[72]

SAFETY ISSUES. There has been no demonstrated toxicity of quercetin in humans or animals.

Medium chain triglycerides (MCT) 1-10 gm
Slows down lean tissue wasting, enhances thermogenesis (making of heat), and augments burning of fat, a fuel source which cancer cells cannot use.

Fatty acids can have a length of anywhere from 2 carbons to 24 carbons. The long chain fats (or triglycerides, called LCT) include most dietary fats of soy oil and beef fat. LCT is difficult to absorb and requires special bile acids and absorption pathways in the lymphatic ducts.[73] Medium chain triglycerides (MCT) are much easier to absorb and are quickly burned in the human system. MCTs are primarily found in coconut oil and smaller amounts in other nuts. Almost like adding kindling (MCT) to a group of logs (LCT), medium chain triglycerides actually promote the burning of the body's fat stores, which helps to encourage thermogenesis (making of heat) in humans.[74] Cancer cells can be selectively destroyed by elevating the body temperature. MCT has been shown to be a useful tool:
◊ in the control of obesity
◊ lowering serum cholesterol
◊ as a concentrated and readily available source of energy
◊ helps to prevent immune suppression in critically ill people[75]
◊ maintains body (visceral) protein stores during wound recovery.[76]

MCT is extremely safe, provides quick energy for the person, does not feed the cancer, protects protein reserves in the body, and helps to slowly melt away unwanted fat stores in the adipose tissue.

L-glycine 1 gm

    Energizer, calmitive agent, detoxifier, controls fat levels in the blood, builds energy stores (glycogen) in the liver, helps in wound recovery and collagen synthesis.

    Glycine's name reflects its sweet flavor. It is considered a non-essential amino acid, since it can be formed from the amino acids threonine and serine. Glycine may help the cancer patient in several ways:

◊   Acts as a preservative in foods

◊   Sweetening agent, tastes much like sugar, does not alter glycemic index

◊   May be converted into glutathione (see that section) for antioxidant and detoxification benefits

◊   May be converted in the body into dimethylglycine (DMG)

◊   Works as a calming agent in the nervous system and also helps to improve spastic conditions[77] and muscular weakness.[78]

◊   Promotes collagen formation, thus possibly helping the body to encapsulate tumors

---

Glucaric acid (cal D glucarate) 500-1000 mg

    Improves detoxification in the gut and liver, escorts estrogen out of the system, may have anti-proliferative activity.

    Calcium D-glucarate, or CDG, is such a non-toxic and potentially helpful substance for cancer patients that it is undergoing Phase I trials sponsored by the National Cancer Institute and held at Memorial Sloan Kettering Hospital in New York. D-glucaric acid is a substance found in certain fruits (oranges) and vegetables (broccoli, potatoes). CDG has been shown to encourage critical phase II detoxification pathways in the gut by inhibiting the counterproductive enzyme produced by intestinal bacteria, beta-glucuronidase.[79] Oral administration of CDG provided a 50% drop in beta-glucuronidase for 5 hours.[80] In animals fed CDG, serum estradiol levels were decreased (a good sign for breast cancer) by 23%.[81] Animals fed CDG experienced a 50-70% reduction in mammary cancers.[82] In cultured cancer cells, D-glucarate combined with retinoid (vitamin A analog) provided a synergistic inhibition of tumor growth.[83] When D-glucaric acid is bound to calcium, the resulting molecule, calcium D-glucarate, becomes a time-released version of glucaric acid in the gut, helping to detoxify poisons and hormones while dampening unregulated cell growth.

PATIENT PROFILE: REVERSING INCURABLE CYTOMA

S.M. was a 44 year old male diagnosed with a rare form of cancer (hemangiopericytoma) that had caused pain and numbness in his back and legs. Began 13 rounds of radiation therapy to spinal region, which produced considerable relief from pain and weakness. One month later, CAT scans and liver biopsy found metastatic disease throughout pancreas, liver, kidneys, lungs, and pressing on spinal cord. Physicians agreed in medical staff meeting that this condition is "refractory to all medical therapy and invariably fatal." Patient began aggressive nutrition program of diet and supplements, along with detoxification (coffee enemas), 3 months chemotherapy (FUDR), and extensive prayer. CAT scans showed 50% shrinkage in tumors on pancreas, lungs and kidneys with elimination of tumors on liver. S.M.'s bloodwork was constantly normal, whereas one would expect declines in white cell count (leukopenia) and red blood cell count (anemia). Three years later, S.M. still has some tumor burden, but has had good quality of life and is well beyond the most optimistic predictions of his original oncologist.

ENDNOTES

[1]. Langsjoen, PH, et al., Int. J. Tiss Reac, vol.12, p.163, 1990
[2]. Folkers, K, et al., International Journal of Vitamin and Nutrition Research, vol.40,p.380, 1970
[3]. Sugiyama, S, Experientia, vol.36, p.1002, 1980
[4]. Gwak, S. et al., Biochem et Biophys Acta, vol.809, p.187, 1985
[5]. Turrens, JF, Biochem J., vol.191, p.421, 1980
[6]. Ham, EA, et al., J. Biol Chem, vol.254, p.2191, 1979
[7]. Nakamura, Y, et al., Cardiovasc Res, vol.16, p.132, 1982
[8]. Folkers, K., Med Chem Res, vol.2, p.48, 1992
[9]. Folkers, K., Biomedical and Clinical Aspects of Coenzyme Q, vol.3,p.399, Elsevier Press, 1981
[10]. Lockwood, K., et al., Biochem and Biophys Res Comm, vol.199, p.1504, Mar.1994
[11]. Budavari, S. (eds), THE MERCK INDEX, p.1591, Merck & Co., Whitehouse Station, NJ 1996
[12]. Packer, L., et al., Free Radical Biol. Med., vol.19, p.227, 1995
[13]. Stoll, S., et al., Ann.NY Acad.Sci., vol.717, p.122, 1994
[14]. Passwater, R., LIPOIC ACID, Keats, New Canaan, CT, 1996
[15]. Nagamatsu, M., et al., Diabetes Care, vol.18, p.1160, Aug.1995
[16]. Podda, M., et al., Biochem.Biophys., Res.Commun., vol.204, p.98, 1994
[17]. Han, D., et al., Biochem.Biophys.,Res.Commun., vol.207, p.258, 1995
[18]. Ou, P., et al., Biochem.Pharmacol., vol.50, p.123, 1995
[19]. Ohmori, H., et al., Jpn.J.Pharmacol., vol.42, p.275, 1986
[20]. Jacob, S., et al., Diabetes, vol.45, p.1024, 1996
[21]. Bray, TM, et al., Biochem.Pharmacol., vol.47, p.2113, 1994
[22]. DeLeve, LD, et al., Pharmac.Ther., vol.52, p.287, 1991
[23]. Bray, TM, et al., Biochem.Pharmacol., vol.47, p.2113, 1994
[24]. Julius, M., et al., J.Clin.Epidemiol., vol.47, p.1021, 1994
[25]. Beutler, E., et al., J.Lab.Clin.Ned., vol.105, p.581, 1985
[26]. Hercbergs, A., et al., Lancet, vol.339, p.1074, May 1992
[27]. DiRe, F., et al., Cancer Chemother.Pharmacol., vol.25, p.355, 1990
[28]. Cascinu, S., et al., J.Clin.Oncol., vol.13, p.26, 1995
[29]. Trickler, D., et al., Nutr.Cancer, vol.20, p.139, 1993

[30]. Shklar, G., et al., Nutr.Cancer, vol.20, p.145, 1993
[31]. Science, vol.212, p.541, May 1981
[32]. Ranek, DK, et al., Liver, vol.12, p.341, 1992
[33]. Lash, LH, et al., Proc.Natl.Acad.Sci., vol.83, p.4641, July 1986
[34]. Donnerstag, B., et al., Int.J.Oncol., vol.7, p.949, Oct.1995
[35]. Witschi, A., et al., Eur.J.Clin.Pharmacol., vol.43, p.667, 1992
[36]. Hagen, TM, et al., Am.J.Physiol., vol.259, p.G524, 1990
[37]. Steenge, GR, J.Nutr., vol.133, no.5, p.1291, May 2003
[38]. Barak, AJ, Alcohol, vol.13, no.5, p.483, Sep.1996
[39]. junnila, M., Vet.Pathol., vol.37, no.3, p.231, May 2000
[40]. Abdelmalek, MF, Am.J.Gastroenterol., vol.96, no.9, p.2711, Sep.2001
[41]. Bremer, J., Physiol.Rev., vol.63, p.1420, 1983
[42]. Borum, PR, et al., J.Am.Coll.Nutr., vol.5, p.177, 1986
[43]. Sachan, DS, et al., Am.J.Clin.Nutr., vol.39, p.738, 1984
[44]. Dragan, GI, et al., Physiologie, vol.25, p.231, 1987
[45]. Furitano, G, et al., Drugs Exp.Clin.Res., vol.10, p.107, 1984
[46]. DeSimone, C., et al, Acta Vitaminol. Enzymol., vol.4, p.135, 1982
[47]. Qureshi, AA, et al., Am.J.Clin.Nutr., vol.53, p.1042S, 1991
[48]. Farrell, PM, et al., in MODERN NUTRITION, Shils, ME (eds), Lea & Febiger, Philadelphia, 1994
[49]. Komiyama, K., et al., Chem.Pharm.Bull., vol.37, p.1369, 1989
[50]. Tan, B., Nutrition Research, vol.12, p.S163, 1992
[51]. Azuine, MA, et al., Nutr. Cancer, vol.17, p.287, 1992
[52]. Havsteen, B., Biochem.Pharmacol., vo.32, p.1141, 1983
[53]. Murray, MT, ENCYCLOPEDIA OF NUTRITIONAL SUPPLEMENTS, p.321, Prima, Rocklin, 1996
[54]. Middleton, E., et al., in ADJUVANT NUTRITION IN CANCER TREATMENT, Quillin, P. (eds), p.319, Cancer Treatment Research Foundation, Arlington Heights, IL 1994
[55]. Middleton, E., et al., in ADJUVANT NUTRITION IN CANCER TREATMENT, Quillin, P. (eds), p.325, Cancer Treatment Research Foundation, Arlington Heights, IL 1994
[56]. Boik, J., CANCER & NATURAL MEDICINE, p.181, Oregon Medical Press, Princeton, MN 1995
[57]. Scambia, G., et al., Cancer Chemother. Pharmacol., vol.28, p.255, 1991
[58]. Wood, AW, et al., in PLANT FLAVONOIDS IN BIOLOG, p.197, Cody, V. (eds), Liss, NY, 1986
[59]. Scambia, G., et al., Anticancer Drugs, vol.1, p.45, 1990
[60]. Afanasev, IB, et al., Biochem.Pharmacol., vol.38, p.1763, 1989
[61]. Suolinna, E., et al., J.Nat.Cancer Inst., vol.53, p.1515, 1974
[62]. Stavric, B., Clin.Biochem., vol.27, p.245, Aug.1994
[63]. Gugler, R., et al., Eur.J.Clin.Pharmacol., vol.9, p.229, 1975
[64]. Berma, AK, et al., Cancer Res., vol.48, p.5754, 1988
[65]. Ranelletti, FO, et al., Int.J.Cancer, vol.50, p.486, 1992
[66]. Kandaswami, C., et al., Anti-Cancer Drugs, vol.4, p.91, 1993
[67]. Bracke, ME, et al., in PLANET FLAVONOIDS, p.219, Cody, E. (eds), Liss, NY, 1988
[68]. Kim, JH, et al., Cancer Research, vol.44, p.102, Jan.1984
[69]. Castillo, MH, et al., Amer.J.Surgery, vol.158, p.351, Oct.1989
[70]. Bauman, J., et al., Prostaglandins, vol.20, p.627, 1980
[71]. Middleton, E, et al., Arch.Allergy Appl.Immunol., vol.77, p.155, 1985
[72]. Busse, WW, et al., J.Allergy Clin.Immunol., vol.73, p.801, 1984
[73]. Bach, AC, et al., Am.J.Clin.Nutr., vol.36, p.950, 1982
[74]. Mascioli, EA, et al., J.Parenteral Enteral Nutr., vol.15, p.27, 1991
[75]. Jensen, GL, et al., J.Parenteral Enteral Nutr., vol.14, p.467, 1990
[76]. Maiz, A., et al., Metabolism, vol.33, p.901, Oct.1984
[77]. Davidoff, RA, Annals Neurology, vol.17, p.107, 1985
[78]. Braverman, ER, et al., HEALING NUTRIENTS WITHIN, p.238, Keats, New Canaan, CT 1987
[79]. Dwivedi, C, et al, Biochem.Med. & Metabolic Biol., vol.43, p.83, 1990
[80]. Dwivedi, C., et al., Biochem.Med.Metabol.Biol., vol.43, p.83, 1990
[81]. Walaszek, Z, et al., Carcinogenesis, vol.7, p.1463, 1986
[82]. Walaszek, Z, Cancer Letters, vol.54, p.1, 1990
[83]. Curley, RW, et al., Life Sciences, vol.54, p.1299, 1994

CHAPTER 24

CHANGING THE UNDERLYING CAUSES OF CANCER

✯

"Whom the gods would destroy, they first make brainless."
Taylor Caldwell, in ROMANCE OF ATLANTIS

No one with a headache is suffering from a deficiency of aspirin. And no one with elevated serum cholesterol is suffering from a deficiency of clofibrate. Arthritis sufferers are not suffering due to lack of cortisone, and cancer patients are not lacking chemotherapy. All of these therapies are short term, symptom-fixing drugs that provide immediate relief, but do nothing to change the underlying causes of a disease.

Studies have proven that patients who undergo coronary bypass surgery have no extension in lifespan, because no one has changed the cause of the disease by replacing 4 inches of plugged up "plumbing" or arteries

ETIOLOGY FOR MOST DISEASES		
pull out the weed by the root		
primary etiology ⟹	secondary etiology ⟹	diagnosed diseases
NUTRITION	INFECTIONS	HEART DISEASE
INFECTIONS	INFLAMMATION	CANCER
EXERCISE	HYPERCOAGUL	DIABETES
ATTITUDE	DYSBIOSIS	STROKE
TOXINS	HYPOTHYROID	AUTO-IMMUNE
ENERGY ALIGN	MALDIGESTION	CHRONIC FATIG
GENETIC VULN	IMMUNE DYSFUN	MENTAL ILLNESS
	HYPERGLYCEMIA	ALZHEIMER'S
	ALLERGIES	PARKINSON'S
	HORMONE IMBAL	et al.
	OXIDATIVE STRES	
	ACIDOSIS	

near the heart. Same goes for other drugs and conditions. Beta-blockers and diuretics for the 60 million Americans with high blood pressure actually INCREASE the risk for a heart attack by causing a loss of the crucial cardio-protective minerals of potassium and magnesium.

The following listing is a very brief description of the underlying causes of disease, listed in order of importance (my professional opinion). These biological, psychological, chemical and electrical factors have been gleaned and synthesized from such classic works as THE TEXTBOOK OF NATURAL MEDICINE by Drs. Pizzorno and Murray, OPTIMAL WELLNESS by Dr. Ralph Golan, and the out-of-print 1957 copyright book CANCER: NATURE, CAUSE AND CURE by Alexander Berglas. The ideal combination therapy for any disease would include short-term relief with minimal drugs, coupled with the long-term goal of changing the underlying causes of the disease. For more information, consult with your health care professional.

FIX WHAT'S BROKE

If you have a zinc deficiency, then a truckload of vitamin C will not be nearly as valuable as giving the body what it needs to end the zinc deficiency. If an accumulation of lead and mercury has crimped the immune system, then removing the toxic metals is more important than psychotherapy. If a low output of hydrochloric acid in the stomach creates poor digestion and malabsorption, then hydrochloric acid supplements are the answer. If a broken spirit brought on the cancer, then spiritual healing is necessary to eliminate the cancer.

The need to "fix what's broke" is a prime limiting factor in studies that examine cancer therapies. In a given group of 100 cancer patients, based upon my experience, 10 may need grief counseling, 10 may need high dose supplements to stimulate the immune system, 5 may need serious detoxification, and the remaining 75 have a complex combination of problems. This issue complicates cancer treatment tremendously and makes "cookbook" cancer treatment an exercise in futility. Our progress against cancer has been crippled not only by the complexity of cancer, but also by the need for Western science to isolate one variable. While it is easier to conduct and interpret research with one or two variables, cancer and the human body are far more complex than that. We will eventually help most cancer patients by fixing whatever bodily function needs repair. This is easier said than done. Finding the underlying problem requires a physician trained in comprehensive medicine.

1) PSYCHO-SPIRITUAL

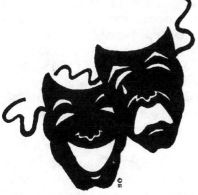

Grief, loss of loved one, lack of purpose, depression, low self esteem, hypochondriasis as means of getting attention, need love for self and others, touching, be here now, sense of accomplishment, happiness, music, beauty, sexual satisfaction, forgiveness, etc..

>SOLUTION: Create a new way of thinking (crisis=opportunity or danger)

It was Hans Selye, MD, who first scientifically showed that animals subjected to stress undergo thymic atrophy (immune suppression), elevations in blood pressure and serum lipids, and erosion of the stomach lining (ulcers).[1]   Since then, literally thousands of human studies have demonstrated that an angry, stressed, or depressed mind can lead to a suppressed immune system, which allows cancer and infections to take over. Drs. Locke and Horning-Rohan have published a textbook consisting of over 1,300 scientific articles written since 1976 that prove the link between the mind and the immune system.

We are finally beginning to accept what philosophers and spiritual leaders have been telling us for thousands of years: the mind has a major impact on the body and health. Proverbs 17:22 tells us "A joyful heart is good medicine, but a broken spirit dries up the bones." Over 100 years ago, observant physicians claimed that significant life events might increase the risk for developing cancer.[2] In the 1800s, emotional factors were related to breast cancer, and cervical cancer was related to sensitive and frustrated women. Loss of a loved one has long been known to increase the risk for breast and cervical cancer. When 2,000 men were assessed and then followed for 17 years, it was found that depression doubled the risk for cancer.

Researchers at the National Institute of Health, spearheaded by Candice Pert, PhD, have investigated the link between catecholamines, endorphins, and other chemicals from the brain as they influence cancer. A reknowned researcher, Jean Achterberg, PhD, has demonstrated a clear link between the attitude of the cancer patient and their quality and quantity of life.[3] In my years of experience, about 90% of the cancer patients I deal with have encountered a major traumatic event 1-2 years prior to the onset of cancer. This is especially true of breast cancer patients. There is even a medical textbook on the subject of "STRESS AND BREAST CANCER"[4]

Not only can mental depression lead to immune suppression and then cancer, but there may be a metaphorical significance to the location of the cancer. Divorced women may lose a breast as they feel a loss of their feminity. One of my patients developed cancer of the larynx a year after his wife left him. He tried to get her to talk about it, but she said there was "nothing left to say". And he developed cancer of the "say" box. Is it merely a coincidence that the great comedians, like Bob Hope (1903-2003), George Burns (1896-1996), and Milton Berle (1908-2002) lived decades longer than the average American male?

The good news is that the mind can be a powerful instrument at eliminating cancer. This is an empowering concept. Helplessness and hopelessness are just as lethal as cigarettes and bullets. Key your eyes on the "prize" of a healing from your cancer.

Norman Cousins cured himself of a painful collagen disease by using laughter and attitude adjustment, along with high doses of vitamin C. Bernie Siegel, MD, a Yale surgeon, noticed that certain mental characteristics in his cancer patients were indicators of someone who would beat the odds: live each moment, express yourself, value your dreams, and maintain an assertive fighting spirit against the disease. Carl Simonton, MD, a radiation oncologist, found that mental imagery and other mind techniques vastly improved the results in his cancer patients. In a National Cancer Institute study conducted at the University of Texas, researchers were able to predict with 100% accuracy which cancer patients would die or deteriorate within a two month period--strictly based upon the patient's attitude.[5] While tobacco products contain carcinogenic substances, mentally handicapped people, many of whom smoke, experience a 4% death rate from cancer, compared to 22% for the population at large.[6] Indeed, there may be a certain amount of bliss in ignorance.

Enkephalins and endorphins, also called "the mind's rivers of pleasure", are brain chemicals that are secreted when the mind is happy. Endorphins improve the production of T cells, which improves the effectiveness of the immune system against cancer and infections. Enkephalins increase the vigor of T-cells attacking cancer cells as well as increasing the percentage of active T-cells. Essentially, your immune system is a well orchestrated army within to protect you against cancer and infections, and your mind is the four-star general directing the battle. Depending on your attitude, your mind either encourages or discourages disease in your body.

The take-home lesson here is: you can take a soup bowl full of potent nutrients to fight cancer while you are being treated by the world's best oncologist, but if your mind is not happy and focused on the immune battle that must occur, then the following program of nutrition will not be nearly as effective as it should be.

We all have to drive over the "bumps in the highway of life". Your "shock absorber system"; like humor, prayer, meditation, music, friends, nature, gardening, sense of purpose, fun, etc; is your coping ability that makes stressful events less damaging to your well being. Depending on whether you perceive cancer as an "opportunity for personal growth" or a "death sentence" may become self-fulfilling.

2) TOXIC BURDEN

In 1996, hundreds of dead seals washed up on the beaches of Denmark and Germany. Scientists determined that a virus had killed these seals. However, the same virus exists in all healthy seals without creating any infection. Actually, it was pollution from the Rhine River that caused the immune systems of the seals to succumb to these normally-non-toxic viruses. At the same time in a forest just east of Los Angeles, California, a normal strain of beetles was decimating a huge stand of virgin pine trees. While these beetles normally live among these pine trees, it was the air pollution from Los Angeles that lowered the immune functions of the pine trees and allowed these innocuous beetles to devastate the forest. Meanwhile, thousands of bass fish are washing up on the shores of lakes in the southern plains of the US. Cause of death? A virus that normally inhabits the fish, but becomes lethal when the fish are exposed to pollutants, which lower immune defenses. Pollutants lower our defenses to everything from the common cold to cancer, while also jamming the body's many intricate biochemical reactions.

INTAKE from:
   Voluntary pollutants of drugs, alcohol, tobacco
   Involuntary toxins of:
⇒ Food (1.2 billion lbs/yr pesticides on fresh produce, 2800 FDA-approved food additives, 5 million lbs/yr of antibiotics to grow animals faster, herbicides, fungicides, wax on produce, parasites, veterinarian drug residue, hormones.
⇒ Water. EPA estimates that 40% of fresh water in US is unusable. 1300 different chemicals exist in the average "EPA-approved" city drinking water. Chlorine and lead are most common, with many industrial volatile organic chemicals ending up in the drinking water. 60,000 chemicals in regular use, according to American Chemical Society, half of these in contact with humans. Farm runoff of herbicides, pesticides, and fertilizer (nitrates combine with amino acids in stomach to form carcinogenic nitrosamines).
⇒ Air. 50 million Americans breathe air that is dangerous for health. Smoking and second-hand smoke are obvious. Millions of tons of known carcinogens are produced annually and legally from paper mills, petrochemical refineries, burning of medical waste (generate dioxin from PVC). Crop dusting, diesel fumes, leaded exhaust, etc.
⇒ Industrial exposure. Workers in factories, vinyl industry, paper mills, refineries, asbestos, etc.
⇒ Other. Mercury amalgams, electromagnetic fields from cellular phone antenna, high voltage power lines.

>SOLUTION: DETOXIFICATION (EXCRETION) VIA:
* Urine. Increase intake of clean water, vitamin C, beans (sulfur amino acids are chelators), garlic, chelation EDTA therapy.
* Feces. 50 billion bacteria/lb fecal matter. 40% of lymphoid tissue is surrounding the GI tract. Common constipation leads to toxic buildup, dysbiosis. Increase fluid, fiber, psyllium seed husk, sena, cascara sagrada, buckthorn, fructo-oligosaccharides, probiotics (lactobacillus, yogurt). Appropriate use of enemas, coffee enemas (every other day during intensive detox).
* Sweat. Skin is the largest organ of body, 2000 pores/square inch skin. Increase sweating through exercise, hot tubs, jacuzzi, sauna. Hyperthermia via far infrared saunas (SmartyHealth.com, Saunas.com, SunlightSaunas.com) can be useful. Bring core body

temperature up to 102 F for 10-30 minutes/day. Do not use anti-perspirants.

* Liver. Most significant detoxifying organ of body, using conjugase (put together), oxidase, reductase, and hydrolase enzymes to neutralize poisons. Increase intake of glutathione (dark green leafy veg), silymarin, garlic, vitamin E, selenium.
* Other. Some chose chelation therapy, mercury amalgam removal, or magnets to neutralize electro-magnetic field pollution.

-Get rid of the garbage.

Everyone is detoxifying their bodies all day throughout their lives--or they would die. But some people don't detox fast enough, and the toxins build up to encumber their bodily processes. One of the favored theories of aging says that eventually the accumulation of these cellular waste products overwhelms the cells, and they begin to die. Similarly, fermenting yeast creates alcohol to a certain point and then dies in its own toxins. Cell cultures of living tissue that are kept in a fresh nutrient solution and changed daily to eliminate toxin buildup will experience slowed aging.

If I was forced to summarize the essence of good health into one simple sentence, it would be: "bring in the right groceries (nutrients) and take out the trash (toxins)." Each of the 60 trillion cells in your body is like a house in your neighborhood. You must bring in the right collection of essential groceries and remove the garbage often. Many cancer patients have erred at both ends of this equation: not enough essential nutrients, coupled with an accumulation of poisons.

Fortunately, humans are not "virgins" at exposure to poisons. The human body, when properly nourished, has an enormous capacity to either excrete or neutralize a certain amount of poisons. Yet 20th century pollution has stretched the limits of our elaborate detoxification systems. We have physical means of eliminating waste products through urine, feces, exhaled air, sweat, and tears. We also possess an elaborate system of chemical detoxification that is mostly concentrated in the liver, where a complex array of enzymes serve to neutralize poisons. Cytochrome P-450, catalase, mixed function oxidase, conjugase, and other enzymes are constantly at work neutralizing and excreting poisons from the body. That is why the liver is often the secondary organ affected after some other part of the body becomes cancerous--like trying to break up a fight and, instead, getting beat up.

Not only do many people voluntarily consume poisons, such as tobacco, alcohol, and prescription and "recreational" drugs, but we are also exposed to an alarming amount of involuntary poisons in our air, food, and water supply. Annually, America alone dumps 90 billion pounds of toxic waste into our 55,000 toxic waste sites, sprays 1.2 billion pounds of pesticides on our food crops[7], and spews forth 600 pounds of air pollutants for every person in America. Scientists have found residues of the lethal industrial solvent PCB (polychlorinated biphenyls) and the pesticide DDT in every human on earth, including mother's milk. And on it goes.

After looking at the toxic burden carried by the average American adult, the question is not "why do 42% of us get cancer?", but a more appropriate question might be "why do only 42% of us get cancer?" A noted professor at the University of Illinois, Dr. Sam Epstein, has profound evidence showing that regardless of other measures taken, our cancer epidemic will not be abated until we get our environmental disaster cleaned up. By increasing the body's ability to purge poisons, detoxification may help the cancer recovery process for some individuals. Toxic burden blunts the immune system, erodes the delicate DNA, changes cellular functions, and encourages cancer growth.

> **A word on coffee enemas.** Enemas are one of the oldest healing modalities in human literature. Milk enemas are still used by noted surgeons and gastroenterologists to stem diarrhea that does not respond to medication. Coffee enemas have been in the Merck Medical Manual for decades, until 1977, when editors of the manual claimed that this revered therapy was eliminated for "lack of space" in the new manuscript. The reality is that coffee enemas became the focal point in criticizing alternative cancer therapies. Coffee enemas help to purge the colon and liver of accumulated toxins and dead tissue. Coffee enemas are prepared by brewing regular organic and caffeinated coffee, let cool to body temperature, then use enema bag as per instructions with 4 to 8 ounces of the coffee solution. Proponents of this therapy use it daily for very sick cancer patients, or weekly for recovering cancer patients.

As a by-product of living, we create our own waste products, which must be eliminated or we die in our own biological sewage. Urine contains a collection of worn out parts, filtered out toxins, and potentially lethal ammonia. The intestines can become a distillation device like the old moonshiner "still", loaded with strange by-products as bacteria ferment food matter into an incredible array of chemicals and gases. Feces contains unabsorbed food matter, about 50 billion bacteria per pound, and many toxins that could cause cancer if allowed to contact the intestinal wall long enough.

Detoxification includes:

-**Urine.** Increasing urinary output and dilution of urine poisons by drinking more clean water, 8-10 cups of fluid daily, which is enough to have urine that is light yellow in color and inoffensive in odor. Drink filtered water, preferably from reverse osmosis. Chelation therapy helps the body to gather up toxic minerals and excrete them via the urine.

-**Feces.** Improve fiber intake until feces are soft in consistency. Also, fix digestive problems, such as low output of hydrochloric acid or digestive enzymes. Take mild herbal purgatives, such as buckthorn, senna, and cascara sagrada. Some people use enemas and colonic irrigation. The typical American diet is low in fiber and loaded with poisons. Colon cleansing, through a variety of methods, is crucial for whole body detoxification.

-**Sweat.** Encourage purging of toxins through sweat glands by taking saunas, far infrared saunas, hot baths, and steam baths, then scrubbing the skin to scrape off the excreted poisons.

-**Reduce intake of poisons**. 25% of Americans and up to 90% of males in other countries still smoke. In my work with hundreds of cancer patients, I have never seen a smoker get better. Ironically, smoking may have a minor benefit for some people, since smoking elevates basal metabolism, which is particularly noticeable in hypothyroid individuals. My hunch is that people who find smoking such an addiction are using nicotine to elevate basal metabolism as a crutch to support their sagging thyroid output. A way to ease the withdrawal for these people is to normalize thyroid output. See "gland or organ insufficiency" section for more details on thyroid help.

According to the National Academy of Sciences, pesticide residues on food crops cause 14,000 new cases of cancer each year out of 1.4 million total cases, which means that about 1% of our cancer comes from pesticide use and abuse. That estimate did not include the more recent findings that pesticides amplify each other's toxicity by 500 to 1,000 fold!! That 1% is fairly insignificant, unless you are one of those 14,000 people.

TO CLEAN YOUR FRESH COMMERCIAL PRODUCE. For those people who do not have easy access to organic produce, which is grown without pesticide use, peeling or washing produce is mandatory. For produce that you consume entirely, like broccoli and apples, soak it in a solution of one gallon of warm water per 2 tablespoons of vinegar for 5 minutes, then rinse and brush.

From tainted water, food, and air; to exposure to carcinogens in the home and work place; to voluntary intake of poisons in drugs, alcohol, and tobacco; to showers of electromagnetic radiation falling on us--Americans are constantly pushing the outer envelope for toxin tolerance. Too many of these common toxins both assault the fragile DNA and blunt immune functions. We need to be more responsible in dealing with our 20th century waste products. Cancer patients need to do everything possible to eliminate accumulated wastes and minimize intake of new toxins.

-**Mercury**. With more than 90% of the American population sporting at least a few mercury fillings in their teeth, the subject of mercury poisoning has become a hot topic. Lewis Carroll's classic book, ALICE IN WONDERLAND, showcased the "mad hatter" as representative of an industry that whimsically used mercury to give stiffness to formal felt hats. Mercury is a deadly poison, and putting it in the mouth to erode over the years and eventually be swallowed is just plain ridiculous. About 1% of the population, or 2 million people, are very sensitive to any exposure to mercury, while most other people would be better off without any mercury in their mouth. Some people have found relief from a wide assortment of diseases, including cancer, by having their mercury fillings replaced with non-toxic ceramic or gold material.[8] Mercury detox can be assisted with Captomer (Thorne 800-228-1966), Detoxosode (HVS 941-643-4636), chlorella, kelp extracts, cilantro, and intravenous DMPS chelation from your doctor.

Half the weight of a "silver" filling is from mercury. According to Doctor's Data Lab, people with mercury fillings have 13 times more mercury in their stools than people without mercury fillings. With the assistance of common bacteria in the mouth, mercury in fillings becomes methylated and is then 100 times more toxic.[9] Roughly 78% of the 200 million adults in America have an average of 8 mercury fillings, which translates into 557 tons (1.1 million pounds) of mercury stored in the mouths of Americans today. For this reason, there are extraordinary levels of mercury gas emitted when cremating patients with the typical 8 mercury fillings. 90% of dentists still use mercury amalgams, adding another 100 million mercury fillings annually to the mouths of Americans.[10] Animal studies show that radioactively-labelled mercury from fillings quickly migrates to the kidneys, brain, and intestinal wall.[11] There are already class action law suits pending against the dental industry for mercury poisoning that will make any previous class action suits look like a socialite tea party.

In a famous case of blatant clinical mercury toxicity, the Chisso factory in Minamata dumped 100 tons (91,000 kilograms) of mercury wastes into the nearby bay in 1980, with the resulting fish being contaminated and the people eating the fish getting very sick. Nearly 500 people died, and thousands were declared severely brain damaged by acute mercury poisoning. But mercury rarely kills anyone outright. It slowly erodes all bodily functions until you wish you were dead. Multiple sclerosis (MS) patients have 800% the mercury levels in the cerebrospinal fluid around the brain and spinal cord as compared to healthy controls. Inorganic mercury is capable of producing symptoms that are identical to MS.[12] Mercury poisoning also can mimic Alzheimer's disease. Over 4 million Americans have Alzheimer's with a tripling (12 million) expected within a decade.

Common symptoms of mercury poisoning include:
Mental: depression, fearfulness, anger, hallucinations, inability to accept criticism, inability to concentrate, indecision, irritability, loss of memory, metallic taste, persecution complex, tremors of hands, etc
Physical: anemia, anorexia, low body temperature, poor vision, drowsiness, excitability, headache, hypersensitive reflexes, insomnia,

poor energy, weight loss, irregular heart beat, low or high blood pressure, allergies, sinusitis, lymph node enlargement, dizziness, ringing in ears (tinnitis), fatigue, muscle weakness, apathy, numbness, hearing loss, speech disorder, joint pains.

American industry still releases 4.3 million pounds of mercury into the atmosphere as gas. Mercury is used in coal-burning facilities, which still generate the majority of electricity in America, to make aluminum, to coat seeds for planting, to make mercury vapor tube lamps, mercury electrical switches, etc. Imagine the mercury that was released when the World Trade Center and its office mercury-rich fluorescent lamps were vaporized by the terrorist attack on September 11, 2001. A surprising 40% of workers at the 9/11 cleanup site have reported physical or mental health problems that could be attributed to mercury poisoning. All sewer plants in the U.S. and sewer sludge have been found by government assays to have high levels of mercury. This sewer sludge is used to fertilize fields, which gets into the plants grown from those fields, and the animals that eat the plants, and so on.

All this mercury has been cumulative. Mercury is immortal. There is no half life. It never decomposes. Mercury in the air returns as mercury in the world's land and waterways, which enters the food chain through fish and seafoods. The World Health Organization (WHO) has conducted studies showing that the more fish you eat, the more mercury you have in your body. The higher the fish on the food chain (shark, tuna, swordfish are higher than salmon, cod, sole, and crab), the more the concentration of mercury in the flesh. States that have a higher mercury load have it in the water and soil, hence the food supply in general. WHO reports that the largest source of mercury in most people is from mercury amalgams.

If you overlay a map of mercury pollution in the US with elevated rates of cancer, they match. Mercury toxicity may be the initial insult which leads to depressed immunity, which leads to fungal and other infections, which leads to inflammation, hypercoagulability, and eventually some serious diagnosed disease like heart disease, stroke, cancer, diabetes, etc. If you want a truly terrifying piece of literature to read before bedtime, never mind the Steven King novels, download the "Mercury Study" from epa.gov on the Internet.

Mercury suppresses the immune system and impairs nerve transmission. Lowered immunity, inability to focus, and other problems are common early warning signs of mercury toxicity. Also, mercury causes fungi to mutate into a more virulent and invasive forms. As the final nail in the coffin, mercury is quick to replace zinc (an essential mineral) in the 80+ different enzyme systems that are crucial to human health. In one fell swoop, mercury turns the villains into super-villains and sends the cops to bed, then puts terrorists in control of all other functions in the city (body). This is a common state of affairs in

Americans and good reasons why mercury amalgam replacement (with bio-compatible material) and mercury detoxification are so crucial for normalizing the immune system and other healing pathways in the body.

-**Chelation of heavy metals**. Lead poisoning is much more common than mercury poisoning. Though our use of lead is starting to be reduced, lead is a clearcut immune poison and has been targeted by the Environmental Protection Agency as a "top priority" cleanup item. Chelation therapy involves injecting chemicals (like EDTA) that put the heavy metal in a molecular "cage" and carry it out of the body in the urine. Chelation therapy may help to reduce heavy metal toxicity, which is assessed by mineral excretion in the urine or by hair/nail analysis.

PATIENT PROFILE: GB was a bright, energetic, successful physician. He fancied himself a "health nut', running, working out with weights, fishing in nearby Lake Michigan, and eating the fresh fish. GB developed cardiomyopathy, or failure of the heart muscle, and was told by his fellow doctors that he needed a heart transplant. He questioned such invasive therapies and set out on a lengthy odyssey to find out why his heart was failing when he seemed to be doing all the healthy lifestyle things. He found he had mercury poisoning by eating fish from Lake Michigan. He commenced mercury detoxification in every conceivable way, including oral and intravenous chelating agents. Eventually, GB lowered his mercury load to a manageable level and used much of what he learned in this bizarre health odyssey to help his many patients. However, his heart gave out 13 years after he was told he needed a heart transplant operation. He added measurably to his life via mercury detox, but never would have had these problems if the fish in Lake Michigan had not been so criminally polluted with mercury.

---

3) EXERCISE

Humans evolved as active creatures. Our biochemical processes depend on regular exercise to maintain homeostasis. A well-respected Stanford physician, Dr. William Bortz, published a review of the scientific literature on exercise and concluded: "our dis-eases may be from dis-use of the body."[13] Cancer patients who exercise have fewer side effects from oncology therapy. Exercise oxygenates the tissue, which slows the anaerobic cancer cell progress. Exercise stabilizes blood sugar levels, which selectively deprives cancer cells of their favorite fuel. Even if exercise is not a possibility for the cancer patient, deep breathing would be invaluable. The most essential nutrient in the human body is oxygen. Sheldon Hendler, MD, PhD, has written an excellent book on the need for oxygenation of tissue in THE OXYGEN BREAKTHROUGH.[14] Westerners typically are sedentary and breath shallowly, which deprives the body of oxygen, which is a perfect environment for cancer.

Exercise is an absolutely essential ingredient for health. It is a primary tool for detoxification, stabilizing blood glucose levels, improving digestion and regularity, proper oxygenation of tissue, stress tolerance, improving hormone output (i.e. growth hormone & DHEA), burning fatty tissue, and eliminating harmful by-products (i.e., estrogen, uric acid).

4) BLOOD GLUCOSE

Sugar in the blood can feed cancer growth. See the chapter on sugar and cancer for more information.

5) REDOX

Life is a continuous balancing act between oxidative forces (pro-oxidants) and protective forces (antioxidants). We want to fully oxygenate the tissue, which generates pro-oxidants, but we also want to protect healthy tissue from excess oxidative destruction, using anti-oxidants. Antioxidants are a sacrificial substance, to be destroyed in lieu of body tissue. Antioxidants include beta-carotene, C, E, selenium, zinc, riboflavin, manganese, cysteine, methionine, N-acetylcysteine, and many herbal extracts (i.e. green tea, pycnogenols, and curcumin).

Tumor tissue does not absorb antioxidants as effectively as healthy host tissue. Hence, loading the patient with therapeutic levels of antioxidants is like giving the good cells bullet-proof vests before you go in with a SWAT unit that opens fire (chemo and radiation), thus killing more cancer cells than healthy cells. Some recent research shows that the destruction of tumor tissue that occurs with administration of EPA fish oil occurs because the tumor cells do not have normal protection against the oxidation of fats. These highly polyunsaturated fats are like grenades going off in cancer cells, but have minimum impact on healthy cells that are able to protect themselves with fat-soluble antioxidants, like vitamin E and CoQ.

>SOLUTION: Use an appropriate mix of mixed antioxidants along with adequate breathing and oxygenation of cells for optimal redox levels to fight cancer.

6) IMMUNE DYSFUNCTIONS

We have an extensive network of protective factors that circulate throughout our bodies to kill any bacteria, virus, yeast, or cancer cells. Think of these 20 trillion immune cells as both your Department of Defense and your waste disposal company. The immune system of the average American is "running on empty". Causes for this problem include toxic burden, stress, no exercise, poor diet, unbridled use of antibiotics and vaccinations, innoculations from world travelers, and less breast feeding.

Most experts now agree to the "surveillance" theory of cancer. Cells in your body are duplicating all day every day at a blinding pace. This process of growth is fraught with peril. When cells are not copied exactly as they should be, then an emergency call goes out to the immune system to find and destroy this abnormal saboteur cell. This process occurs frequently in most people throughout their lives. Fortunately, only one in three people will actually develop detectable cancer, yet most experts agree that everyone gets cancer about 6 times per lifetime. It is the surveillance of an alert and capable immune system that defends most of us from cancer. See the chapter on immune functions.

7) GLAND OR ORGAN INSUFFICIENCY

As we age, many glands and organs produce less vital hormones and secretions.

* Stomach (hydrochloric acid)
* Pancreas (digestive enzymes)
* Thyroid (thyroxin)
* Adrenals (DHEA, cortisol)
* Thymus (thymic extract)
* Spleen (spleen concentrate)
* Joints (glucosamine sulfate)
* Pineal (melatonin)
* Pituitary (growth hormone).

Replacing missing secretions often dramatically improves health.
>**Thyroid check**.

METABOLIC REPLACEMENT THERAPY
due to aging, stress, toxins, disease, & malnutrition

melatonin (pineal)

thymus concentrate

digestive enzymes
(small intestines)

testosterone (gonads)

thyroxin (thyroid)

HCl (stomach)

DHEA (adrenal)
estrogen, progesterone
(ovaries)

CONDITIONALLY ESSENTIAL NUTRIENTS

EPA, DHA, GLA, carnitine
CoQ, choline, lecithin,
inositol, bioflavonoids, DNA,
RNA, lipoic acid, probiotics

After protein-calorie malnutrition, the second most common malnutritive condition in the world is iodine deficiency, with about 400 million people suffering from this condition. The mineral iodine feeds the thyroid gland, a small walnut-shaped gland in the throat region that produces a mere one teaspoon of thyroxin annually. But that thimble-full of thyroxin can make a huge difference in whether you will be bright or dull, fat or lean, healthy or sick, energetic or always tired. There are some regions of the world, particularly inland and mountainous areas, where iodine deficiency (goiter) is so common that the few people who do not have goiter are called "bottlenecks" for their abnormally slim necks. While the United States has made progress against goiter by adding iodine to salt, there are unsettling results from studies showing that about 33% of children with seemingly adequate iodine intake still have goiter.[15]

What does all this have to do with cancer? There is compelling evidence that low thyroid output substantially elevates the risk for cancer.[16] Based upon the groundbreaking work by Broda Barnes, MD, PhD, from 1930 through 1980, it is clear that about 40% of the population suffers from chronic hypothyroidism. Dr. Barnes earned his doctorate in physiology and medical degree from the University of Chicago. His primary interest was the thyroid gland. He found that people with a basal temperature of less than 97.8 F. were probably suffering from low thyroid. Symptoms include coldness; easy weight gain; constipation; sexual dysfunctions of infertility, frigidity, heavy periods, regular miscarriages, or impotence; elevated serum lipids to induce heart disease; mental confusion and depression; hypoglycemia and diabetes; and cancer. This may sound like an improbable grocery list of diseases that can all stem from one simple cause. But realize that the thyroid gland regulates energy metabolism throughout the body, which is the basis for all other functions.

Work with your physician on this issue. Blood tests for thyroid function are not valid indicators of thyroid problems. Body temperature is the best way to detect hypothyroidism. Take your temperature first thing in the morning before getting out of bed. If your temperature is below 97.8 F., then you may have a problem that can be easily resolved. Dessicated thyroid supplements are inexpensive and non-toxic. For some people, raw thyroid (Premier Labs, available from U.S. Health 800-935-8743), ginseng, kelp, homeopathic preparations for stimulating thyroid function, exercise, chromium picolinate, L-carnitine, and/or medium chain triglycerides (MCT) will slowly bring thyroid function up to normal. People who consume kelp, or sea vegetables, often have healthier thyroid functions, which indicates that sea vegetables or kelp tablets should be consumed by cancer patients. Here is another area of "simple solutions for major problems".

8) MALDIGESTION

After a lifetime of high fat, high sugar, overeating, too much alcohol, stress, drugs, indigestible foods (i.e., pizza), many Americans have poor peristalsis, insufficient stomach and intestinal secretions, damaged microvilli, and imbalances of friendly (probiotic) vs unfriendly (anaerobic, pathogenic) bacteria. One must remove, repair, replace, and re-inoculate. Food separation (combinations) may be of value for a brief time until the GI tract recuperates. Digestive enzymes and/or hydrochloric acid taken with meals may help.

As many people mature, they can lose their ability to produce hydrochloric acid in the stomach (hypochlorhydria) or digestive enzymes in the intestines (pancreatic insufficiency), or their intestines become inhabited by hostile bacteria (dysbiosis), or their intestines become more permeable to food particles, which causes allergies to surface.

To determine the health of the digestive tract, you will probably need the help of a holistically-oriented physician. There are laboratory companies, like Metametrix (800-221-4640) or Great Smokies Lab (800-522-4762), that are skilled at detecting the problem in a compromised GI tract. If you cannot find professional help, then here are some tips to help you determine if you have a problem with digestion. If your GI tract is working well, then you should have:

- a sensation of stomach emptying about 30-60 minutes after a meal.
- no excessive gas or discomfort.
- daily soft bowel movements that do not have greasy appearance or terribly offensive odor.
- bowel movements that do not have undigested food matter within.

If you do not have this "ideal" GI tract, then read on.

1) Hypochlorhydria. If you have a sense of stomach fullness for more than 30 minutes after eating, then you may be suffering from insufficient hydrochloric acid flow. To test this hypothesis, take 2 capsules of betaine hydrochloride (derived from beets), available at most health food stores, with your meal. If this therapy improves symptoms, then hypochlorhydria was indeed your problem. If this does not improve symptoms, then add 1 more pill with each meal until you get to five pills. If you have heartburn, then decrease dosage next time. If you find no relief, then discontinue altogether.

2) Pancreatic insufficiency. If you have cramps, heartburn, or your food appears relatively undigested or greasy in the stools, then you may not be making enough digestive enzymes to break down your food. For enzyme replacement therapy, use digestive enzymes from Enzymatic Therapy (800-558-7372), called BioZyme. You may need 2-3 pills with each meal. If symptoms improve, then you may need to continue this therapy for the foreseeable future.

3) Parasites. Most of us have intestinal parasites. In some of us, these worms and bacteria are causing serious harm to the lining of the intestinal tract, such as a permeable gut, which allows allergies to form. Our ancestors developed many de-worming techniques that they used seasonally, such as fasting while consuming purgative herbs or regular flushing out with garlic. In order to confirm whether you have a problem, you send a stool sample to a lab (Metametrix, Great Smokies) capable of detecting the myriad of microorganisms that inhabit the GI tract.

9) pH (potential hydrogens)

Acid alkaline balance (7.41 ideal in human veins) brought about by:

- ♦ proper breathing
- ♦ exercise (carbonic buffer from carbon dioxide in blood)
- ♦ diet (plant foods elevate pH, animal foods and sugar reduce pH)
- ♦ water (adequate hydration improves pH).
- ♦ other agents, such as cesium chloride, citric acid, sodium bicarbonate
- ♦ yeast infections that generate a collection of acids that lower pH

Cancer is acidic (low pH) tissue.[17] It is clear from all human physiology textbooks that pH in the blood, saliva, urine, and other areas is a critical factor for health. Blood pH is usually 7.35-7.45, with 7.41 thought to be ideal. Acceptable pH for saliva is 6.0-7.5, stomach 1.0-3.5, colon 5.0-8.4, and urine 4.5-8.4. pH is a logarithmic scale, meaning that moving from a healthy pH of 7.41 in the veins to 6.41 in the tumor tissue is a 10-fold (1,000 times) deterioration in the number of hydrogen ions influencing all chemical reactions. Most foods influence pH-- pushing toward either acid or alkaline. Clinicians will spend much time adjusting parenteral feedings to achieve a proper pH in the blood. Meanwhile, there have been many alternative health books that attempt to treat various diseases by adjusting the body pH via the diet.

Potential hydrogens (pH) refers to the acid or alkaline nature of a chemical. If you mix a mild acid, like vinegar, with a mild alkaline substance, like baking soda, then the resulting reaction produces a salt-- they neutralize one another by exchanging hydrogens. Just about everything that goes in your mouth can alter pH, including oxygen. The acidic pH of cancer cells also decreases the oxygen-carrying capacity of the surrounding blood so that tissue can become somewhat anaerobic-- which are perfect conditions for cancer to thrive. Deep breathing has an alkalizing effect on the blood. An alkalizing diet of lots of plant food also helps to encourage removal of toxic heavy metals.

The macrobiotic book claims that pH adjustment is one of the more crucial objectives of their diet.[18] Yet, I have worked with a few cancer patients who got worse on the macrobiotic program. Remember our discussion of biochemical individuality--not everyone will thrive on the same diet. Nick Gonzales, MD, sometimes uses a diet high in red meat to adjust the cancer patient's pH into a normal range. It appears that some people are prone toward extreme acid or alkaline metabolism. For these people on the edge of acceptable biological pH, diet provides a counterbalance to bring serum pH back toward normal. Think of sailing a small boat where you may have to use your body as a counterbalance to prevent the boat from being tipped over by the wind. If your metabolism is in jeopardy of "tipping over" toward extreme pH, then diet and breathing become your counterbalances that keep metabolism upright.

While this area may be absolutely essential for some cancer patients, a trial and error method may be the only way to find out which direction your pH needs adjusting. If your condition improves on the macrobiotic program, then you are pushing your pH in the right direction. If your condition worsens on the macrobiotic program, then you must push your pH in the opposite direction.

About 8% of the population must have acid-forming foods to counterbalance their extremely alkalotic pH. Some people can eat anything they want and their internal mechanisms compensate to find an acceptable pH. For many people, an alkalizing diet (toward the left) will help to neutralize their acidifying tendencies, which can invite cancer.

Venous pH is the most accurate indicator of your overall body pH. Yet blood tests are invasive, expensive, and not practical for regular use. A rough indicator of your body pH is your saliva and urinary pH, since one of the functions of the kidneys is to filter out excess hydrogen ions (acid) to keep the blood mildly alkaline. When these acids are concentrated in the urine, then there is a good chance that the body is struggling to keep the blood at a healthy pH. You can purchase Nitrazine paper from your local druggist and follow the directions for measuring saliva or urine pH. Test your saliva at least one hour after any food or drink. If your saliva is strongly acidic, then you may need to emphasize this part of my program.

10) HYPOXIA

Humans are aerobic organisms. All cells thrive when there is proper oxygenation to the tissue. Red blood cell production is dependent on iron, copper, B-6, folate, B-12, protein, and zinc. Adequate exercise and proper breathing help. Cofactors, like CoQ, and B-vitamins improve aerobic energy metabolism in cell mitochondria. Fatty acids in diet dictate "membrane fluidity" of all cells and their ability to absorb oxygen.

One of the most prominent differences between healthy cells and cancer cells is that cancer is an anaerobic cell, fermenting rather than metabolizing food and living in the absence of oxygen. Professor Otto Warburg received two Nobel prizes, in 1931 and 1944, for his work on cell bioenergetics, or how the cell extracts energy from food. In 1966, Professor Warburg spoke to a group of Nobel laureates regarding his work on cancer cells: "...the prime cause of cancer is the replacement of the respiration of oxygen in normal body cells by a fermentation of sugar."

Cancer cells are more like primitive yeast cells, extracting only a fraction of the potention energy from sugar by fermenting food substrates down to lactic acid.

This singular difference is both the strength and weakness of cancer. Cancer slowly destroys its host by using up fuel inefficiently and thus causing lean tissue wasting, in which the patient begins to convert protein to sugar in order to maintain a certain level of blood sugar. Cancer also hides in its oxygen-deficit pockets. The denser and more anaerobic the tumor mass, the more resistant the tumor is to radiation therapy.

Aerobic-enhancing nutrients. Yet, by oxygenating the tissue, you can exploit the "Achilles heel" of cancer. Cancer shrinks from oxygen like a vampire shrinking from daylight. Fuel is burned in the cellular furnaces, called mitochondria. As long as the mitochondrial membrane is fluid and permeable, oxygen flows in and carbon dioxide flows out and the cell stays aerobic. With a diet high in fat, saturated fat, and cholesterol, the mitochondrial membrane becomes more rigid and less permeable to the flow of gases and electrons, which are essential to aerobic metabolism.

Nutrient factors that heavily influence aerobic metabolism include the B-vitamins, including biotin, B-1 thiamin, B-2 riboflavin, and B-3 niacin. Numerous herbal extracts, including ginseng and ginkgo biloba, can enhance the aerobic capacity of the cell. Coenzyme Q-10 is a nutrient that is the rate-limiting step in aerobic metabolism, not unlike the bridge that ties up traffic going into the city during rush hour. Most people are low in their levels CoQ.

Breathing is a lost art in our modern world. Ancient scholars and spiritual teachers taught us that breath is the essence of life. Modern Americans breathe shallowly, or try the military breathing stance with chest thrust out and stomach sucked in--all of which leaves the tissue oxygen-starved. Proper breathing should include stomach and diaphragm deep breathing. Lay flat on your back on the floor. Place a book on your stomach. Begin inhaling through the nose and push out the stomach. Raise the book as high as you can, then complete inhalation by filling the chest with air. Exhale through the mouth slowly. This is diaphragm breathing, which more thoroughly oxygenates tissue and can be done by the most bed-ridden patient.

11) EFFECTS OF AGING

By age 65, the average American has eaten 100,000 lb (50 tons) of food. Poor diet accumulates in chronic sub-clinical malnutrition, such as calcium and osteoporosis, chromium and diabetes, vitamin E and heart disease, vitamin C and cancer. Toxins accumulate in fatty tissue and liver. Chronic exposure to unchecked pro-oxidants eventually creates arthritis, Alzheimer's, heart disease, stroke, cancer, etc. Organ reserve is used up in stress and poor diet. Errors in DNA replication become more common as we age. Telomeres become shortened. The risk for cancer doubles with every 5 years of age. Although only 12% of the US population are over 65 years of age, 67% of US cancer patients are over 65. Gland/organ insufficiencies can be partially compensated. Ill health consequences of aging may be slowed down.

12) PHYSICAL ALIGNMENT

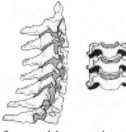

Spinal vertebrae must be in proper alignment. Chiropractic and osteopathic manipulations on spine, joints, and skull plates can be helpful. Accidents, poor muscle tone, and aging create alignment problems. Nerves and blood vessels radiate from the spinal column, which can become misaligned and cause compression on these vital channels of energy. Exercise, inversion, and physical manipulations from chiropractic or osteopathic physicians may solve these problems.

13) ENERGY ALIGNMENT

Meridians, chakras, and energy pathways were discovered by metaphysicians in ancient India. Use magnets, acupuncture, electro-acupuncture, and acupressure to correct these problems. Homeopathy probably works on this level.

14) MECHANICAL INJURY

Chronic injury requires hyperplasia, or the growth of new cells. If not properly nourished, new cell growth can become erratic and error-prone, leading to arthritis, cancer, and Alzheimer's.

CONQUERED BREAST CANCER

A.R. was a 48 year old female diagnosed with advanced breast cancer. After her bilateral radical mastectomy, doctors discovered 14 positive lymph nodes. Prognosis: less than 2 years to live, even with medical therapy. Patient began 6 rounds of chemo in her home town. Became violently ill. "Camped out in the bathroom" with nausea and vomiting. Eight months later, went to another hospital where she refused chemo, but received 6 weeks of radiation therapy twice daily to the chest and underarm lymph nodes that were positive. At same time began an aggressive nutrition program including lean and clean meat (elk, deer, fish), lots of vegetables and water, abundant prayer, and a wide assortment of nutrition supplements. One month later, she was considered "disease free". Four years later, she was still in complete remission.

ENDNOTES

[1]. Selye, H, STRESS WITHOUT DISTRESS, JB Lippincott, NY, 1974

[2]. Newell, GR, Primary Care in Cancer, p.29, May 1991

[3]. Achterberg, J., IMAGERY IN HEALING, New Science, Boston, 1985

[4]. Cooper, CL (ed.), STRESS AND BREAST CANCER, John Wiley, NY, 1988

[5]. National Cancer Institute, NCI# NO1-CN-45133, National Institute of Health, Washington, DC 1977

[6]. Achterberg, J, IMAGERY IN HEALING, New Science Library, Boston, 1985, p. 177

[7]. Quillin, P, SAFE EATING, M. Evans, NY, 1990

[8]. Huggins, HA, IT'S ALL IN YOUR HEAD, Life Sciences Press, Colorado Springs, 1989

[9]. Heintze, G, et al., Scan.J.Dent.Res., vol.91, p.150, 1983

[10]. Berry, TC, et al., J.Am.Dent.Assn., vol.120, p.394, 1994

[11]. Zalups, RK, Pharmacol.Rev., vol.52, no.1, p.113, Mar.2000

[12]. Ahlrot, U., Nutrition Research, suppl. p.403, 1985, Second Nordic Symposium on Trace Elements in Human Health & Disease, Odense, Denmark, Aug.1987

[13]. Bortz, WM, Journal American Medical Association, vol.248, no.10, p.1203, Sept.10, 1982

[14]. Hendler, SS, THE OXYGEN BREAKTHROUGH, Simon & Schuster, NY, 1989

[15]. Ziporyn, T., Journal American Medical Association, vol.253, p.1846, Apr.1985

[16]. Langer, SE, et al., SOLVED: THE RIDDLE OF ILLNESS, Keats, New Canaan, 1984

[17]. Newell, K, et al., Proceedings of National Academy of Sciences, vol.90, no.3, p.1127, Feb.1993

[18]. Aihara, H., ACID & ALKALINE, Macrobiotic Foundation, Oroville, CA, 1971

CHAPTER 25

IS CANCER AN INFECTION?

"I have been wrong.   The bacteria is nothing.   The terrain is everything."   *Louis Pasteur 1822-1895*

Ignaz Semmelweis (1818-1865) was an Austrian physician who found that washing hands with a dilute chlorine solution before delivering a baby would cut down the incidence of infections (puerperal fever) and mortality in the mother and newborn infant.   His

INFECTIONS COME IN DIFFERENT SIZES
ALL ARE FORMIDABLE PATHOGENS
(INCREASING SIZE OF PATHOGENS)

parasites, worms, flukes

yeast

bacteria

mycobacteria
virus
bacteriophage (virus that attacks bacteria)
stealth pathogens
mycoplasma
prion
?? miasm

successes in his clinic in the 1840s were profoundly better than other physicians, who would go straight from the autopsy room without washing their hands to delivering an infant.   Dr. Semmelweis had a logical, non-toxic, inexpensive, clinically-proven solution to a horrible problem of that era.   His technique reduced mortality in mothers and newborns to

1.3% which was a 90% reduction from his colleagues' results of 11% mortality.

Unfortunately, his simple solution was rejected because his critics asked: "So, Dr. Semmelweis, what is causing these women to die?" "I don't know." replied Semmelweis. "And are we to suspect that 'spooks' are involved?" they laughingly chided. When Louis Pasteur peered into a microscope and cooked (pasteurized) bacteria to death, he presented his data to his colleagues: "I have found Dr. Semmelweis's spooks."

Semmelweis died a broken man, yet many hospitals in Europe are named after this brilliant and courageous physician. How many people died because critics of Semmelweis refused to accept his solution? How many cancer patients die because we are stuck in a half-century battle with cancer using outdated methods and theories? Many cancers are probably infections, with the infectious organism (fungi, virus, bacteria) becoming an intracellular pathogen, creating a hybrid DNA from the weaving of the pathogen with host human DNA. Let's look at the facts.

➢ The most conservative estimates show that 10% of all cancers are caused by infections.[1]
➢ Human papilloma virus (HPV) is associated with at least 80% of all cervical cancer. Virus is a piece of DNA or RNA that is wrapped in protein and invisible to standard microscopes. (See sketch to right).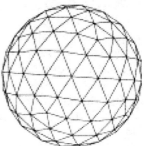
➢ The bacteria Helicobacter pylori is a major risk factor for stomach cancer.[2]
➢ Infection with the AIDS virus often leads to the cancer lymphoma. Infection with Epstein-Barr virus often leads to Burkitt lymphoma.[3]
➢ Chronic infection with hepatitis B virus usually leads to liver cancer.[4]
➢ Any exposure to the fungal poison aflatoxin or extensive exposure to the fungal by-product alcohol will often cause liver cancer.[5]
➢ Researchers have long known that C-reactive protein (CRP) is a marker in the blood that detects heart disease and probably diabetes. Now researchers at the Cleveland Clinic have found that CRP is a valuable marker for the progression of cancer.[6] CRP measures inflammation as a by-product of infection.
➢ A National Science Foundation grant winner, Professor David Hess, has written a fascinating book linking infections as the underlying cause of many cancers.[7]
➢ Ketoconazole is an anti-fungal drug that is commonly used to treat prostate cancer.[8] While researchers speculate that ketoconazole works against prostate cancer through a hormonal pathway, it may work by killing fungal cells disguised as cancer cells.[9]

> Researchers in Taiwan have found that Griseofulvin, an antifungal drug, killed human colon cancer cells in a culture dish by inducing apoptosis, or programmed cell death.[10]
> Milton White, MD found evidence that cancer is a blend (hybrid) of human DNA with spores of plant bacterial conidia.[11]

I have seen many an end-stage cancer patient with an opportunistic yeast infection, like a bully picking on a person who is already down on the pavement. Many patients told me of their thrush (oral candidiasis, coating of white yeast on the tongue) and incredible bloating in the intestinal region, not unlike a brewery where yeast ferments any reasonable carbohydrate into gas and alcohol.

Mainstream physicians scoff at the notion of fungal infections in anyone but the most immune-compromised person. In the academic textbook on fungal infections in humans, PRINCIPLES AND PRACTICES OF CLINICAL MYCOLOGY, researchers note that 46% of patients with fungal bone infections had known risk factors for lowered immunity via diabetes, corticosteroids, or other immunosuppressive drugs.[12] Which means that in the majority of cases, 54% of systemic fungal infections, there are no good explanations for the immuno-compromised status in the patient. Lung cancer oftentimes spreads to the brain. So does the fungal infection Aspergillosis.[13]

PATIENT PROFILE: LUNG CANCER OR FUNGAL INFECTION? D.M. came to me in 1998 in the end-stages of lung cancer. He was 75 years old and had failed the best chemo and immune protocols from his home town in Florida, the Harvard Deaconness Hospital and the National Cancer Institute. He had a sweet tooth, a history of toenail fungal infections, and the needle biopsy of his lung cancer was "indeterminate". I asked him to follow an anti-fungal diet, supplements, and for his physician to prescribe an antifungal medication (Diflucan) for his toenail fungal infection. Within 3 months, his lung cancer had shrunk by 40% based on CAT scans. Unfortunately, the congestive heart disease he had developed as a consequence of many cardiotoxic chemo agents caused his death. But the anti-fungal program was reversing his lung cancer.

PATIENT PROFILE: LUNG CANCER OR FUNGAL INFECTION? C.T. was diagnosed with lung cancer and scheduled for a lobectomy, or surgical removal of a lobe of her lung. Another physician, who also held a doctorate in mycology (the study of fungi) examined the patient and found possibilities of a fungal infection in the lungs. The oncologist for C.T. was enraged that someone would have such a ludicrous idea that a board-certified oncologist did not know the difference between lung cancer and fungal infection in the lungs. The patient felt more comfortable with the possibility of fungal infection and went on anti-fungal medication rather than going in for surgery the next day. The patient recovered fully from her "lung cancer".

DIAGNOSIS
YOU CANNOT FIND WHAT YOU ARE NOT LOOKING FOR.

I have worked shoulder-to-shoulder with many very bright physicians. When I mentioned concern about a possible fungal infection in a patient, the doctor would invariably reply: "Fine. Then we will perform a blood culture to determine the presence of fungi." Yet, again in the definitive textbook on fungal infections, the experts tell us: "Despite uniformly negative blood cultures, necrotizing vasculitis and infarction are characteristic of zygomycosis." Meaning, you cannot pick up fungal infections from blood cultures, aka fungemia, until the patient is nearly dead.

In 1999, doctors at the Mayo Clinic released a study showing that 96% of the chronic sinusitis patients they analyzed were suffering from a fungal infection.[14] Millions of American sinusitis patients have taken antibiotics over the past half century because doctors assumed the problem was due to a bacterial infection. These Mayo Clinic researchers used the sophisticated tool of PCR (polymerase chain reaction) to look for DNA fingerprints of fungi, which could not be found before without this valuable tool.

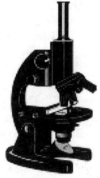

Realize that when doctors give the diagnosis of cancer, in many cases it is not as clear cut as it may sound. Pathologists, surgeons, radiologists, and other experts confer to assess this abnormal tissue. If, under a microscope or on a CAT scan, all the cancer cells were blue and all healthy cells were red, then diagnosis would be easy. But that is not the case. Cancer cells, infected cells, aging cells, and fungal colonies can become an indistinguishable blur. As Thomas Cox, MD wrote in *Journal of Family Practice*: "Although artificial categories have been set up to divide a continuum of abnormal cells, nature's paintbrush is not as specific as we would like." There is a great deal of subjectivity, discretion, judgment, and professional guessing that goes into the diagnosis of cancer. Cancer is sometimes misdiagnosed.

Enter the 2001 textbook CELL WALL DEFICIENT FORMS: STEALTH PATHOGENS, in which a Yale-trained microbiologist explains how microorganisms, including fungi, mutate throughout their life cycle into many different shapes (pleomorphism) and even shed their cell wall coating to become almost invisible under the microscope. Pathologists routinely ignore a common staining technique when they are trying to assess tissue for a cancer diagnosis. Acridine Orange will find traces of nucleic acid from nearby cell wall deficient microorganisms. But it is not used. The only way you are going to see sparrows is to look up. If you don't look up, then you won't see any sparrows. Unless you stain the slide properly for microscopic evaluation, you won't find any pleomorphic cell wall deficient fungi in the cancer patient's tissue. Of all the agents that cause microorganisms to shed their cell wall and become "invisible", antibiotics are the most powerful. The scary part is that modern medicine disregards the importance of systemic fungal infections: "Discovery of aspergillosis is often made at autopsy".[15]

ANTIBIOTICS: PART OF THE PROBLEM OR THE SOLUTION?

True story. While working in his Scottish fields one day, Mr. Fleming rescued a young boy from the bogs, or Scottish swamps. Next day, the boy's father arrives in a lavish coach with his boy in tow. "You saved my son's life. How can I repay you?" asked the wealthy gentleman Churchill. "I cannot take money for saving your son's life" replied farmer Fleming. "I notice that your son seems to be about the same age as my son. I will have your son educated at the finest schools, along with my son." said Mr. Churchill. Many years later farmer Fleming's now well-educated son, Alexander Fleming (1881-1955), discovered penicillin, which was used to save the life of Winston Churchill (1874-1965), the same boy who had been saved in the bogs decades ago.

It was 1928 when Alexander Fleming noticed that a gray furry mold in his petri dish killed all the surrounding bacteria.[16] The chemical from the mold (Penicillium notatum) produced the first successful antibiotic (meaning "against life"), penicillin, for which Fleming was awarded the shared Nobel prize in medicine in 1945. Just ask any physician who remembers the 1950s, when medicine was shifting from sulfa drugs and colloidal silver to antibiotics. Doomed patients with bacterial infections were sometimes pulled from the brink of death by antibiotics. In ancient Ayurvedic medicine, the healer would apply a piece of moldy bread (rich in antibiotics) to a wound to prevent infection. Unfortunately, this warm and fuzzy story does not end here.

Antibiotics are chemical "no trespassing" borders that are excreted by fungi and some bacteria. Most of the nearly one thousand antibiotics, or mycotoxins, that have been tested proved to be so toxic that they could not be used without killing the patient. One mycotoxin, aflatoxin B, is the most carcinogenic substance on the planet earth. Streptozotocin is an antibiotic that is too toxic for human use except as a chemotherapy drug for cancer patients, but is used in research because it kills the pancreas in all experimental animals and generates insulin-dependent diabetes.[17] Now the researchers can produce all the diabetic animals they need for experiments.

The FDA must consider the risk-to-benefit ratio of all antibiotics, since there is a thin line between killing the bacterial infection and killing the patient. After bee venom, the most hyper-allergenic substance in the world is penicillin. Today, Americans use about 17 million pounds (7.7 million kilograms) of antibiotics to make the 8 billion animals raised for human consumption grow faster.[18] Most European countries do not allow antibiotics to be given at "sub-therapeutic" levels to make animals grow faster. In the 1950s, American farmers would add 5-10 parts per million of the antibiotic tetracycline to animal feed to accelerate the rate of growth by about 20%. Today, farmers need to use 50-200 ppm (10 to 40 times more than previous dosage) to get the same effect.

Bacteria carry within them little mysterious forms of life called plasmids. These "hitchhikers" get free room and board in exchange for their ability to "hack" the code on chemical poisons in the environment. Plasmids somehow figure out how to bypass the biochemical pathways of antibiotics, which makes the bacteria immune to the effects of this poison.[19] Bacteria exchange plasmids frequently, like a convention of hackers trying to beat the code. Antibiotics are extremely stable to heat, sun, and even passing through the digestive tract of an animal, which means they remain active in the environment in raw sewage and all the more likely to allow the plasmids an opportunity at hacking the chemical combination that allows the bacteria to be immune to the drug's effects. We now have drug-resistant "bullet-proof" microbes that thrive in spite of our best drugs, including the "big stick" of antibiotics, vancomycin. Even the American Medical Association endorses this viewpoint. From 20-50% of patients now exhibit bacterial infections that are resistant to one or more once-effective antibiotics.

We also consume 20 million pounds of antibiotics annually as prescription drugs, oftentimes for people who do not have a bacterial infection. Of the 100 million

ANNUAL PRODUCTION OF ANTIBIOTICS IN AMERICA
millions of pounds

prescriptions for antibiotics given in America each year, half are considered "inappropriate" by medical officials, with 40 million of those antibiotic prescriptions given to people with a viral cold. According to one study published in the *Journal of the American Medical Association*, 44% of children going to the doctor for a cold were given antibiotics, which is inappropriate therapy.[20] In a separate study, researchers observed 250 adults being treated for a fever that lasted less than a week. The physicians were wrong 50% of the time in assessing whether the patient had a viral or bacterial infection.[21] Intussusception is the leading cause of intestinal obstruction in young children in America. Antibiotic use triples the risk for intussusception in children. The antibiotic Cephalosporin increases the risk for intestinal obstruction by 20 fold.[22]

Antibiotics are useless against a virus, but may induce a fungal infection in the process. Antibiotics are given before, during and after nearly all medical and dental procedures; from a tooth cleaning to routine chemotherapy to bone marrow transplantation. Antibiotics are among the most toxic of all cancer therapy drugs, including adriamycin and bleomycin. Antibiotics can control certain bacterial infections, but do nothing to kill viruses or most other infectious agents. This rampant misuse of antibiotics has turned the gift from the angels into a gift from the devils. Antibiotics kill most or all bacteria that they encounter, including the good bacteria (probiotics) in the digestive tract.

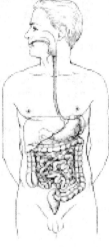

The average human has about 4 pounds of microorganisms in the gut. Good bacteria in the gut help us to make vitamins (biotin, K, etc.), digest food, encourage regularity, and compete with or eat the unfriendly yeast that can overrun the gut. A healthy human gut is like a balanced ecosystem of a garden in which the birds eat the bugs, and the bugs do minimal damage to the vegetable garden. When we kill off the birds (friendly bacteria), the bugs (harmful yeast) have no predators and quickly overrun the garden. When we overuse antibiotics, we kill ALL the bacteria in the gut and commonly end up with a yeast infection that can become systemic.[23] All major clinical textbooks on fungal infections agree that antibiotic use is a leading cause of fungal infections in humans.[24] "Candida overgrowth and bloodborne dissemination are favored by...multiple antibiotics, catheters, and tubes."[25]

IN SUMMARY. Antibiotics, if used appropriately, can save lives. Unfortunately, antibiotics are being wildly overused today with the net effect of:

- ➢ lowering the chance of the antibiotic working in a truly appropriate case
- ➢ raising the risk for some pandemic drug-resistant plague sweeping the globe
- ➢ wiping out the friendly bacteria in the gut to induce malnutrition, constipation, diarrhea, etc.
- ➢ inducing fungal infections and the myriad of diseases that can occur from mycotoxins
- ➢ as outright poisons, antibiotics can shut down any number of organs or systems in the body

PATIENT PROFILE: LC was a reasonably healthy 25 year old woman when she came down with a cold in 1975. After a few days of misery, she went to her doctor who gave her a prescription for antibiotics, having never taken a throat culture to see if the infection was bacterial. A week later, LC was still sick. More and different antibiotics were prescribed. Eventually, LC recovered from the cold. Three months later, LC began discharging blood in her stools. As the "solution" to this problem, her doctor performed an ileostomy, or removal of the colon and ileocecal valve and placed a plastic bag on her hip. No more normal toilet pooping. A few years later, LC developed vaginal bleeding. Her doctor surgically removed all of her female organs by hysterectomy and ovariectomy. She has since experienced hot flashes and chronic fatigue syndrome that would flatten anyone. It is quite possible that her nearly 30 years of health problems could have been avoided by not using antibiotics for a cold, or dealing with the inevitable yeast overgrowth from the antibiotics in ways other than removal of "elective" organs.

In 1908, the Nobel laureate, Elie Metchnikoff, PhD (1845-1916), who discovered the bacteria (Lactobacillus acidophilus) that makes yogurt, said "Death begins in the colon." Once the balance of power in the gut swings from healthy bacteria to unhealthy yeast overgrowth, illness in the body is inevitable and death is quite possible.

Orian Truss, MD is a well-respected internist in Alabama who wrote the seminal book on the subject of yeast infections, THE MISSING DIAGNOSIS. He describes a half century of his own medical practice and the bewildering collection of conditions produced in patients who had taken antibiotics.[26] Dr. Truss was working in New York City in the 1950s when antibiotics were being prescribed with great enthusiasm for

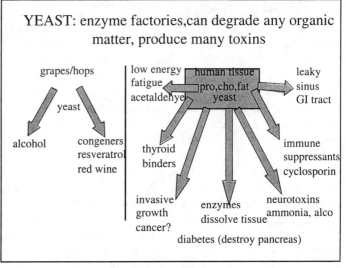

many inappropriate conditions. Patients would return a few months later with chronic fatigue syndrome, or Crohn's disease, or irritable bowel syndrome, or multiple sclerosis. Dr. Truss was the first one to link antibiotic side effects to yeast overgrowth and the limitless diseases that can be produced through fungal by-products, or secondary metabolites.

The immune system is a collection of 20 trillion highly specialized warrior cells that patrol the human body looking for bad guys. You are either with us or against us. Recognize self from non-self. This is truly an amazing feat. When the immune system is suppressed, we get infections or cancer. When the immune system is overstimulated, we get auto-immune diseases as the immune system begins to attack our own tissues. When antibiotics were first discovered in the 1930s, there were no auto-immune diseases known to modern medicine. Today there are 80 and counting. Arthritis, juvenile diabetes, multiple sclerosis, scleroderma, ankylosing spondylitis, lupus erythematosus, Crohn's disease, and many others are growing exponentially in numbers. Overuse of antibiotics may generate systemic fungal infections. Fungi can either slow down the immune system to allow more infections and cancer[27], or can upregulate the immune system to trigger an autoimmune attack.[28] Now the body is literally eating itself alive.

So if antibiotics are not the answer to all infections, then what is? A healthy immune system. When our immune system is properly fortified with nutrients, and not impaired by toxins or stress, then our immune system can recognize and destroy the most evasive of microbes. Lymphocytes, Natural Killer cells, helper and suppressor cells, antibodies, and immunoglobulins constitute the world's most sophisticated army to repel invaders in our body.

The worst plague to hit the human race was the Black Plague of 1347, in which about half of Europe, or nearly 75 million people, died. Yet half survived, because of their healthy immune system. Every year about 62,000 Americans die from the flu and pneumonia, of which 90% are older people with compromised immune systems.[29] Cancer is the second leading cause of death among Americans. A compromised immune system is partly at fault in our cancer "epidemic".

WHERE DO THE FUNGI COME FROM?
"The majority of exogenous fungi causing serious invasive disease are acquired by inhalation." C.C. Kibbler, in PRINCIPLES AND PRACTICES OF CLINICAL MYCOLOGY, p.16, Wiley, UK, 1996

For 50 years, American physicians have routinely prescribed antibiotics (only useful for some bacterial infections) for the 45 million Americans who suffer from chronic sinus infections. In 1999, researchers at the Mayo Clinic found that 96% of all sinus infections were caused by fungi. Where else can fungi find ideal conditions for growth: warm, dark, wet, full of sugar (mucus is a sweet molecule of mucopolysaccharides)?

Doctors at Georgetown Medical Center in Washington, DC found that patients with unexplained chronic fatigue were nine times (900%) more likely to be suffering from sinusitis than the population at large. Patients with chronic pain were 6 times (600%) more likely to be suffering from sinusitis than the control group.[30] Maybe the fungi enters the body through the sinus cavities, creates an infection there, then spreads throughout the body to create pain, fatigue, and possibly eventually cancer.

One study found that 69% of healthy young humans who had fasted from food for 3 hours and abstained from alcohol for 24 hours and were then fed 50 grams of glucose (about the sugar present in a soft drink) showed a measurable amount of alcohol in the bloodstream within 1 hour.[31] Many of us have yeast in our guts waiting to ferment simple sugars into alcohol and a bewildering assortment of congener by-products. Given the 140 pounds per year of refined sugar consumed by the average American, coupled with 50 million pounds of antibiotics that we consume directly as drugs or indirectly through our meat and milk supply, coupled with the multiple nutrient deficiencies in the American population, it is no stretch of the imagination to envision a high percentage of Americans with mild to raging fungal infections.

> **GUT FERMENTATION "AUTO BREWERY" SYNDROME**
> Hunnisett, A., J.Nutr.Med., vol.1, p.33, 1990
>
> STUDY DESIGN:
> Group 1: 36 healthy adults, 3 hr no food, 24 hr no alcohol, 50 gram oral glucose load, blood glucose and ETOH measured 1 hour after glucose load
> RESULTS: 69% (25/36) positive ETOH in blood (+3.7 mg%)
>
> Group 2: 510 "unwell" patients, same except 5 gm oral glucose,
> RESULTS: 61% (311/510) positive ETOH in blood (+2.5 mg%)
>
> SUGGESTS THAT: Yeast and bacteria reside in the stomach and small intestine and ferment simple sugars to alcohol within minutes. Yeast grow well on simple refined carbohydrates. Alcohol increases intestinal permeability for toxin absorption. Alcohol can be degraded to acetaldehyde, general toxin.

Fungi are so prolific and so fecund as to defy the imagination. A wood decay fungus (Ganoderma) sends out 5.4 trillion spores per season. Corn smut fungi produces 25 billion fungal spores per ear of corn. In one experiment, researchers on the first floor of a building took the lid off of a culture dish with fungi. Within 10 minutes, these unique fungi had traveled through the ventilation system, up to the 4th floor, and were measured in thousands per square yard.[32]

The Government Accounting Office tells us that 20% of the 80,000 public schools in America have an air quality problem, usually including fungi, which cause breathing problems and more in school children. Close up a school for 3 months of a hot humid summer with plenty of food (books) for the fungi, and the possibility of mold-causing health problems in school children escalates. Americans have been to the moon, built the Panama Canal and the Internet, and have more Nobel laureates than any other country on earth, yet we are only beginning to look at one of the most powerful and potentially destructive creatures on the planet earth: fungi. Never mind Jaws or the Predator. Fungi can make these two horror films look like cartoons.

The definitive textbook on fungal infections in humans, PRINCIPLES AND PRACTICES OF CLINICAL MYCOLOGY, by world renowned physicians and researchers, says that fungal infections in the bone are virtually identical to bone cancer (i.e. leukemia, multiple myeloma) on an X-ray machine: "Differentiation of blastomycotic bone disease from tuberculosis, malignant disease, or other fungal disease is difficult." A.V. Costantini, MD, former professor at the University of California San Francisco Medical School and former head of the World Health Organization, has amassed an impressive amount of data showing that mycotoxins in our food supply can and do cause many forms of cancer, including breast and prostate.[33]

Where do the fungi come from? They come from the air around us and the fungi that live within our gut, mouth, sinuses, vaginal tract, and other body cavities.

THE ECOLOGIST AND UNDERTAKER.

Let's have a *Reader's Digest* quick look at fungi, aka the kingdom Mycota. Fungi (also known as yeast, mold, rust, and mushrooms) are on top of the food chain on earth, because they degrade all organic matter once dead. When the minister cites "ashes to ashes and dust to dust" at the funeral, we are talking about the job of fungi. Fungi turn us and everything else into dirt. There are over 400,000 species of fungi recognized by mycologists, with an estimated 1.5 million different species on earth, of which 400 species can cause diseases in humans. Candida is the species most often associated with human fungal infections, yet there are

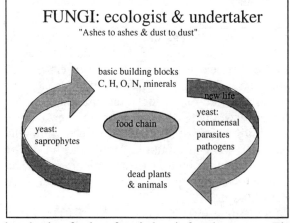

FUNGI: ecologist & undertaker
"Ashes to ashes & dust to dust"

basic building blocks
C, H, O, N, minerals

new life

yeast:
commensal
parasites
pathogens

food chain

yeast:
saprophytes

dead plants
& animals

hundreds of other fungi that infect humans. The fungi, Aspergillus, "eat" damp grains and nuts in the field and give off aflatoxins, one of the most toxic and cancer-causing agents on the planet earth. Fungi are, basically, enzyme factories. They make enzymes to digest any organic matter on earth. When all the people, bugs, poop, and leaves have fallen, then fungi step in to degrade this organic matter back to the basic elements of carbon, hydrogen, nitrogen, oxygen, and minerals. Unfortunately, sometimes fungi are too eager to perform their duties. Fungi are at their best working to turn your back yard compost pile into rich soil and at their worst in a dying patient.

WHAT IS YOUR VITALITY SCORE?

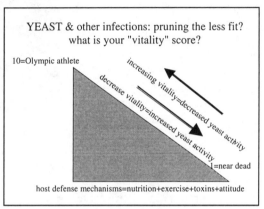

YEAST & other infections: pruning the less fit? what is your "vitality" score?

10=Olympic athlete

increasing vitality=decreased yeast activity

decrease vitality=increased yeast activity

1=near dead

host defense mechanisms=nutrition+exercise+toxins+attitude

Why do we have so many Americans suffering from systemic fungal infections? Bacteria, yeast, virus, parasites are abundantly present all around us. What keeps you well is "your terrain", or your "non-specific host defense mechanisms". How does anyone recover from the flu, a laceration of the skin, or a broken bone? You recover through the miraculous healing properties within your body.

What is your "vitality score"? How healthy are you? If vitality exists as a continuum, with 0 meaning dead, 1 being very ill, and 10 being an Olympic athlete, then where are you on this scale? If we drop below 7 or so on the scale, fungi become eager to perform their duties in us. This is where the bubble bursts on the American dream of a "magic bullet" drug to kill all disease-causing organisms in our body, while we consume 140 pounds per year of sugar, tiny portions of our mercury fillings, routine antibiotics, the only exercise that we get is coughing, and an endless stream of stress hormones from unhappy spirits. A malnourished, sugar-drenched, toxically-compromised, exhausted, and stressed-out person is an easy target for a fungal infection. When we are well, the fungi live as "commensal" organisms, creating small amounts of uric acid as an antioxidant to slow down the aging process. As our vitality score drops, yeast switch into saprophytic mode, or begin to decay any available fuel in our body. When things really get ugly, the yeast becomes a parasite and can cause a slow torturous death with a bewildering assortment of medical labels. The typical American lifestyle generates a very low vitality score. Fungi are there to do their job. If you want to get well, then begin a healthy lifestyle that discourages the presence of fungal infections.

IF CANCER IS REALLY FUNGI, THEN..

In the hundreds of medical staff meetings and tumor boards that I have attended, brilliant physicians have presented their most puzzling cancer cases. How does a cancer cell secrete enzymes to break through the various epithelial barriers and eventually metastasize throughout the patient's body? Why does a cancer feed primarily on sugar (glucose), which is why we use a PET scan to find the cancer? How does a cancer cell generate a wide assortment of chemicals that mimic the human fetus, as if to create a regional immune suppression or "stealth coating"? 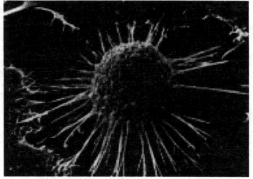 How does cancer create substances (like lactic acid) that cause havoc with energy metabolism of the patient? How does cancer send out roots to burrow into the flesh of the host. Fungi can do all of this, and more.

Fungi is a formidable invader in the human body for many reasons. For instance, bacteria are prokaryotic cells that lack a membrane around the nucleus. It is easier for human immune cells to "smell" the difference between human and bacterial cells. Fungal cells mimic human cells as eukaryotic cells that do have a membrane around the nucleus, making it more difficult for the immune system to detect "good guys from bad guys".

GETTING WELL. Stop taking indiscriminate antibiotics. Cut back on sugar intake dramatically. Eat lean and clean fish, chicken, poultry, and wild game with plenty of fresh vegetables. Add reasonable amounts of fruit, grains, legumes, nuts, and seeds in their natural state. Avoid processed foods. Detoxify the poisons from your body.

CONDITIONS THAT ENCOURAGE YEAST:
- toxins (i.e. mercury, petrochemicals, pesticides, etc.)
- stress
- malnutrition (excess, deficiency, or imbalance or any nutrient)
- chronically-elevated blood glucose
- sedentary lifestyle
- mold overload (working around mold, like autumn leaves, animal dung, moldy attics)
- antibiotics

TO DETECT YEAST OVERGROWTH:

organic acid urine analysis, Great Plains Labs, 913-341-8949

TO REVERSE YEAST OVERGROWTH:

1) Starve it. Diet must be high in live whole food. Meat, chicken, fish and colorful vegetables are the core. Small amounts of nuts, seeds, beans, little whole grains. Very little fresh fruit. No sugar. Reduce blood sugar to 60-90 mg%. Buy and use a home blood glucose testing kit, available at your local pharmacy. Avoid moldy food, i.e. blue cheese dressing.

2) Kill it.
➢ prescription anti-fungals include diflucan, sporonox, ketoconazole, nystatin (only useful in the gut due to poor absorption). May require 6-12 months on medication. May initially feel worse with yeast die off (Herxheimer reaction).
➢ garlic, oil of oregano, grapefruit seed extract, Essiac tea, castor oil, capryllic acid, medium chain triglycerides, olive oil
➢ purge yeast sanctuaries (such as wherever it is dark, warm, wet, with a fuel source, and compromised host defenses): sinus, colon, vagina, ears, mouth, feet. Use tongue scraper, vaginal douche using dilute boric acid, maintain bowel regularity.

3) Change the conditions that allow yeast to thrive. Add probiotics (yogurt, lactobacillus), biotin (5 mg/day), detoxify heavy metals, endorphins (peace and happiness), exercise, immune stimulation, lots of greens (chlorella, spirulina, barley green), healthy prostaglandin mix through less omega 6 oils (corn, soy, safflower) and more omega 3 oils (fish), MSM (sulfur).

Alright, you have read this far in this chapter. We all must be careful to distinguish facts from hunches. I have presented many relevant scientifically-based facts in this chapter. My hunch regarding cancer as an infection? We have a certain level of vitality in our cells that is driven by nutrition, exercise, attitude, toxins, and energy alignment. If we play our cards right and live a healthy lifestyle, then our cells percolate with adequate vitality to resist the onslaught of pathogens. If our lifestyle is less than ideal, then pathogens are drawn to our compromised cells, like ants to dead flies on the sidewalk. The pathogens become infections in our body, sometimes regional (such as the gut or sinuses) and sometimes systemic, meaning throughout the body. Some pathogens invade the cell membrane and "mate" with our DNA, creating a new cell that begins to take over the body and is diagnosed as cancer. Your mission, should you choose to accept it, is to make your body so full of wellness through lifestyle, that there is no room for illness, such as cancer.

My sincere appreciation to Orian Truss, MD, Milton White, MD, A.V. Costantini, MD, William Crook, MD, and Doug Kaufmann for making the rest of the world more aware of an underdiagnosed problem: mycotoxins in our food supply and fungal infections in our bodies.

PATIENT PROFILE: "Doc" Pennington was an oil magnate who developed end-stage non-resectable (cannot be surgically removed) colon cancer at the age of 70 in 1972. His doctors told him to "get his affairs in order". Pennington got his physician to write a prescription for Griseofulvin, an anti-fungal drug. Three months later, his oncologist found that Doc Pennington had no more colon cancer. Remember, Pennington had no medical therapy. Pennington died at age 92 in 1994, but not before spending $125 million of his own money to found the Pennington Biomedical Center to study the link between yeast, nutrition, and cancer. Researchers in Taiwan have found that Griseofulvin induced suicide, or apoptosis, in human colon cancer cells in a culture dish.[34]

ENDNOTES

[1] . Dollinger, M., EVERYONE'S GUIDE TO CANCER THERAPY, p.8, Andrews McMeel, Kansas City, 2002

[2] . Sugiyama, T, Med.Electron.Microsc., vol.37, no.3, p.149, Sep.2004
[3] . Cheung, TW, Cancer Invest.vol.22no.5, p.787, 2004
[4] . Brechot,C., Gastroenterology, vol.127,5 suppl.1, p. S56
[5] . Williams, JH, Am.J.Clin.Nutr., vol.80, no.5, p.1106, Nov.2004
[6] . Mahmoud, FA, Curr.Oncol.Rep., vol.4, no.3, p.250, May 2002
[7] . Hess, DJ, CAN BACTERIA CAUSE CANCER?, New York Univ.Press, 1997
[8] . Peehl, DM, Urology, vol. 58, 2 suppl. 1, p.123, Aug.2001
[9] . Bok, RA, Drug Saf., vol.20, no.5, p.451, May 1999
[10] . Yuan-Soon, H., Int.J.Cancer, vol.91, p.383, 2001
[11] . White, MW, Medical Hypotheses, vol.55, no.4, p.302, 2000
[12] . Kemper, CA, PRINCIPLES AND PRACTICES CLINICAL MYCOLOGY, p.58, Wiley, NY, 1996
[13] . Graybill, JR, PRINCIPLES AND PRACTICES CLINICAL MYCOLOGY, p.96, Wiley, NY, 1996
[14] . Ponikau, JU, Mayo Clin.Proc., vol.74, p.877, 1999
[15] . Graybill, JR, ibid.
[16] . Mitchell, J. (ed.), RANDOM HOUSE ENCYCLOPEDIA, p.2191, Random House, NY, 1983
[17] . Mavrikakis, ME, et al., Exp.Clin.Endocrinol.Diabetes, vol.106, no.1, p.35, 1998
[18] . Levy, S., ANTIBIOTIC PARADOX,p. 149, Perseus Publ, Cambridge, MA, 2002
[19] . Levy, SB, THE ANTIBIOTIC PARADOX, Perseus Publ, Cambridge, MA, 2002
[20] . JAMA, vol.279, p.875, 1998
[21] . Brit.J.Gen.Practice, vol.51, p.998, 2001
[22] . Spiro, DM, et al., vol.157, no.1, p.54, Jan.2003
[23] . Verduyn, L, Diagn.Microbiol.Infect.Dis., vol.34, no.3, p.213, Jul 1999
[24] . Kibbler, CC, et al., PRINCIPLES AND PRACTICES OF CLINICAL MYCOLOGY, Wiley, NY, 1996; see also Calderone, RA, CANDIDA AND CANDIDIASIS, ASM Press, Washington, 2002
[25] . Graybill, JR, p.97, ibid.
[26] . Truss, O., THE MISSING DIAGNOSIS, Missing Diagnosis, Inc., Birmingham, AL, 1985
[27] . Boutrif, E., et al., Global Significance of Mycotoxins, in MYCOTOXINS AND PHYCOTOXINS, p.3, deKoe, Netherlands, 2001
[28] . Norred, WP, et al., Toxicology and mechanisms of action of selected mycotoxins, in MYCOTOXINS AND PHYCOTOXINS, deKoe, Netherlands, 2001
[29] . US Mortality Public Use Data Tape, National Center for Health Statistics, Centers for Disease control and Prevention 2003
[30] . Chester, AC, Arch.Intern.Med., vol.163, no.15, p.1832, Aug11, 2003
[31] . Hunnisett, A., J.Nutritional Med., vol. 1, p.33, 1990
[32] . Hudler, GW, MAGICAL MUSHROOMS, MISCHIEVOUS MOLDS, Princeton Press, 1998
[33] . Costantini, AV, PREVENTION OF BREAST CANCER, Oberlin Verlag, Germany, 1996
[34] . Yuan-Soon, H., Int.J.Cancer, vol.91, p.383, 2001

CHAPTER 26

RATIONAL CANCER TREATMENT
✯
IF I HAD CANCER,
WHAT WOULD I DO?

"Humor is the balancing stick that allows us to walk the tightrope of life."   John F. Kennedy, 35th president of US

> I would use an appropriate combination of:
> 1) restrained cytotoxic therapies to reduce tumor burden
> 2) an aggressive collection of naturopathic (cell-restorative) therapies to re-regulate the body and bolster host defense mechanisms.

The combination of changing the underlying conditions that brought on the cancer (naturopathic) and attacking the cancer with therapies that kill cancer, but do not harm the host (cytotoxic), can be incredibly effective.

Chemotherapy, radiation, and surgery may be appropriate in certain cancers and for certain people. But make sure that the physician understands the concept of "restrained" medical therapies against cancer. I have worked with cancer patients who were devastated by unrestrained chemo, radiation, or surgery.

If you threw a hand grenade into your garage to get rid of the mice, then you may have accomplished the goal of killing the mice, but you don't have a garage anymore. Similarly, too many cancer patients are exposed to "maximum sub-lethal" therapies, which may provide an initial "response" or tumor shrinkage, but in the end may reduce the quality and quantity of life for the cancer patient by suppressing immune functions, damaging the heart and kidneys, and creating a tumor that is "drug resistant", or virtually bullet-proof.

There are other cancer therapies that may be more effective at killing cancer and less toxic to the cancer patients, such as hyperthermia, Burzynski's anti-neoplastons, PolyMVA, enzymes, Cell Specific Cancer Therapy, Ukrain, Govallo's vaccine, and others.

COMPREHENSIVE CANCER TREATMENT INCLUDES:

1↓

change underlying cause(s) of disease
NUTRITION
DETOXIFICATION
DYSBIOSIS
HORMONE BAL.
HYPERGLYCEMIA
INFECTIONS
STRESS
EXERCISE
ENERGY PATHWAYS
ETC.

2↓

restrained tumor debulking
CHEMO?
RADIATION
SURGERY
BURZYNSKI
HYPERTHERM
PHOTO-CYTO
HERBALS
APHERESIS
LYMPH.INFUS.

3↓

symptom management
PAIN**
NAUSEA
ANOREXIA
ANEMIA
LEUKOPENIA
DEPRESSION
CACHEXIA
HAIR LOSS

PATIENT PROFILE: SPIRIT OVER NUTRIENTS

H.G. was a fun-loving, guy who enjoyed cigarettes, wine, and a good laugh. He developed prostate cancer with bone metastasis while in his mid 50s. His doctor said: "Get your affairs in order." H.G. went to a psycho-neuroimmunology clinic to help him use his mind as a healing tool in his advanced untreatable cancer. He felt that he had been burdened with an endless procession of responsibilities, from high school to the Marines, to a profession, family, and more. He wanted to be free of all of this. He left his wife and his cancer went into remission. Meanwhile, his wife, B.G. was a non-smoker, drank very little, hiked, was in good shape, and ate a very good diet. One year after H.G. left her, B.G. developed advanced brain cancer and died within 6 weeks of diagnosis. Nutrition is an important factor in cancer outcome. But as a nutritionist, I must admit that what you are eating you is not as important as what's eating you--as H.G. and his wife illustrated.

★

CHAPTER 27

BEATING CANCER SYMPTOMS

"What cancer cannot do: It cannot cripple love, or shatter hope, or corrode faith, or destroy peace, or kill friendship, or suppress memories, or silence courage, or invade the soul, or steal eternal life, or conquer the Spirit." anonymous, from Ann Landers column

For many cancer patients, the side effects can be worse than facing a life-threatening disease. This concise guide may help to minimize many of the complications from cancer or the cytotoxic treatment. My gratitude to Marge Affleck, RN, and Rebecca Wright, RD, for their invaluable assistance in completing this chapter.

PATIENT PROFILE: MIND OVER NUTRIENTS

S.H. was a cute 33 year old Colorado farmer's wife and mother of 2 small children when she was diagnosed with breast cancer in 1992. She had a radical bilaterial mastectomy along with chemo and radiation at her nearby hospital. The cancer metastasized to her internal organs, liver, and bone, and she was told to "get her affairs in order." She failed therapy at an alternative clinic in Mexico. She came to our hospital in such advanced state of disease that our doctors did not expect her to live 2 months. She began the nutrition program, coupled with detoxification, psycho-spiritual counseling, fractionated chemotherapy, and radiation. In 2 months, she not only wasn't dead, she was off her pain medication. In 6 months, her hair had grown back, her disease was markedly diminished, and she was having an excellent quality of life. After 14 months, the cancer has been reduced to tiny shadows on her CAT scans. By then, her husband thought she had beat the disease, and, after supporting her throughout her 3 year battle with cancer, decided that he had enough. He left her. One month later, she died of coronary arrest, quite possibly a "broken heart." We need to pay homage to the importance and the majesty of our human spirit. Vitamins will not cure a broken heart or give us a reason to live.

BEATING CANCER SYMPTOMS		
SYMPTOMS	**ALLOPATHIC**	**NATUROPATHIC**
NAUSEA	Zofran, Compazine	enzymes, ginger, acupressure wrist band, acupuncture
VOMITING	Phenergan, Tigan	suck on ice cubes, yogurt, ginger tea or caps, ginger ale, acupuncture
ANOREXIA	Megace, Marinol	enzymes, small meals, ginger, dining with others, zinc, B vitamins
MALNUTRITION	TPN, Advera, Impact	hydrazine sulfate, Dragon Slayer shake, enzymes, high protein meals
DIARRHEA	Lomotil, Imodium, Questran	yogurt, probiotics, SeaCure, glutamine, milk enemas, Pepto Bismol, acupuncture,blueberries
MALDIGESTION	enzymes, Hcl, Pancrease	SeaCure, enzymes, probiotics, betaine HCl, ginger, mustard, Zymarine
LYMPHEDEMA		lymph drainage therapy (iahe.com), rebounder (trampoline), massage, topical castor oil
CONSTIPATION	Senacote, Milk Magnesia, Mag Citrate, glycerin suppositories	probiotics,psyllium,Perfect7,sena, buckthorn,cascara sagrada, epsom salts,fiber, water, walking, aloe
GAS	Phyzeme, Propulsid, Reglan, Zantac	enzymes, probiotics, soil-based organisms, ginger, mustard, onions; walking,; avoid beans, nuts, broccoli
ANEMIA	Epogen, Procrit (erythropoietin)	liquid liver extract, B-12, B-6, chelated iron supplements, folate, copper, beet juice, shark liver oil
LEUKOPENIA	Newpogen	ImmunoPower, PCM4, ImmKin, bovine cartilage, garlic, ginseng, propolis, olive leaf, shark liver oil, echinecea, vit. C, E, A, betacarotene, selenium, zinc, colloidal silver, astragalus, colostrum, golden seal, ginkgo
HAIR LOSS		1600 iu vit.E 1-2 weeks prior to beginning chemo, aloe, vit.D ointment
FATIGUE	Megace, antidepressants, i.e. Prozac	B vit., B-12 sublingual, ginseng, mahuang , bee pollen, chromium, DHEA, caffeine from tea, high protein diet
ORAL MUCOSITIS	Mylanta ,Maalox, Zylocaine Benadryl,Nystatin	vit.E oil from capsule topically applied 3x daily with cotton swab, prophylactic antioxidants
YEAST INFECTIONS	Diflucan, Ketoconazole, Sporonox, Amphotericin, Vitrex, Nystatin, DMSO with diflucan	grapefruit seed extract, topical Australian tea tree oil, garlic, undecenoic acid (castor), caprylic acid, MCT, probiotics, biotin, Essiac tea, vaginal suppository of gentian violet or boric acid capsules
DEPRESSION	Prozac, etc.	St. John's wort, SAMe, TMG, tryptophan, niacinamidesunlight, ginkgo, DHEA except for hormonal cancers
ANXIETY	Xanax, Ativan	hops, valerian, kava, homeopathic, 5HTP
INSOMNIA	Ambien, Xanax	melatonin, 5HTP, kava, hops, valerian
PAIN	Tylenol, morphine, colchicine	acupuncture, hypnosis, magnets, white willow, DL phenylalanine

CHAPTER 28

PARTING COMMENTS

✳

"If I have seen, for then it is by standing upon the shoulders of giants."
Sir Isaac Newton (1642-1727) father of modern science

From my cancer patients I have learned of the incredible tenacity of the human body and spirit; of the immeasurable dignity and generosity that is waiting to be expressed by all of us; of the undying passion and commitment shown by a dedicated mate when a loved one is failing; and above all-of the preciousness of life. In our increasingly callous world, it is easy to drift away from the true pleasures in life: love, enthusiasm, laughter, freedom, meaningful work, skills developed, helping one another, and savoring the beauty in this emerald paradise planet. For many people, cancer has become the ultimate "truth serum" in helping them to establish real priorities.

While the scope of the book is to offer helpful advice on using nutrition to improve outcome in cancer treatment, there are some fundamental flaws in the structure of our health care system and governmental surveillance that impair our ability to investigate and use rational cancer treatments. In the state of California, chemotherapy, radiation, and surgery are the only LEGAL options for cancer patients. Physicians have lost their licenses and even gone to jail for venturing outside the narrow confines of this allopathic model for cancer. There are 7 states in the U.S. that have passed an AMTA bill, or Access to Medical Treatment Act, meaning the licensed health care professional can offer whatever therapies the doctor and the patient agree to be appropriate. Such freedom is desperately needed if we are to truly win the war on cancer. I strongly encourage all Americans to voice your opinion with your representative in state and federal legislatures regarding the need for more freedom and options in cancer treatment. Why do cancer patients have to leave the country or visit some "underground" clinic to seek alternative cancer treatment? How can we possibly consider the FDA protecting cancer patients when much of what is FDA approved is either ineffective or barbaric?

"Unless we put medical freedom into the Constitution, the time will come when medicine will organize itself into an undercover dictatorship." Dr. Benjamin Rush, signer of the Declaration of Independence

FIND A "CO-PATIENT" TO HELP YOU

Cancer is a difficult disease to treat. And it gets even more difficult to overcome when you are doing it all on your own. Find a "co-patient" to help. Someone who has faith, hope, and sense of humor, and encourages you. Spend as much time as you can with that person. It could be a spouse, family member, friend, neighbor, or member of your church or synagogue. Tell him or her that they will get as much out of this journey together as you, the patient, will receive. Bask in the glow of their enthusiasm and optimism. I find that cancer patients who have a "co-patient" are much more likely to beat the odds.

MAKING A DIAMOND OUT OF COAL

You are the pro-active and assertive cancer victor. You have been through some or all of the phases that come with the disease: anger, denial, rejection, isolation, withdrawal, and more. While the bulk of this book is spent providing nutritional facts to change the biochemistry of your body, my final parting comments are directed more at your soul, because cancer is a disease of the mind, body, and spirit.

Today, we wage full-scale chemical warfare on ourselves with potent agricultural and industrial carcinogens, while stripping our once-benevolent food supply of any vestige of nutritional value. We are subjected to intolerable stress from work and dissolving family structures, thousands of murders per year on TV and movies, and an endless procession of gut-wrenching stories on the nightly news.

Nourish your body, mind, and spirit. Take every opportunity to say: "I love you." Give away smiles with reckless abandon. Practice random acts of kindness and beauty. Savor each day as though it may be your last, because the same holds true for all of us. You have the opportunity to be born again with a renewed vigor and purpose in life.

My prayer for you is the same thought that began this book--that you will soon be able to say: "Cancer is the best thing that ever happened to me." Since you have cancer, you might as well turn this ultimate challenge into the ultimate victory, to make your life into a masterpiece painting.

Other Information Services

-Greg Anderson, Cancer Recovery Foundation of America, Box 238, Hershey, PA 17033, 800-238-6479 or 717-545-7600, fax -7602, www.CancerRecovery.org

-Orthomolecular Oncology, The Estate Office, Ashton, Nr Oundle, Northamptonshire, PE8 5LE, United Kingdom, www.canceraction.org.gg/index2.htm

-Center for the Study of Natural Oncology, 437 S. Hwy. 101, Ste. 201, Solana Beach, CA 92075, 800-557-2944 or 858-523-9144, fax -0919, www.natural-oncology.org

-Us Too! International, 5003 Fairview Ave, Downers Grove, IL 60515, (630) 795-1002, fax (630) 795-1602, www.ustoo.org

MIND & BODY CONNECTION

-Center for Mind-Body Medicine, 5225 Conn. Ave. NW Ste 414, Washington, DC 20015, 202-966-7338, fax -2589, www.cmbm.org

-Healing Journeys, 2011 P St., Ste. 301, Sacramento, CA 95814, 800-423-9882 or 916-930-9040, fax -9042, www.healingjourneys.org

INTERNET USERS

www.healthy.com

search google.com, overture.com, askjeeves.com

National　　　　　Library　　　　　of　　　　　Medicine: http://www.ncbi.nlm.nih.gov/entrez/query.fcgi

American Cancer Society: Cancer.org

American Hospice Foundation: AmericanHospice.org

American Institute for Cancer Research: AICR.org

American Society of Clinical Oncology: ASCO.org

R.A. Bloch Cancer Foundation: BlochCancer.org

BOOKS AND TAPES ON PSYCHOLOGICAL HEALING

Leshan, Lawrence L. CANCER AS A TURNING POINT (2nd ed.).

Ryan, Regina Sara (2000). AFTER SURGERY, ILLNESS, OR TRAUMA: 10 STEPS TO RENEWED ENERGY AND HEALTH. Prescott, AZ: Hohm Press.

Siegel, Bernie S. (1988). LOVE, MEDICINE AND MIRACLES. New York:HarperCollins.

Simonton, O. Carl et al. (1978). GETTING WELL AGAIN. New York: Bantam

CDs and Audiotapes of visualizations for healing cancer:

Rossman, Martin, FIGHTING CANCER FROM WITHIN FightCancerWithin.com

Collinge, William (1998) A Guide To Self-Healing Techniques For Cancer (www.healthynet.net/collinge; Audio Renaissance Tapes 800-452-5589)

Naparstek, Belleruth Cancer Guided Imagery - "Enhance your spiritual connection and optimize your healing energy." $12; 800-759-1294; www.touchstarpro.com

Naparstek, Belleruth For People with Cancer (Health Journeys). Time Warner Audio Books.

Siegel, Bernie Getting Ready: Preparing for Surgery, Chemotherapy & Other Treatments "Enjoy empowering meditations and inspiring inner journeys that combine guided imagery and self-hypnosis for enhancing your treatments." www.touchstarpro.com

Simonton, Carl (1987). Getting Well: A step-by-step, self-help guide to overcoming cancer for patients and their families. Audio Renaissance Tapes 800-452-5589 (St. Martin's Press).

Most of the above audiotapes (and many other cancer-healing visualization tapes) can be ordered at the following:
www.marilynjoyce.com/products.html; 800-352-3443
Simonton Cancer Ctr: 800-459-3424 or 310-457-3811;
www.simontoncenter.com
Hay House (Louise Hay) 800-654-5162 www.hayhouse.com
Audio Renaissance Tapes 800-452-5589
www.healthjourneys.com
www.innertalk.com; 800-964-3551
www.touchstarpro.com
Academy Guided Imagery: 800-726-2070 www.interactiveimagery.com

CANCER RETREAT CENTERS
Commonweal.org
Smith Farm Cancer Help Program (CHP)
1229 15th St. NW, Washington DC 20005, ph 202-483-8600
www.smithfarm.com,
smithfarm1@aol.com

Healing Journeys
2011 P Street, Suite 301
Sacramento, CA 95814, (800) 423-9882 or (916) 930-9040
Fax (916) 930-9042,
jan@healingjourneys.org
www.healingjourneys.org

Hawaii Naturopathic Retreat Center

Pahoa, Hawaii 96778, ph 808 965 7243

www.mindyourbody.info;
Email: nd@mindyourbody.info

Mind-Body Wellness Center
18201 Conneaut Lake Road
Meadville, Pennsylvania 16335
phone (814) 333-5060
fax (814) 333-5067
www.mind-body.org
info@mind-body.org

Harmony Hill Cancer Retreats
E. 7362 Hwy 106
Union, WA 98592
360-898-2363
www.harmonyhill.org

APPENDIX

✴

MAIL ORDER NUTRITION PRODUCTS

If you have a health food store nearby, then it would be a good idea to develop a relationship with a knowledgeable salesperson. If you do not have a health food store nearby, or do not have the time to shop, then the following companies can give you good service and value.

INTERNET SHOPPING
LEF.org
vitamins.com
wholepeople.com
mothernature.com
allherb.com
wizcitybotanicals.com
healthshop.com
gainesnutrition.com
enutrition.com
vitaminshoppe.com

BULK FOODS
Organic produce sent overnight: Diamond Organics 800-922-2396
Allergy Resources Inc., 195 Huntington Beach Dr., Colorado Springs, CO 80921, ph 719-488-3630
Deer Valley Farm, RD#1, Guilford, NY 13780, ph. 607-674-8556
Diamond K Enterprises, Jack Kranz, R.R. 1, Box 30, St. Charles, MN 55972, ph. 507-932-4308
Gravelly Ridge Farms, Star Route 16, Elk Creek, CA 95939, ph. 916-963-3216
Green Earth, 2545 Prairie St., Evanston, IL 60201, ph. 800-322-3662
Healthfoods Express, 181 Sylmar Clovis, CA 93612, ph. 209-252-8321
Jaffe Bros. Inc., PO Box 636, Valley Center, CA 92082, ph. 619-749-1133

Macrobiotic Wholesale Co., 799 Old Leicester Hwy, Asheville, NC 28806, ph. 704-252-1221
Moksha Natural Foods, 724 Palm, Watsonville,CA, 95076, 408-724-2009
Mountain Ark Co., 120 South East Ave., Fayetteville, AR, 72701, ph. 501-442-7191, or 800-643-8909
New American Food Co., PO Box 3206, Durham, NC 27705, ph. 919-682-9210
Timber Crest Farms, 4791 Dry Creek, Healdsburg, CA, 95448, ph. 707-433-8251, FAX -8255
Walnut Acres, Penns Creek, PA 17862, ph. 717-837-0601

MAIL ORDER VITAMINS
Bronson, 800-235-3200
NutriGuard, 800-433-2402
Health for Living, 813-566-2611
Vitamin Research , 800-877-2447
Vitamin Trader, 800-334-9310
Terrace International, 800-824-2434
Willner Chemists, 800-633-1106

SELLING HERBS
Gaia Herbals, 800-994-9355
Frontier Herbs 800-786-1388
Blessed Herbs 800-489-HERB
Trout Lake Farm 509-395-2025
San Francisco herb fax 800-227-5430
Star West 800-800-4372

APPENDIX

NUTRITION & CANCER BOOKS
✯

Available through Tattered Cover Bookstore, Denver, CO, 800-833-9327; or Mail Order Books 800-233-5150; or Discount Books 800-833-0702 or the Internet via www.amazon.com.

Bendich, A., and Chandra, RK, MICRONUTRIENTS AND IMMUNE FUNCTION, New York Academy of Sciences, vol.587, ISBN 0-89766-575-9

Boik, J. (2001). NATURAL COMPOUNDS CANCER THERAPY. Princeton, MN:

Bump, EA, RADIOPROTECTORS, CRC, Boca Raton, Fl, 1998

Cilento, R., HEAL CANCER, Hill Publishers, Australia, 1993, ISBN 0-85572-213-4

Congress of United States, Office of Technology Assessment, UNCONVENTIONAL CANCER TREATMENTS, U.S. Government Printing Office, Washington, DC, 1990, GPO # 052-003-01208-1, (ph. 800-336-4797)

Diamond, WJ, et al, DEFINITIVE GUIDE TO CANCER, Future Medicine, Tiburon, CA, 1997, ISBN 1-887299-01-7

Fischer, William L. (1994). HOW TO FIGHT CANCER AND WIN (2nd ed.).

Frähm, Anne E., with Frähm, David J. (1992). A CANCER BATTLE PLAN.

Frähm, David J. (2000). A CANCER BATTLE PLAN: SOURCEBOOK.

Hoffman, EJ, CANCER AND THE SEARCH FOR SELECTIVE BIOCHEMICAL INHIBITORS, CRC, Boca Raton, FL, 1999

Jacobs, M., VITAMINS AND MINERALS IN THE PREVENTION AND TREATMENT OF CANCER, CRC Press, Boca, FL, 1991, ISBN 0-8493-4259-7

Kaminski, MV, HYPERALIMENTATION, Marcel Dekker Press, NY, 1985

Laidlaw, SA, and Swendseid, ME, VITAMINS AND CANCER PREVENTION, Wiley & Sons (ph.800-225-5945), 1991, ISBN 0-471-56066-9

Lerner, M. (1994). CHOICES IN HEALING. Cambridge, MA: MIT Press.

Machlin, LJ, HANDBOOK OF VITAMINS, Marcel Dekker, NY, 1991

McKinnell, RG, BIOLOGICAL BASIS OF CANCER, Cambridge, NY 1998

Meyskens, FL, and Prasad, KN, MODULATION AND MEDIATION OF CANCER BY VITAMINS, S. Karger Publ., Basel, Switzerland, 1983, ISBN 3-8055-3526-0

Moss, RW, ANTIOXIDANTS AGAINST CANCER, Equinox, Brooklyn, 2000

Murray, Michael et al. (2002) HOW TO PREVENT AND TREAT CANCER WITH NATURAL MEDICINE. Riverhead Books.

National Academy of Sciences, DIET, NUTRITION, AND CANCER, National Academy Press (ph.800-624-6242), 1982, ISBN 0-309-03280-

Papas, AM, ANTIOXIDANT STATUS, DIET, CRC, Boca Raton, FL, 1999
Poirier, LA, et al., ESSENTIAL NUTRIENTS IN CARCINOGENESIS, Plenum Press, NY, 1986; ISBN 0-306-42471-1
Prasad, KN, and Meyskens, ML, NUTRIENTS AND CANCER PREVENTION, Humana Press, Clifton, NJ, 1990, ISBN 0-89603-171-3
Prasad, KN, VITAMINS AGAINST CANCER, Healing Arts Press, Rochester, VT, 1984, ISBN 0-89281-294
Quillin, P and Williams, RM (eds), ADJUVANT NUTRITION IN CANCER TREATMENT, Cancer Treatment Research Found, Arlington Heights, IL, 1994
Simone, CB, CANCER AND NUTRITION, Avery Publ., Garden City, NY, 1992
Stoff, Jesse (2000) THE PROSTATE MIRACLE. Kensington. Tarcher/Putnam.
U.S. Dept. Health & Human Services, SURGEON GENERAL'S REPORT ON NUTRITION AND HEALTH, U.S. Government Printing (ph. 800-336-4797), 1988
Werbach, MR, NUTRITIONAL INFLUENCES ON ILLNESS, Third Line Press, Tarzana, CA, 1996, ISBN 0-9618550-5-3
Yance, D. R. (1999). HERBAL MEDICINE, HEALING & CANCER. New Canaan,

GOOD NUTRITION REFERENCES:
Anderson, WELLNESS MEDICINE, Keats, 1987
Balch, James F., and Balch, Phyllis A. (1997). PRESCRIPTION FOR NUTRITIONAL HEALING (2nd ed.). Garden City Park, NY: Avery.
Burton Goldberg Group (Eds.). (1993). ALTERNATIVE MEDICINE.
Duke, James A. (1992). HANDBOOK OF BIOLOGICALLY ACTIVE PHYTOCHEMICALS. Boca Raton, FL: CRC Press.
Eaton, PALEOLITHIC PRESCRIPTION, Harper & Row, 1988
Fallon, Sally (2001). NOURISHING TRADITIONS (2nd ed.).
Golan, R., OPTIMAL WELLNESS, Ballantine, NY 1995
Haas, STAYING HEALTHY WITH NUTRITION, Celestial, 1992
Hendler, DOCTOR'S VIT AND MIN ENCYCLOPEDIA, Simon & Schuster,1990
Hendler, PDR FOR NUTRITIONAL SUPPLEMENTS, Medical Economics, 2001
Lieberman, S. et al., REAL VITAMIN & MINERAL BOOK, Avery, 1990
Life Extension, DISEASE PREVENTION & TREATMENT, Life Extension 2003
Lininger, S., et al., THE NATURAL PHARMACY, Prima, Rocklin, CA 1998
Marion, Joseph B. (2003). ANTI-AGING MANUAL: THE ENCYCLOPEDIA OF NATURAL HEALTH (3rd ed.). South Woodstock, CT.
Murray, M, et al., ENCYCLOPEDIA OF NATURAL MEDICINE, Prima, 1990
National Research Council, RECOMMENDED DIETARY ALLOWANCES, Nat Academy, 1989
Price, NUTRITION AND PHYSICAL DEGENERATION, Keats, 1989
Quillin, P., HEALING NUTRIENTS, Random House, 1987
Ronzio, RA, ENCYCLOPEDIA NUTRITION & HEALTH, Facts, NY 1997
Shils, ME, et al., MODERN NUTRITION, Lea & Febiger, 1994
Werbach, M, NUTRITIONAL INFLUENCES ON ILLNESS, Third Line, 1997

COMPREHENSIVE CANCER TREATMENT

ZIP CODE, NAME, CREDENTIALS, ADDRESS, CITY, STATE, PHONE

04410 Moshe Myerowitz, DC, CCN, 1570 Broadway,Bangor, ME 04401; 800-649-2873

08648 Charles Simone MD, 123 Franklin Corner Rd, Lawrenceville, NJ 609-896-2646

10021 Nicholas Gonzalez, MD, 737 Park Ave., NY, NY 212-535-3993

10901 Michael Schachter,MD, Suffern, NY, 845-368-4700, www.mbschachter.com

11203 John Casey, MD,142 E. 56th St.,Brooklyn, NY; 718-498-5010

11576 Thomas Lodi, MD, 55 Lumber Rd.,Roslyn, NY, 800-246-8730

12572 Ken Bock, MD, 108 Montgomery St., Rhinebeck, NY 914-876-7082

28031 Rashid Buttar, DO, 20721 Torrence Chapel Rd, Cornelius, NC ph 704-895-9355

30342 Stephen Edelson MD, 3833 Roswell Rd #110, Atlanta, GA 404-841-0088

33133 Victor Marcial-Vega MD, 4037 Poinciana Av, Coconut Grove,FL 305-442-1233

33160 Martin Dayton, MD, 18600 Collins Ave., Sunny Isles Beach, FL ph 305-931-8484

38834 Arnold Smith, MD, 1401 River Rd.,Greenwood, MS 38930; ph.800-720-8933

48103 James Arond-Thomas, MD, 220 Collingwood St., Ann Arbor, MI 734-995-4999

60008 Jack Taylor DC, 3601 Algonquin Rd, #801, Rolling Meadows, IL 847-222-1192

60099 Midwest Regional Med Ctr, 2501 Emmaus Ave., Zion, IL 60099; 800-322-9183,

60201 Keith Block MD, 1800 Sherman Ave, #515, Evanston, IL 847-492-3040, fax 3045,

67219 Ron Hunninghake, MD,Ctr Human,3100 N. Hillside,Wichita, KS ; 316-682-3100

74133 Southwest Med Ctr,10109 E. 79th St.,Tulsa, OK 800-577-1255 cancercenter.com

77082 Stan Burzynski MD, PhD,Houston, TX,713-335-5697,www.cancermed.com

80246 Jack Taylor DC, CCN, 4803 E Kentucky Ave. #217, Denver, CO, 727-418-0218,

80303 Robert Rountree MD, 4150 Darley Ave, #1, Boulder, CO 303-499-9224

85032 Christian Issels, ND,13832 N. 32nd St.#126, Phoenix, AZ,602-493-2273, fax –2159,

89502 James Forsythe MD, 75 Pringle Way, #909, Reno, NV 702-826-9500

89502 John Diamond MD, 4600 Kietzke Ln, M-242, Reno, NV 702-829-2277

89509 Douglas Brodie MD,6110 Plumas #B, Reno, NV, 775-829-1009 www.drbrodie.com

89511 Phillip Minton, MD, 521 Hammill Ln, Reno, NV 775-324-5700

91724 James Privitera,MD, NutriScreen, 256 W. San Bernardino Rd., Covina, CA

91902 Geronimo Rubio MD, Bonita, CA 619-267-1107, www.ami-health.com

91935 David Getoff, CCN, Box 803, Jamul, CA , ph. 619-468-6846

92024 Mark LaBeau,DO, Ctr Med,4403 Manchester.#107,Encinitas,CA, 760-632-9042

92075 Vincent Gammill ScD,ND,Natural Oncology, Solana Beach CA,858-523-9144,

92143 Bio-Medical Ctr (Hoxsey Clinic), Box 433654, San Ysidro CA, 52-6-684-9011

92143 Ernesto Contreras MD, P.O. Box 43-9045, San Ysidro, CA 800-700-1850

92153 Francisco Contreras,MD, Oasis Hosp, Box 530478, San Diego, CA, 619-690-8400

92154 Geronimo Rubio MD, 555 Saturn Blvd,Bld B, San Diego,CA 619-267-1107

92648 Dr. Fereshteh Akbarpour,18800 Delaware St,Huntington Beach, CA 714-842-1777

95060 Michael Tierra OMD,912 Cente, Santa Cruz,CA, 831-429-8066

97209 Tori Hudson ND, 2067 NW Lovejoy, Portland, OR 503-222-2322

97214 Martin Milner ND, 1330 SE 39th Ave, Portland, OR 503-232-1100

98004 Dietrich Klinghardt MD, 1200 112th Ave.NE #A-100, Bellevue WA, 425-688-8818,

98112 Cancer Treat Ctr,122 16th Avenue E,Seattle, WA 800-577-1255 cancercenter.com

WIN1AA Etienne Callebout MD, 10 Harley St., London ENGLAND 44-207-255-2232

AUSTRALIA Ruth Cilento, MD 1 Trackson St., Alderly, Brisbane 4051; ph. 07-352-6634

V5S4C6 Jim Chan ND, Vancouver,CANADA 604-435-3786, www.drjimchan.com

V8T4E5 Abram Hoffer MD, Victoria, BC CANADA 250-386-8756,orthomolecular.org

BAHAMAS ITL Cancer Clinic, Freeport, Grand Bahama, 242-352-7455, www.iatclinic.com

MEXICO RodriguezMD, Intl BioCare Hosp, 52-664-681-31-71 www.ibchospital.com

MEXICO Filiberto Muñoz, MD,San Diego Clinic,52-66-46-83-13-98, wwwsdiegoclinic.com

MEXICO Frank J Morales, MD, 956-592-5586; fax 544-4439, frankstaf@hotmail.com

GERMANY Wolfgang Woeppel, MD, Hufeland Kiinik, 49-7931-5360, www.hufeland.com

GERMANY Friedrich Douwes, MD, Bad Aibling, 49(0)8061-398-0, klinik-st-georg.de

ENGLAND Fritz Schellander, MD, Tunbridge Wells, Kent TN4 9LT, 01892 543535,

DOCTORS USING NUTRITION AS PART OF MEDICAL PRACTICE

01060, Barry D. Elson, MD, 295 Pleasant Street, Northampton, MA, ph 413-584-7787
01583, N. Thomas La Cava, MD, 360 West Boylston St., #107, West Boylston, MA, ph 508-854-1380
01701, Carol S. Englender, MD, 160 Speen Street #203, Framingham, MA, ph 508-875-0875
01742, Janet Beaty, ND, 56 Winthrop St., Concord, MA, ph 978-287-5352
01824, Tara Greaves, ND, 6 Courthouse Lane, Ste. 16, Chelmsford, MA, ph 978-452-4512
01844, Paul Giordano, DC, ND, 460 Broadway, Rt. 28, Methuen, MA, ph 978-688-7100
02134, Ruben Oganesov, MD, APCT, 39 Brighton Ave., Boston, MA, ph 617-783=5783
02140, Guy Pugh, MD, BPCT, 2500 Massachusetts Ave., Cambridge, MA, ph 617-661-6225
02148, George Milowe, MD, APCT, 11 Bickford Road, Malden, MA, ph 781-397-7408
02210, Earl Robert Parson, MD, 495 Summer Street, Boston, MA, ph 617-753-3113
02421, James Belander, ND, 442 Marrett Rd., Ste. 8, Lexington, MA, ph 781-274-6190
02459, Martha Stark, MD, 3 Ripley Street, Newton Centre, MA, ph 612-244-7188
02460, Jeanne T. Hubbuch, MD, 288 Walnut, Ste. 420, Newton, MA, ph 617-965-7770
02474, Glenn Rothfeld, MD, 180 Massachusetts Ave., #303, Arlington, MA, ph 781-641-1901
02474, Michael Janson, MD, FACAM, 180 Massachusetts Ave., Arlington, MA, ph 617-547-0295
02493, Barry Taylor, 270 Winter St., Weston, MA, ph 781-237-8505
02631, Lorraine Hurley, MD, 210 Griffith's Pond Rd., Brewster, MA, ph 508-896-1142
02664, Kimberlee Allen, PA-C, CNN, 23 H. White's Path, S. Yarmouth, ME, ph 508-760-2423
02720, Paul Giordano, DC, ND, 101 President Ave., Fall River, MA, ph 508-324-9999
02828, Zofia Laszewski, MD, 3 W. Prospect St., Greenville, RI, ph 401-949-2334
02840, Dariusz J. Nasiek, MD, 17 Friendship Street, Newport, RI, ph 401-846-1230
02906, Sheila Frodermann, ND, MA, 144 Waterman St., Providence, RI, ph 401-455-0546
03031, Michael Janson, MD, FACAM, 1 Overlook Drive, Ste. 11, Amherst, NH, ph 603-673-7910
03079, Luke Huber, ND, 53 Stiles Road, Ste. 101, Salem, NH, ph 603-890-9900
03264, David Olarsch, ND, 572 Tenney Mountain Hwy., Plymouth, NH, ph 603-536-4888
03801, Ian Bier, ND, Ph.D., Lac, 44-46 Bridge St., Portsmouth, NH, ph 603-430-7600
03801, James D'Adamo, ND, DC, 44-46 Bridge St., Portsmouth, NH, ph 603-430-7600
03801, Leon Hecht III, ND, BS, 500 Mark St., Ste. 1F, Portsmouth, NH, ph 603-427-6800
03894, Stephen Clark, ND, 376 N. Main St., Wolfeboro, NH, ph 603-569-6318
03903, Dayton Haigney, MD, 46 Dow Hwy, Eliot, ME, ph 207-439-1046
04032, Merrit Armstrong, DC, 30 Bow Street, Freeport, ME, ph 207-865-3649
04039, Raymond Psonak, DO, 51 West Gray Rd., #1A, Gray, ME, ph 207-657-4325
04043, Teresa A. Caprio, DO, 68 Main Street, Ste. 1, Kennebunk, ME, ph 207-985-1806
04096, David Markowitz, 3 Marine Rd., Yarmouth, ME, ph 207-846-6163
04096, Dixie Mills, MD, 3 Marina Rd., Yarmouth, ME, ph 207-846-6163
04101, Alan N. Weiner, DO, CCN, Four Milk Street, Portland, ME, ph 207-828-8080
04101, Devra M. Krassner, ND, 4 Milk Street, Portland, ME, ph 207-773-2517
04103, Christopher Maloney, ND, 796 Forest Ave., Portland, ME, ph 207-712-0725
04106, Priscilla Skerry, ND, PA, 260 Western Ave., South Portland, ME, ph 207-772-5227
04401, Moshe Myerowitz, DC, CCN, 1570 Broadway, Bangor, ME, ph 207-947-3333
04769, Eva Shay, DO, 1 Second St., Presque Isle, ME, ph 207-764-6880
04769, Narayana M. Prasanna, MD, 181 Academy Street, Ste. 5, Presque Isle, ME, ph 207-760-8100
04901, Arthur Weisser, Do, APCT, 81 Grove Street, Waterville, ME, ph 207-873-7721
05055, Susan Kowalsky, ND, 16 Beaver Meadow Road, Norwich, VT, ph 802-649-1064
05255, Kathleen Audette, ND, 185 North St., Bennington, VT, ph 802-442-7000
05446, Charles Anderson, MD, 65 Creek Farm Road #7, Colchester, VT, ph 802-879-6544
05482, Lorilee Schoenbeck, ND, 33 Harbor Road, Schelburne, VT, ph 802-985-8250
05482, William Warnock, ND, 33 Harbor Rd., Schelburne, VT, ph 802-985-8250
05534, Todd McGillick, DC, 311 5th Street, Gaylord, MN, ph 507-237-2454
05602, Donna Caplan, ND, 172 Berlin St., Montpelier, VT, ph 802-229-2635
05753, Karen Miller-Lane, ND, Lac, 50 Court St., Middleburg, VT, ph 802-989-9068
05851, Kathleen Meeker, ND, 1545 Darling Hill Road, Lyndonville, VT, ph 802-274-0808

06001, Mitchell Kennedy, ND, P.O. Box 778, Avon, CT, ph 860-673-9954
06015, Richard Duenas, DC, 557 Prospect Ave., W. Hartford, CT, ph 860-523-5833
06040, Stephen T. Sinatra, MD, FACC, 483 West Middle Tpke, Manchester, CT, ph 860-643-5101
06105, Mary Guerrera, MD, ABHM, 99 Woodland St., Hartford, CT, ph 860-714-6520
06119, Sharon Hunter, ND, 777 Farmington Ave., West Hartford, CT, ph 860-232-0000
06250, Fran Storch, ND, 203 Storrs Rd., Munsfield Center, CT, ph 860-423-2759
06340, Jordan Goetz, MD, ABHM, 1057 Poquonnock Rd., Groton, CT, ph 860-445-2130
06430, K. Vishvanath, ND, LCEH, PA, 2324 Post Rd., Fairfield, CT, ph 203-259-2700
06437, Jeffrey Klass, ND, 5 Durham Road Bldg. 2, Ste. B6, Gilford, CT, ph 203-453-1906
06443, Robert Lang, MD, PC, 11 Woodland Road, Madison, CT, ph 203-318-5200
06447, Mark Breiner, DDS, 325 Post Rd. #3A, Orange, CT, ph 203-799-8353
06457, Gregory Shields, MD, ABHM, 90 S. Main St., Middletown, CT, ph 860-358-3500
06470, Vicky Crouse, ND, 50 Deepbrook Rd., Newton, CT, ph 203-270-0830
06473, Ginger Nash, ND, 2 Washington Ave., North Haven, CT, ph 203-234-9780
06477, Robban A. Sica, MD, 370 Boston Post Road, Orange, CT, ph 203-799-7733
06518, Robert Lang, MD, PC, 60 Washington Ave., #105, Hamden, CT, ph 203-248-4362
06604, Sherry Stemper, ND, 2270 Park Ave., Bridgeport, CT, ph 203-579-4261
06610, Tadeusz A. Skowron, MD, 50 Ridgefield, Ave., #317, Bridgeport, CT, ph 203-368-1450
06615, Jennifer Brett, ND, 80 Ferry Blvd. Ste. 220, Stratford, CT, ph 203-377-1525
06702, Decio M. de Escobar, MD, 80 Phoenix Ave., Ste. 306, Waterbury, CT, ph 203-757-9336
06716, Paul M. DiDomizio, DC, 444 Wolcott Road, Wolcott, CN, ph 203-879-4695
06757, Bradford J. Harding, MD, ABHM, 64 Maple Street, Kent, CT, ph 860-927-1855
06776, Tamara M. Sachs, MD, 17 Poplar St., New Milford, CT, ph 860-350-6797
06783, Mary I. Miller, MD, FACP, ABHM, P.O. Box 312, Roxbury, CT, ph 203-262-6900
06790, Jerrold N. Finnie, MD, APCT, 333 Kennedy Dr., #204, Torrington, CT, ph 860-489-8977
06795, Ronald F. Schmid, ND, 48 Sperry Rd., Watertown, CT, ph 860-945-7444, www.DrRons.com
06820, Joel Evans, MD, ABHM, 1500 Boston Post Rd., Darien, CT, ph 203-656-6635
06820, Victoria Zupa, ND, 397 Post Rd., Darien, CT, ph 203-656-4300
06831, D. Barry Boyd, MD, FACP, 239 Glenville Rd., Greenwich, CT, ph 203-532-0600
06840, Richard Cooper, ND, 72 Park Street, Ste. 105, New Canaan, CT, ph 203-972-6800
06851, Marvin Schweitzer, ND, 1 Westport Ave., Norwalk, CT, ph 203-847-2788
06877, David L. Johnston, MD, ABHM, 40 Mallory Hill Rd., Ridgefield, CT, ph 203-438-9915
06877, George P. Zabrecky, MD, DC, 424a Main Street, Ridgefield, CT, ph 203-438-4762
06877, Marcie Wolinsky-Friedland, MD, 31 Bailey Avenue, Ridgefield, CT, ph 203-431-6165
06877, Mitchell Hubsher, DC, ND, 77 Chestnut Hill Rd., Ridgefield, CT, ph 203-431-3222
06883, Barry Kerner, MD, ABHM, 331 Goodhill Rd., Weston, CT, ph 203-222-5110
06890, Darin Ingels, ND, 2425 Post Road, Ste. 100, Southport, CT, ph 203-254-9957
06897, Warren Levin, MD, 13 Powderhorn Hill, Wilton, CT, ph 203-834-1174
06902, Alan R. Cohen, MD, BPCT, 80 Mill River St., #2200, Stamford, CT, ph 203-363-1547
06905, Henry C. Sobo, MD, 111 High Ridge Rd., Stamford, CT, ph 203-348-8805
06907, Andrea Gordon, MD, ABHM, 95 Columbus Place #3, Stamford, CT, ph 203-353-2154
07003, Richard L. Podkul, MD, 1064 Broad Street, Bloomfield, NJ, ph 973-893-0282
07009, Robert Steinfeld, MD, 912 Pompton Ave., Ste. 9B1, Cedar Grove, NJ, ph 973-571-0572
07029, Norma Migoyo, MD, P.O. Box 512, Harrison, NJ, ph 201-991-5522
07041, Daniel Zacharias, MD, BPCT, 68 Essex Street, Millburn, NJ, ph 973-912-0006
07041, Sharda Sharma, MD, 131 Millburn Ave., Millburn, NJ, ph 973-376-4500
07050, Shashi Agarwal, MD, 290 Central Ave., Orange, NJ, ph 973-676-1234
07087, Simon Santos, MD, 410 – 36th Street, Union City, NJ, ph 201-863-7744
07092, Albert Rose, DC, 615 Sherwood Parkway, Mountainside, NJ, ph 908-233-4774
07095, David M. Strassberg, MD, 1 Woodbridge Center, #245, Woodbridge, NJ, ph 732-855-7700
07103, Stephen Holt, MD, APCT, 105 Lock Street, Ste. 405, Newark, NJ, ph 973-824-8800
07105, Herbert Smyczek, MD, 132 Van Buren St., Newark, NJ, ph 973-690-5513
07202, Gennaro Locurcio, MD, BPCT, 610 Third Ave., Elizabeth, NJ, ph 908-351-1333
07204, Yulius Poplyansky, MD, BPCT, 236 E. Westfield Ave., Roselle Park, NJ, ph 908-241-3800
07410, Anthony M. Giliberti, DO, 14-01 Broadway, Fair Lawn, NJ, ph 201-797-8534
07417, Stuart Weg, MD, BPCT, 498 Island Way, Franklin Lakes, NJ, ph 201-447-5558
07423, Irene Catania, ND, 119 First Street, Ho-Ho-Kus, NJ, ph 201-444-4900
07424, Nancy Lentine, DO, 96 E. Main Street, Little Falls, NJ, ph 973-237-0700

07450, Arie Rave, MD, BPCT, 1250 E. Ridgewood Ave., Ridgewood, NJ, ph 201-689-1900
07450, Kenneth Y. Davis, DC, PC, 60 West Ridgewood Ave., Ridgewood, NJ, ph 201-652-2554
07601, Robin Leder, MD DPL, 235 Prospect Ave., Hackensack, NJ, ph 201-525-1155
07601, Robin Leder, MD, APCT, 235 Prospect Ave., Hackensack, NJ, ph 201-525-1155
07628, Jack Larmer, ND, 34 Bussell Court, Dumont, NJ, ph 201-385-7106
07631, Center for Nutrition & Preventative Medicine, 66 N. Van Brunt St., Englewood, NJ
07631, Gary Klingsberg, DO, APCT, 66 North Van Brunt St., Englewood, NJ, ph 201-503-0007
07652, Thomas A. Cacciola, MD, BPCT, 403 Farview Ave., Paramus, NJ, ph 201-261-8386
07702, Neil Rosen, DO, 555 Shrewsbury Ave., Shrewsbury, NJ, ph 732-219-0894
07712, Robert H. Sorge, ND, Ph.D., 208 Third Ave., Asbury Park, NJ, ph 732-775-7575
07748, David Dornfeld, DO, 18 Leonardville Rd., Middletown, NJ, ph 732-671-3730
07823, M. G. Reddy, MD, 234 Greenwich St., Belvedere, NJ, ph 908-475-2391
07834, Majid Ali, 95 E. Main St., #101, Denville, NJ, ph 973-586-4111
07960, Esra S. Onat, MD, 26 Madison Ave., Morristown, NJ, ph 973-889-0200
07960, Faina Munits, MD, 4 Boxwood Drive, Morristown, NJ, ph 973-292-3222
08003, Allan Magaziner, DO, APCT, 1907 Greentree Rd., Cherry Hill, NJ, ph 856-424-8222
08003, Scott R. Greenberg, MD, BPCT, 1907 Greentree Rd., Cherry Hill, NJ, ph 856-424-8222
08033, Roberta Morgan, DO, BPCT, 124 Kings Highway West, Haddonfield, NJ, ph 856-216-9001
08050, Mark J. Bartiss, MD, BPCT, 24 Nautilus Drive, #5, Manahawkin, NJ, ph 609-978-9002
08053, Debrah Harding, ND, 16 N. Maple Ave., Marlton, NJ, ph 609-970-2240
08053, Vivienne Matalon, MD, 230 N. Maple Ave., Crispin Square, Marlton, NJ, ph 856-985-0590
08109, Jennifer Phillips, ND, 41 West Chestnut Ave., Merchantville, NJ, ph 856-488-7067
08203, Michael J. Dunn, MD, 1311 East Shore Drive, Brigantine, NJ, ph 609-266-0400
08215, Perry Ricci, DC, 5734 Pleasant Mills Road, Egg Harbor City, NJ, ph 609-965-4404
08225, Barry D. Glasser, MD, 1907 New Road, Northfield, NJ, ph 609-646-9600
08260, John G. Costino, DO, 404 Surf Avenue, North Wildwood, NJ, ph 609-522-8358
08332, Charles Mintz, MD, 10 E. Broad Street, Millville, NJ, ph 609-825-7372
08559, Stuart H. Freedenfeld, MD, 56 S. Main St., #A, Stockton, NJ, ph 609-397-8585
08619, Robert J. Peterson, DO, 2239 Whitehorse-Mercerville Rd., #4, Trenton, NJ, ph 215-579-0330
08648, Charles Simone, MD, 123 Franklin Corner Rd., Lawrenceville, NJ, ph 609-896-2646
08690, Imtiaz Ahmad, MD, 1760 Whitehorse Hamilton Sq. Rd., #5, Trenton, NJ, ph 609-890-2966
08701, Gloria Freundlich, DO, 12 Hope Chapel Road, Lakewood, NJ, ph 732-961-9217
08816, James Lynch, Jr., MD, 150 Tices Lane, East Brunswick, NJ, ph 732-254-5553
08837, James A. Neubrander, MD, 15 South Main St., Ste. 6, Edison, NJ, ph 732-634-3666
08837, Richard B. Menashe, DO, 15 South Main St., Edison, NJ, ph 732-906-8866
08873, Marc Condren, MD, 7 Cedar Grove Lane, #20, Somerset, NJ, ph 908-469-2133
09170, Carol Rainville, ND, 8 Naples Road, Salem, MA, ph 617-699-0812
10002, Lawrence Young, MD, 19 Bowery Street, Rm. 1, New York, NY, ph 212-431-4343
10003, Jeffrey A. Morrison, MD, BPCT, 103 Fifth Ave., 6th Floor, New York, NY, ph 212-989-9828
10003, Sabina Barbara Ostolski, 200 Park Ave. S, Ste. 914, New York, NY, ph 212-253-5501
10011, Serafina Corsello, MD, 119 W. 23rd Street, Suite 400, New York, NY, ph 212-727-3600
10016, Eric R. Braverman, MD, APCT, 185 Madison Ave., 6th Fl., New York, NY, ph 212-213-6155
10016, Fred Pescatore, MD, BPCT, 274 Madison Ave., #402, New York, NY, ph 212-779-2944
10016, Gennaro Locurcio, MD, BPCT, 112 Lexington Ave., New York, NY, ph 212-696-2680
10016, Raymond Y. Chang, MD, FACP, 102 E. 30th St., New York, NY, ph 212-683-1221
10016, Ronald Hoffman, MD, FACAM, APCT, CNS, 40 E. 30th St., New York, NY, ph 212-779-1744
10019, Patrick Fratellone, MD, 24 West 57th Street, #701, New York, NY, ph 212-977-9870
1002, Thomas Bolte, MD, 141 East 55th St., #8H, New York, NY, ph 212-588-9314
10020, John P. Salerno, DO, One Rockerfeller Pl., #1401, New York, NY, ph 212-582-1700
10021, Claudia M. Cooke, MD, 133 East 73rd St., #506, New York, NY, ph 212-861-9000
10021, Richard N. Ash, MD, 800-A Fifth Ave. 61st St., New York, NY, ph 212-758-3200
10021, Wellington S. Tichenor, MD, 642 Park Ave., New York, NY, ph 212-517-6611
10022, Alexander N. Kulick, MD, 625 Madison Avenue, #10-A, New York, NY, ph 212-838-8265
10022, Cancer Research Institute, 681 Fifth Avenue, New York, NY, ph 800-992-2633
10022, Gary Ostrow, DO, 625 Madison Ave., #10-A, New York, NY, ph 212-838-8265
10023, Majid Ali, MD, 140 West End Ave., Ste. I-H, New York, NY, ph 212-873-2444
10028, Morton M. Teich, MD, 930 Park Ave., New York, NY, ph 212-988-1821
10032, Heather Greenlee, ND, MPH, 722 W. 168th St., 7th Fl., New York, NY, ph 212-342-4130

10312, Thomas K. Hand, DC, 3676 Richmond Avenue, Staten Island, NY, ph 718-984-5869

10459, Richard Izquierdo, MD, BPCT, 1070 Southern Blv., Lower Level, Bronx, NY, ph 718-589-4541

10509, Jeffrey C. Kopelson, MD, 221 Clock Tower Commons, Brewster, NY, ph 914-278-6800

10514, Savely Yurkovsky, MD, 37 King Street, Chappaqua, NY, ph 914-861-9161

10549, Neil C. Raff, MD, 213 Main Street, Mt. Kisco, NY, ph 914-241-7030

10708, Joseph S. Wojcik, MD, 525 Bronxville Rd., Ste. 1G, Bronxville, NY, ph 914-793-6161

10803, Erika Krauss, DO, 4662 Boston Post Rd., Pelham Manor, NY, ph 914-738-7100

10901, Michael B. Schachter, MD, 2 Executive Blvd., #202, Suffern, NY, ph 845-368-4700

10941, Levi H. Lehv, MD, 825 Rt. 211 East, Middletown, NY, ph 914-692-8338

10956, Arthur Landau, MD, BPCT, 10 Esquire Road, New City, NY, ph 845-638-4464

10962, Neil L. Block, MD, 14 Prel Plaza, Orangeburg, NY, ph 914-359-3300

10964, Rima E. Laibow, MD, 348 Rt. 9 W, Palisades, NY, ph 845-680-0700

10968, Isadora Guggenheim, ND, MS, 105 Shad Row, Ste. 1B, Piermont, NY, ph 845-358-8385

10977, Evan Fleischmann, ND, 747 Chestnut Ridge Rd., #102, Chestnut Ridge, NY, ph 845-425-5233

11042, Maurice Cohen, MD, 2 ProHealth Plaza, Lake Success, NY, ph 516-608-2806

11203, John Casey, MD, 142 E. 56th St., Brooklyn, NY, ph 718-498-5010

11204, Pavel Yutsis, MD DPL, 6413 Bay Parkway, Brooklyn, NY, ph 718-621-0900

11215, Sabrina Ostolski, DO, 525 4th St., Brooklyn, NY, ph 718-832-1454

11218, Gloria W. Freunclich, DO, 575 Ocean Parkway, Brooklyn, NY, ph 718-437-4459

11234, Robert Weiner, MD, 2352 Ralph Ave., Brooklyn, NY, ph 718-251-0200

11235, Igor Ostrovsky, MD, 3120 Brighton 5th Street, #1-C, Brooklyn, NY, ph 718-934-1920

11377, Fira Nihamin, MD, 39 – 65 52nd Street, Woodside, NY, ph 718-429-0039

11414, Christopher Cimmino, DO, 157-05 Crossbay Blvd., Howard Beach, NY, ph 718-845-5252

11414, Delfino Crescenzo, MD, 161-50 92nd Street, Howard Beach, NY, ph 718-848-0425

11414, William Miller, DO, 157-95 Crossbay Blvd., Howard Beach, NY, ph 718-845-5252

11507, Steven Rachlin, MD, 927 Willis Avenue, Albertson, L.I., NY, ph 516-873-7773

11554, Kathryn Calabria, DO, BPCT, 30 Merrick Ave. #111, East Meadow, NY, ph 516-542-9090

11559, Mitchell Kurk, MD, APCT, 310 Broadway, Lawrence, NY, ph 516-239-5540

11566, Susan Groh, MD, 2916 Frankel Blvd., Merrick, NY, ph 516-867-5132

11733, Johnny Slade, MD, 100 North Country Rd., Setauket, NY, ph 631-941-3137

11733, William Flader, MD, 100 North Country Road, Setauket, NY, ph 631-941-3137

11803, Sharon Stills, ND, 641C Old Country Road, Plainview, NY, ph 516-935-1334

11901, Ashley Lewin, ND, CDN, 906 Pond View Rd., Riverhead, NY, ph 631-722-2246

12134, Ruben Oganesov, MD, 39 Brighton Ave., Allston, MA, ph 617-783-5783

12203, Steven Bock, MD, 10 McKown Road, #210, Albany, NY, ph 518-435-0082

12498, Karen Fuller, ND, 15 Pine Grove Street, Woodstock, NY, ph 845-679-5763

12572, Kenneth A. Bock, MD, 108 Montgomery St., Rhinebeck, NY, ph 845-876-7082

12572, Michael Compain, MD, 108 Montgomery St., Rinebeck, NY, ph 845-876-7082

12572, Steven Bock, MD, 108 Montgomery St., Rhinebeck, NY, ph 845-876-7082

12572, Thomas Francescott, ND, 6384 Mill Street, Rhinebeck, NY, ph 845-876-5556

12801, Andrew W. Garner, MD, APCT, 8 Harrison Avenue, Glens Falls, NY, ph 518-798-9401

13220, Sherry A. Rogers, MD, P.O. Box 2716, Syracuse, NY, ph 315-488-2856

13501, Margarita Schilling, MD, 2305 Genesee Street, Utica, NY, ph 315-797-3799

13501, Richard O'Brien, DO, 2305 Genesee Street, Utica, NY, ph 315-724-8888

13820, Richard Ucci, MD DPL, 521 Main St., Oneonta, NY, ph 607-432-8752

13850, Jeanette Kleger, ND, 400 Plaza Dr., Ste. D, Vestal, NY, ph 607-729-0591

13850, Kristin Stiles, ND, 400 Plaza Dr., Ste. D, Vestal, NY, ph 607-729-0591

14047, Robert F. Barnes, DO, BPCT, 7008 Erie Rd., Derby, NY, ph 716-679-3510

14075, Ronald P. Santasiero, MD, 5451 Southwestern Blvd., Hamburg, NY, ph 716-646-6075

14150, Marshall Lim, ND, MSOM, 4080 Delaware Ave., Tonawanda, NY, ph 716-873-8700

14150, Raffaella Marcantonio, ND, 4080 Delaware Ave., Tonawanda, NY, ph 716-873-8700

14150, William H. Stephan, MD, 4080 Delaware, Tonawanda, NY, ph 716-875-7399

14225, Kalpana Patele, MD, ABCT, 65 Wehrle Drive, Buffalo, NY, ph 716-833-2213

14301, Paul Cutler, MD, APCT, 652 Elmwood Ave., Niagara Falls, NY, ph 716-284-5140

14432, Bonnie Cronin, ND, Lac, 2 Coulter Rd., Clifton Spring, NY, ph 315-462-0390

14432, Les Moore, ND, MSOM, Lac, 2 Coulter Road, Clifton Springs, NY, ph 315-462-0390

14626, Paul Cutler, MD DPL, 1081 Long Pond Rd., Rochester, NY, ph 716-720-1980

14626, Paul Cutler, MD, APCT, 1081 Long Pond Rd., Rochester, NY, ph 716-284-5140

14850, Deanna Berman, ND, LM, 210 West State Street, Ithaca, NY, ph 607-227-0833

15017, Dennis Courtney, MD, 533 Washington Rd. #207, Bridgeville, PA, ph 412-221-5562

15061, Simmon L. Wilcox, MD, 3428 Brodhead Rd., Monaca, PA, ph 724-774-7745

15068, Louis K. Hauber, MD, 2533 Leechburg Rd., Lower Burell, PA, ph 724-334-0966

15220, Dominic A. Brandy, MD, 2275 Swallow Hill Road, #2400, Pittsburgh, PA, ph 412-429-1151

15237, David Goldstein, MD, 9401 McKnight Rd., #301-B, Pittsburgh, PA, ph 412-366-6780

15601, Ralph A. Miranda, MD, APCT, RD 12, Box 108, Greensburg, PA, ph 724-838-7632

15644, R. Christopher Monsour, MD, 70 Lincoln Way East, Jeannette, PA, ph 724-527-1511

15666, Mamduh El-Attrache, MD, 20 E. Main St., Mt. Pleasant, PA, ph 412-547-3576

15680, Louis K. Hauber, MD, BPCT, 2533 Leechburg Rd., Lower Burrell, PA, ph 724-334-0966

15857, Daniel Jones, DC, 129 North Michael Street, St. Mary's, PA, ph 814-834-3217

16051, Roy E. Kerry, MD, 160 East Portersville Road, Portersville, PA, ph 724-368-3558

16055, Donald Mantell, MD, 589 Ekastown Rd., Sarver, PA, ph 724-353-1100

16121, Robert D. Multari, DO, 2120 Likens Lane, #101, Farrell, PA, ph 412-981-3731

16125, Roy Kerry, MD, 17 Sixth Avenue, Greenville, PA, ph 724-588-2600

16335, Paul Peirsel, DPL, 505 Poplar St., Meadville, PA, ph 814-337-7429

16365, James Hickey, DDS, 33 Main Dr., Warren, PA, ph 814-726-4409

16915, Bruce M. Fink, DC, 303 S. Main Street, Coudersport, PA, ph 814-274-8486

17055, John M. Sullivan, MD, APCT, 1001 S. Markt St., #B, Mechanisburg, PA, ph 717-697-5050

17078, Adrian J. Hohenwarter, MD, 741 S. Grant Street, Palmyra, PA, ph 717-832-5993

17356, Frederic A. Osterberg, DC, 718 S. Main Street, Red Lion, PA, ph 717-244-8504

17545, Kenneth F. Lovell, DO, 76 Doe Run Rd., Manheim, PA, ph 717-665-6400

17701, Francis M. Powers, Jr., MD, 1201 Grampian Blvd., #3-A, Williamsport, PA, ph 570-322-6450

17837, George C. Miller II, MD, 3 Hospital Dr., Ste. 216, Lewisburg, PA, ph 570-524-4405

18013, Francis J. Cinelli, DO, 153 N. 11th Street, Bangor, PA, ph 610-588-4502

18018, Sally Ann Rex, DO, 1343 Easton Ave., Bethlehem, PA, ph 610-866-0900

18201, Martin Mulders, MD, 53 West Juniper Street, Hazelton, PA, ph 570-455-4704

18335, Michael Loquasto, DC, P.O. Box 1187, Marshallis Creek, PA, ph 717-223-0140

18505, Kyung Lee, MD, BPCT, 1027 Pittston Ave., Scranton, PA, ph 570-961-0200

18509, Blanche Grube, DMD, 801 Green Ridge St., Scranton, PA, ph 570-343-1500

18901, Steven C. Halbert, MD, APCT, 52 East Oakland Ave., Doylestown, PA, ph 215-348-4002

18923, Harold H. Byer, MD, Ph.D., 5045 Swamp Rd., #A-101, Fountainville, PA, ph 215-348-0443

18940, Robert J. Peterson, DO, 1614 Wrightstown Rd., Newtown, PA, ph 215-579-0330

18951, Denise C. Kelley, MD, 5724 Clymer Road, Quakertown, PA, ph 215-536-1890

18951, Harold E. Buttram, MD, 5724 Clymer Road, Quakertown, PA, ph 215-536-1890

18951, William G. Kracht, DO, BPCT, 5724 Clymer Rd., Quakertown, PA, ph 215-536-1890

18954, John La Hoda, DC, 130 Almshouse Road, Ste. 502, Richboro, PA, ph 215-364-0364

18954, Michael DiPalma, ND, 778 Second Street Pike, Richboro, PA, ph 215-942-2850

19004, Howard Posner, MD, aaa Bala Ave., Bala Cynwyd, PA, ph 610-667-2927, www.docposner.com

19023, Lance Wright, MD, 112 S. 4th Street, Darby, PA, ph 610-461-6225

19047, Eric R. Braverman, MD, APCT, 142 Bellevue Ave., Penndel, PA, ph 215-702-1344

19053, Robert J. Peterson, DO, 4616 Street Road, Trevose, PA, ph 215-579-0330

19063, Arthur K. Balin, MD, Ph.D., FACP, 110 Chesley Dr., Media, PA, ph 610-565-3300

19064, Walter W. Schwartz, DO, 471 Baltimore Pike, Springfield, PA, ph 610-604-4800

19072, Andrew Lipton, DO, APCT, 822 Montgomery Ave., #315, Narberth, PA, ph 610-667-4601

19083, Domenick Braccia, DO, 2050 West Chester Pike, Havertown, PA, ph 610-924-0627

19095, Steven C. Halbert, MD, APCT, 1442 Ashbourne Rd., Wyncote, PA, ph 215-886-7842

19104, Patrick J. Lariccia, MD, 51 N. 39th Street, Philadelphia, PA, ph 215-662-8988

19138, John Bowden, DO, 1738 W. Cheltenham, Philadelphia, PA, ph 215-548-3390

19147, Alan F. Kwon, MD, 211 South Street, #345, Philadelphia, PA, ph 215-629-5633

19147, Sarah M. Fisher, MD, BPCT, 530 South 2nd St., #108, Philadelphia, PA, ph 215-627-3001

19151, K. R. Sampathachar, MD, 6366 Sherwood Rd., Philadelphia, PA, ph 215-473-4226

19151, P. Jayalakshmi, MD, 6366 Sherwood Rd., Philadelphia, PA, ph 215-473-4226

19342, Robert J. Peterson, DO, 2 Woodland Drive, Glen Mills, PA, ph 610-558-8225

19403, Anthony J. Bazzan, MD, BPCT, 2505 Blvd. Of Generals, Jeffersonville, PA, ph 610-630-8600

19403, Journeal Alexandre, MD, 1701 Pheasant Ln., Norristown, PA, ph 610-272-1686

19403, Martin Mulders, MD, 2505 Blvd. Of the Generals, Jeffersonville, PA, ph 610-630-8600

19454, Domenick Braccia, DO, BPCT, 1146 Stump Road, North Wales, PA, ph 215-368-2160

19562, Conrad G. Maulfair, Jr., DO, 403 N. Main Street, Topton, PA, ph 800-733-4065
19713, Gerald Lemole, MD, 4745 Ogletown-Stanton Rd., #205, Newark, DE, ph 302-738-0448
19720, Jeffrey K. Kerner, DO, BPCT, 200 Bassett Ave., New Castle, DE, ph 302-328-0669
20006, Stephanie Becker, ND, 900 19ᵗʰ St. NW, Ste. 250, Washington, DC, ph 202-457-8282
20008, George H. Mitchell, MD, 2639 Connecticut Ave. NW, Washington, DC, ph 202-264-4111
20015, Aldo M. Rosemblat, MD, 5225 Wisconsin Ave. NW, #401, Washington, DC, ph 202-237-7000
20015, Barbara A. Solomon, MD, 5225 Wisconsin Ave., Washington, DC, ph 202-237-7000
20015, Bruce Rind, MD, 5225 Wisconsin Ave. NW, 4ᵗʰ Fl., Washington, DC, 20015, ph 202-237-7000
20016, Ali Safayan, MD, 4801 Wisconsin Ave. NW, Washington, DC, ph 301-816-0500
20017, Mahlon Davis, ND, 1409 Lawrence St. NE, Washington, DC, ph 202-497-9113
20170, Karen Threlkel, ND, 429A Carlisle Dr., Herndon, VA, ph 703-481-6004
20707, Ahmad Shamin, MD, Steward Towers, 200 Ft. Meade Rd., Laurel, MD, ph 301-776-3700
20708, Paul V. Beals, MD, BPCT, 9101 Cherry Lane Park, Ste. 205, Laurel, MD, ph 301-490-9911
20770, Frank Mclograna, MD, 7755 Belle Point Drive, Greenbelt, MD, ph 301-474-3636
20817, Ali Safayan, MD, 5602 Shields Drive, Bethesda, MD, ph 301-897-8090
20850, Norton Fishman, MD, CNS, 15235 Shady Grove Rd., #102, Rockville, MD, ph 301-330-9430
20852, L. J. Leo, 6321 Executive Blvd., Rockville, MD, ph 301-770-6650
20878, Alan R. Vinitsky, MD, 902 Wind River Lane, Ste. 201, Gaithersburg, MD, ph 301-840-0002
21017, Philip W. Halstead, MD, 1200 Brass Mill Road, Belcamp, MD, ph 410-272-7751
21093, Elisabeth Lucas, MD, 1205 York Road, Ste. 30A, Lutherville, MD, ph 410-823-3101
21093, Kenneth B. Singleton, MD, 2328 W. Joppa Rd., #310, Lutherville, MD, ph 410-296-3737
21209, Binyamin Rothstein, DO, APCT, 2835 Smith Ave., #203, Baltimore, MD, ph 410-484-2121
21286, Paul Faust, ND, 521 E. Joppa Rd., Ste. 205, Towson, MD, ph 410-821-1788
21401, Jacob E. Teitelbaum, MD, 466 Forelands Road, Annapolis, MD, ph 410-573-5389
21401, Kevin Passero, ND, 528C College Parkway, Annapolis, MD, ph 410-349-9043
21401, Richard A. Bernstein, MD, 133 Defense Hwy. Ste. 109, Annapolis, MD, ph 410-224-5558
21401, Stephenie Becker, ND, 100 Annapolis St., Annapolis, MD, ph 410-626-0045
21620, Robert L. Henderson, MD, 100 Brown Street, Chestertown, MD, ph 410-788-5170
21666, Paul V. Beals, MD, BPCT, 133 Log Canoe Circle, Stevensville, MD, ph 410-604-6344
21702, Nicola Michael C. Tarauso, MD, 7051 Poole Jones Rd., Frederick, MD, ph 301-662-6726
22001, Norman Levin, MD DPL, P.O. Box 1013, Aldie, VA, ph 703-327-2434
22027, Robert Duca, DC, 2136-D Gallows Road, Dunn Loring, VA, ph 703-641-4966
22030, Karen Davis, ND, 10640 Main St., Ste 300, Fairfax, VA, ph 703-246-9355
22044, Aldo Rosemblat, MD DPL, 6316 Castle Place #200, Falls Church, VA, ph 703-241-8989
22201, Marie Schum-Brady, MD, 3500 N. 14ᵗʰ Street, Arlington, VA, ph 703-527-5384
22207, Denise Bruner, MD, 5015 Lee Highway #201, Arlington, VA, ph 703-558-4949
22312, Manjit R. Bajwa, MD, 6391 Little River Turnpike, Alexandria, VA, ph 703-941-3606
22314, Scott Muzinski, 300 S. Washington Street, #200, Alexandria, VA, ph 703-836-3901
22601, James B. Hutt, Jr., MD, 423 W. Cork Street, Winchester, VA, ph 540-347-0474
22831, Harold Huffman, MD, APCT, P.O. Box 197, Hinton, VA, ph 540-867-5254
22901, Suzanne A. Coffey, DC, 689 Berkmar Cr., Charlottesville, VA, ph 434-975-4434
22958, Mitchell A. Fleischer, MD, Rockfish Ctr, Ste. 1, Nellysford, VA, ph 434-361-1896
23005, Pamela Hannaman-Pittman, MD, 13074 Fairway Lane, Ashland, VA, ph 804-798-4133
23093, David G. Schwartz, MD, P.O. Box 532, Louisa, VA, ph 540-967-2050
23112, Theresa Collier, ND, 4905 Court Ridge Terrace, Midlothian, VA, ph 804-744-4927
23113, Kevin Harrison, DO, 2621 Promenade Parkway, Richmond, VA, ph 804-897-8566
23321, Ernest Aubrey Murden Jr., MD, 4020 Raintree Rd., #C, Chesapeake, VA, ph 757-488-9900
23462, Robert Nash, MD DPL, 5589 Greenwich Rd. #175, Virginia Beach, VA, ph 757-490-9311
23464, Lambert Parker, MD, 917 Dunhill Dr., Virginia Beach, VA, ph 757-963-2969
23507, Vincent Speckhart, MD, 902 Graydon Ave. #2, Norfolk, VA, ph 804-622-0014
23703, Emile S. Sayegh, MD, 3104 Garland Dr., Portsmouth, VA, ph 757-484-3710
24014, Joan M. Resk, DO, 5249 Clearbrook Lane, Roanoke, VA, ph 540-776-8331
24019, J. Michael Becker, DC, 6206 Peters Creek Road, Roanoke, VA, ph 540-563-0334
24378, Eduardo Castro, MD, 799 Ripshin Rd., Trout Dale, VA, ph 276-677-3631
24378, Elmer M. Cranton, MD, APCT, 799 Ripshin Road, Trout Dale, VA, ph 540-677-3631
24701, Albert J. Paine, MD, 2120 Mountain View Ave., Bluefield, WV, ph 304-325-9577
25301, Steve M. Zekan, MD, 1208 Kanawha Blvd. E, Charleston, WV, ph 304-343-7559
25309, William Joardan, DC, 4024 MacCorkle Ave. SW, S. Charleston, WV, ph 304-768-7671

25526, Dallas B. Martin, DO, BPCT, 1401 Hospital Dr., #302, Hurricane, WV, ph 304-757-8090
25526, John P. MacCallum, MD, 3855 Teays Valley Road, Hurricane, WV, ph 304-757-3368
25801, Prudencio Corro, MD, BPCT, 251 Stanaford Rd., Beckley, WV, ph 304-252-0775
26104, Byron Folwell, DC, 3211 Emerson Avenue, Parkersburg, WV, ph 304-485-9124
27103, Walter Ward, MD, PA, 1411 Plaza West Dr. #B, Winston-Salem, NC, ph 336-760-0240
27114, Todd A. Smith, DC, P.O. Box 24506, Winston-Salem, NC, ph 336-760-9355
27278, Dennis W. Fera, MD, BPCT, 1000 Corporate Dr., #209, Hillsborough, NC, ph 919-732-2287
27511, Sharon M. DeFrain, DC, 1363 SE Maynard Rd., Cary, NC, ph 919-467-5552
27603, John Pittman, MD DPL, 4505 Fair Meadow Ln. #111, Raleigh, NC, ph 919-571-4391
27606, Beverly Goode-Kanawati, DO, 6511 Creedmoor Road #101, Raleigh, NC, ph 919-844-4552
27607, Carolina Center for Integrative Medicine, 4505 Fair Meadow La Ste. 111, Raleigh, NC
27607, John C. Pittman, MD, APCT, 4505 Fair Meadow Lane, #111, Raleigh, NC, ph 919-571-4391
27607, Maurice Werness, ND, 4601 Lake Boone Trail, Ste. 2E, Raleigh, NC, ph 919-781-3978
27609, Thomas Spruill, MD, 3900 Browning Place, #201, Raleigh, NC, ph 919-787-7125
27704, Robert E. taylor, MD, 2609 N. Duke Street, Ste. 304, Durham, NC, ph 919-220-0691
27803, Lemuel Kornegay, MD, 500 Shady Circle, Rocky Mount, NC, ph 252-442-7017
27870, Bhaskar D. Power, MD, 1201 East Littleton Road, Roanoke Rapids, NC, ph 252-535-1411
28031, Rashid Ali Buttar, DO, 20721 Torrence Chapel, #101-102, Charlotte, NC, ph 704-895-9355
28083, James Litaker, DC, 206 N. Cannon Blvd., Kannapolis, NC, ph 704-933-2266
28105, Philip Amone, DC, 10610 Independence Pt Pkwy, Matthews, NC, ph 704-849-9393
2817, Anthony J. Castiglia, MD, BPCT, 570 Williamson Rd., Ste. C, Mooresville, NC, ph 704-799-9740
28207, F. Keels Dickson, MD, 2315 Randolph Road, Charlotte, NC, ph 704-366-7921
28207, Mark O'Neal Speight, MD, BPCT, 2317 Randolph Rd., Charlotte, NC, ph 704-334-8447
28207, Michael Stadtmauer, ND, 2040-B Randolph Rd., Charlotte, NC, ph 704-373-9976
28207, Neil Speight, MD, 2317 Randolf Road, Charlotte, NC, ph 704-334-8447
28226, Tyler Freeman, MD, 3135 Springbank Lane, #100, Charlotte, NC, ph 704-716-7979
28226, William Pierce, ND, 3135 Springbank La. #100B, Charlotte, NC 28226, ph 704-716-7979
28227, Dennis C. Schoen, DC, 8108 Idlewild Road, Ste. 200, Charlotte, NC, ph 704-568-8844
28374, Kenneth L. Vieregge II, DC, 5 Regional Cr. Suite C, Pinehurst, NC, ph 910-295-8157
28428, Keith E. Johnson, MD, 1009 N. Lake Park Blvd., Carolina Beach, NC, ph 910-695-0335
28557, Donald Brooks Reece II, MD, BPCT, #2 Medical Park, Morehead City, NC, ph 252-247-5177
28711, Laura K. Frey, DC, P.O. Box 1233, Black Mountain, NC, ph 828-669-8220
28732, Stephen W. Blievernicht, MD, BPCT, 242 Old Concord Rd., Fletcher, NC, ph 828-684-4411
28782, Connie G. Ross, MD, BPCT, 590 South Trade Street, Tryon, NC, ph 828-859-0420
28782, Mack Stuart Bonner Jr., MD, BPCT, 590 South Trade St., Tryon, NC, ph 828-859-0420
28801, Ronald R. Parks, MPH, MD, 245 B South French Broad Ave., Asheville, NC, ph 828-225-1812
28801, Salvatore D'Angio, MD, 25 Orange Street, Asheville, NC, ph 828-253-3140
28803, James Biddle, MD, APCT, 832 Hendersonville Rd., Asheville, NC, ph 828-252-5545
28804, John Davis, Ph.D., ND, 959 Merriman Ave., Ste. 8, Asheville, NC, ph 828-232-0701
28805, Ronald Parks, MD, 1070-1 Tunnel Rd., #252, Asheville, NC, ph 828-225-1812
28806, Eileen Wright, MD DPL, 1312 Patton Ave., Asheville, NC, ph 828-252-9833
28806, John L. Wilson, Jr., MD, APCT, 1312 Patton Ave., Asheville, NC, ph 828-252-9833
28906, Robert E. Moreland, MD, 75 Medical Park Lane, #C, Murphy, NC, ph 828-837-7997
29170, James M. Shortt, MD, BPCT, 3901 Edmund Hwy. #A, W. Columbia, SC, ph 803-755-0114
29356, Mitchell Ghen, DO, 1000 E. Rutherford Rd., Landrum, SC, ph 864-457-4141
29356, Theodore Rozema, MD DPL, 1000 E. Rutherford Rd., Landrum, SC, ph 864-457-4141
29403, Robert Pascal, DC, 119 Spring Street, Suite 4, Charleston, SC, ph 803-723-6475
29406, Arthur LaBruce, MD, 9231A Medical Plaza Dr. #A, Charleston, SC, ph 843-572-1771
29412, Peter W. Kfoury, DC, 13 Clamshell Row, Charleston, SC, ph 843-795-9333
29420, Allan D. Lieberman, MD, 7510 Northforest Dr., North Charleston, SC, ph 843-572-1600
29501, Jon Bergrin, DC, 1927A West Palmette Street, Florence, SC, ph 803-662-4341
29575, Sid Noor, MD, 4301 Hwy 544, Myrtle Beach, SC, ph 803-215-5000
29588, Donald Tice, DO, 4301 Highway 544, Myrtle Beach, SC, ph 803-215-5000
29687, Patricia S. Rowe, DC, 3575 Ritherford Rd. Ext. Ste C, Taylors, SC, ph 864-292-1961
29805, Bernard John Kule, 1847 Hatchaway Bridge Rd., Aiken, SC, ph 803-644-7033
29902, Kenneth Orbeck, DO, 9A Rue du Bois Rd., Beaufort, SC, ph 843-322-8050
30040, American Wellness Clinic, 104 Colony Park Dr., Ste. 800, Cumming, GA, ph 789-679-0632
30040, Rhett Bergeron, MD, 104 Colony Park Dr., Ste. 800, Cumming, GA, ph 789-679-0632

30045, Susan L. Tanner, MD, 44 South Clayton Street, Lawrenceville, GA, ph 770-277-8030
30060, Ralph C. Lee, MD, 110 Lewis Dr. #B, Marietta, GA, ph 770-423-0064
30060, Ralph Lee, MD, 110 Lewis Dr., Ste. B, Marietta, GA, ph 770-423-0064
30075, Marcia V. Byrd, MD, 11050 Crabapple Rd., #105-B, Roswell, GA, ph 770-587-1711
30076, Victoria Anderson, MD, 51 Creekline Dr., Roswell, GA, ph 770-641-6558
30080, Donald Ruesink, MD, 1004 Lincoln Trace Cir. SE, Smyrna, GA, ph 770-818-9908
30092, Cheryl Burdette, ND, 4711 Peachtree Industrial Blvd., Norcross, GA, ph 770-416-8180
30103, Donald Ruesink, MD, 6247 JFH. Pkwy., Adairsville, GA, ph 770-773-7700
30103, Joyce Cream, Phy.D., 6247 JAH Pkwy., Adarasville, GA, ph 770-773-7700
30114, William Early, MD, BPCT, 320 Hospital Rd., Canton, GA, ph 770-479-5535
30120, Claude R. Poliak, MD, APCT, 17 Bowens Court SE, Cartersville, GA, ph 770-607-0220
30281, Dan Bartoli, ND, ImmunoLife Wellness Clinic, Stockbridge, GA, ph 770-474-4029
30281, Michael Rowland, MD, 130 Eagle Springs Ct., Ste. A, Stockbridge, GA, ph 770-507-2930
30281, T. R. Shantha, MD, Ph.D., 115 Eagle Spring Dr., Stockbridge, GA, ph 770-474-4029
30327, William Richardson, MD, APCT, 3280 Howell Mill Rd., #205, Atlanta, GA, ph 404-350-9607
30329, John Davis, Ph.D., ND, 1610 La Vista Rd. #11, Atlanta, GA, ph 404-325-7734
30338, Ben Johnson, 4488 N. Shallowford Rd., #200, Atlanta, GA, ph 770-455-6100
30338, Donovan Christie, MD, 4514 Chamblee-Dunwoody Rd. #262, Atlanta, GA, ph 404-761-2766
30338, Susan E. Kolb, MD, 4370 Georgetown Square, Atlanta, GA, ph 770-390-0012
30342, M. Truett Bridges, Jr., MD, BPCT, 4920 Roswell Rd., #35, Atlanta, GA, ph 404-843-8880
30342, Stephen B. Edelson, MD, APCT, 3833 Roswell Rd., #110, Atlanta, GA, ph 404-841-0088
30360, Milton Fried, MD, APCT, 4426 Tilly Mill Road, Atlanta, GA, ph 770-451-4857
30501, John L. Givogre, MD, BPCT, 655 Jesse Jewell Pkwy., Ste. D, Gainesville, GA, ph 770-297-0356
30503, Kathryn Herndon, MD, 530 Spring St., Gainesville, GA, ph 770-503-7222
30534, Lance Brubaker, MD, 90 Chappell Rd., Dawsonville, GA, ph 706-265-7449
30534, Rhett Bergeron, MD, 90 Chappell Rd., Dawsonville, GA, ph 706-265-7449
30736, Robert Burkich, MD DPL, 148 Scruggs Rd., Ringgold, GA, ph 706-891-1200
30742, Charles C. Adams, MD, BPCT, 100 Thomas Rd., Fort Oglethorpe, GA, ph 706-861-7377
31204, James T. Alley, MD, 2518 Riverside Dr., Macon, GA, ph 478-745-3727
31520, Edward Kaszans, DC, 1613 Union St., Brunswick, GA, ph 912-264-1841
31525, Ralph G. Ellis, Jr., MD, APCT, 158 Sdranton Connector, Brunswick, GA, ph 912-280-0304
31792, John Mansberger, MD, 2705 E. Pinetree Blvd., Ste. C, Thomasville, GA, ph 229-228-7008
31794, Lora Efaw, MD, 1807 Old Ocilla Rd., Tifton< GA, ph 229-388-9393
31906, Jan McBarron, MD, 2904 Macon Rd., Columbus, GA, ph 706-322-4073
32117, John Ortolani, MD, 1430 Mason Ave., Daytona Beach, FL, ph 386-274-3601
32134, George Graves, DO, 11512 County Road 316, Ocala, FL, ph 352-236-2525
32159, Nelson Kraucak, MD, FAAFP, 1501 US Hwy 441 N., The Villages, FL, ph 352-750-4333
32169, William C Douglass III, MD, 2111 Ocean Dr., New Smyrna Beach, FL, ph 386-426-8803
32174, Hana Chaim, DO, 595 W. Granada Blvd. #D, Ormond Beach, FL, ph 386-672-9000
32216, Norman S. Cohen, MD, APCT, 4237 Salisbury Road, #110, Jacksonville, FL, ph 904-296-1116
32250, Stephen Grable, MD, 1504 Roberts Drive, Jacksonville, FL, ph 904-247-7455
32256, Linda A. Woodard, 9765 Southbrook Dr. #2114, Jacksonville, FL, ph 904-646-9348
32404, Samir M.A. Yassin, MD, 516 S. Tyndall Pkwy. #202, Panama City, FL, ph 850-763-0464
32405, James W. De Ruiter, MD, 2202 State Ave., #311, Panama City, FL, ph 850-747-4963
32405, Naima Abdel-Ghany, MD, Ph.D., 2424 B Frankford Ave., Panama City, FL, ph 850-872-8122
32504, R. W. Lucey, MD, 710 Underwood Ave., Pensacola, FL, ph 850-477-3453
32570, William N. Watson, MD, 5536 Stewart St., Milton, FL, ph 850-623-3836
32605, Robert A. Erickson, MD, 905 NW 56th Terrace #B, Gainesville, FL, ph 352-331-5138
32606, Hanoch Talmor, MD, 4140-C NW 27th Lane, Gainesville, FL, ph 352-377-0015
32646, Carlos F. Gonzalez, MD, 7989 S. Suncoast Blvd., Homosassa Springs, FL, ph 352-382-2900
32707, Donald Mayfield, ND, 5023 South Hwy 17-92, Casselberry, FL, ph 407-260-1269
32712, Allan Zubkin, MD, 424 N. Dpark Ave., Apopka, FL, ph 407-886-0611
32714, Kenneth S. Ross, DC, 908 Red Fox Road, Altamonte, FL, ph 407-682-6041
32714, Manuel Faria, DC, 195 S. Westmonte Dr., Ste H, Altamonte Springs, FL, ph 407-862-2287
32724, Jeremy M. Gordon, DC, 339 E. New York Ave., Deland, FL, ph 904-734-4490
32724, John Gaffney, DC, 339 E. New York Ave., Deland, FL, ph 904-734-4490
32746, Jeffrey Mueller, MD, BPCT, 635 Primera Blvd., #111, Lake Mary, FL, ph 407-833-3881
32757, Jack E. Young, MD, Ph.D., 2260 W. Old US Hwy 441, Mount Dora, FL, ph 352-385-4400

32763, Travis L. Herring, MD, MD(H), 106 West Fern Dr., Orange City, FL, ph 386-775-0525
32778, David Frerking, DC, 915 E. Alfred Street, Tavares, FL, ph 352-343-9275
32778, Nelson Kraucak, MD DPL, 204 N. Texas Ave., Tavares, FL, ph 352-742-1116
32779, Robert J. Rogers, MD, 2170 West State Rd. 434, #190, Orlando, FL, ph 407-682-5222
32784, Louis Radnothy, DO, 390 S. Central, Umatilla, FL, ph 352-669-3175
32789, Joya Lynn Schoen, MD, BPCT, 1850 Lee Road, Ste. 240, Winter Park, FL, ph 407-644-2729
32789, Joya Schoen, MD, 1850 Lee Rd., Winter Park, FL, ph 407-644-2729
32795, Diab Ashrap, MD, P.O. Box 951957, Lake Mary, FL, ph 407-805-9222
32819, Katherine Clements, ND, 6651 Vineland Rd., Ste. 150, Orlando, FL, ph 407-355-9246
32819, Kirti Kalidas, MD, 6651 Vineland Rd., #150, Orlando, FL, ph 407-355-9256
32901, Rajiv Chandra, MD, BPCT, 20 E. Melbourne Ave., #104, Melbourne, FL, ph 321-951-7404
32903, Glen Wagner, MD, BPCT, 121 – 6th Ave., Indialantic, FL, ph 407-723-5915
32935, Neil Abner, MD, APCT, 1270 N. Wickham Rd., Melbourne, FL, ph 321-253-2009
32937, Daniel B. Hammond, MD, 1413 South Patrick Dr., Indian Harbour Beach, FL, ph 321-777-9923
32953, Glenn R. Johnston, MD, 585 N. Courtney Pkwy., Merritt Island, FL, ph 321-454-4428
32958, Peter Holyk, MD, CNS, BPCT, 600 Schumann Dr., Sebastian, FL, ph 772-338-5554
33004, E. K. Schandl, Ph.D., Center for Metabolic Disorders, Box 1134, Dania, FL, ph 954-929-4814
33004, Sigmund Ringoen, DC, 308 SE 5th Str., Dania Bch, FL, ph 954-929-4883
33012, Francisco Mora, MD, 1490 West 48th Place, #398, Hialeah, FL, ph 305-820-6211
33020, Emile K. Schandl, Ph.D., 1818 Sheridan St., Ste. 102, Hollywood, FL, ph 954-929-4814
33021, Michelle Morrow, DO, 5821 Hollywood Blvd., Hollywood, FL, ph 954-436-6363
33065, Jerald H. Ratner, MD, 9750 NW 33rd St., #211, Coral Springs, FL, ph 954-752-9450
33071, Anthony J. Sancetta, DO, BPCT, 8217 W. Atlantic Blvd., Coral Springs, FL, ph 954-757-1211
33134, Victor A. Marcial-Vega, MD, 2916 Douglas Rd., Coral Gables, FL, ph 800-771-0255
33149, Sam Baxas, MD, 30 West Mashta Drive, Ste. 200, Key Biscayne, FL, ph 305-361-9249
33160, Martin Dayton, MD, 18600 Collins Ave., Sunny Isles Beach, FL, ph 305-931-8484
33162, Stefano DiMauro, MD, 16695 NE 10th Ave., N. Miami Beach, FL, ph 305-940-6474
33162, Wynne A. Steinsnyder, DO, 17291 NE 19th Ave., N. Miami Beach, FL, ph 305-947-0618
33165, Ivonne F. Torre-Coya, MD, 2580 SW 107th Ave., Miami, FL, ph 305-223-0132
33166, Angelique Hart, MD, 1 South Drive, Miami, FL, ph 305-882-1442
33169, Emmanuel Junard, DC, 18921 WW 2nd Ave., Suite B, Miami, FL, ph 305-770-0607
33176, Joseph G. Godorov, DO, 9055 SW 87th Ave., Ste. 307, Miami, FL, ph 305-595-0671
33317, Alvin Stein, MD, 4104 NW 4th St., #401, Plantation, FL, ph 954-581-8585
33317, Cristino C. Enriquez, MD, BPCT, 767 S. State Road 7, Fort Lauderdale, FL, ph 954-583-3773
33317, Kenneth N. Krischer, MD, Ph.D., 910 SW 40th Ave., Plantation, FL, ph 954-584-6655
33319, Herbert R. Slavin, MD, 7200 W. Commercial Blvd., Ste. 210, Lauderhill, FL, ph 954-748-4991
33321, George A. Lustig, MD, 7401 N. University Dr., #101, Tamarac, FL, ph 954-724-0090
33322, Adam Frent, DO, 1741 N. University Drive, Plantation, FL, ph 954-474-1617
33324, Richard Keller, DDS, 8251 W. Broward Blvd. #201, Plantation, FL, ph 954-473-5020
33401, Daniel N. Tucker, MD, 1411 N. Flagler Dr., #6700, West Palm Beach, FL, ph 561-835-0055
33401, Michael Constantine, ND, 1900 S. Olive, West Palm Beach, FL, ph 561-540-1429
33406, Louis Klionsky, DC, 1840 Forest Hill Blvd., Ste 105, West Palm Beach, FL, ph 561-439-5555
33407, John S. Findlay, DC, 1717 N. Flagler Drive #10, West Palm Beach, FL, ph 561-659-1001
33410, Neil Abner, MD, APCT, 10333-A N. Military Trail, Palm Beach Gardens, FL, ph 561-630-3696
33426, Kenneth Lee, MD, 1501 Corporate Dr., #240, Boynton Beach, FL, ph 561-736-8806
33426, Sherri W. Pinsley, DO, 1325 S. Longress, #207, Boynton Beach, FL, ph 561-752-5776
33432, Albert F. Robbins, DO, MSPH, 400 S. Dixie Hwy., Bldg. 2, Boca Raton, FL, ph 561-395-3282
33432, Dean R. Silver, MD, 24 SE 6th Street, Boca Raton, FL, ph 561-391-1884
33461, Sherri W. Pinsley, DO, 2290 10th Ave., Lake Worth, FL, ph 561-220-1697
33469, R. J. Oenbrink, DO, 396 Tequesta Drive, Tequesta, FL, ph 561-746-4333
33477, D. J. Rubin, DC, 229 E. RiverPark Drive, Jupiter, FL, ph 561-936-3517
33487, Leonard Haimes, MD, BPCT, 7300 N. Federal Hwy. #100, Boca Raton, FL, ph 561-995-8484
33510, Erika Bradshaw, MD, 1209 Lakeside Drive, Brandon, FL, ph 813-661-3662
33525, Edward Harshman, MD, 38047 Pasco Ave., Dade City, FL, ph 352-518-0725
33541, Mark B. Frank, DC, 4900 Allen Rd., Zephyrhills, FL, ph 813-788-0496
33604, Daniel Pia, DC, 1907 W. Sligh Ave., Tampa, FL, ph 813-935-7125
33606, Eugene H. Lee, MD, 1804 W. Kennedy Blvd. #A, Tampa, FL, ph 813-251-3096
33607, Edward Harshman, MD, 1710 West MLK Blvd., Tampa, FL, ph 352-518-0725

33611, Jean M. Allen, DO, 4212 S. Manhattan Ave., Tampa, FL, ph 813-837-8591

33616, Carlos M. Garcia, MD, APCT, 4710 Havana Ave., #107, Tampa, FL, ph 813-350-0140

33661, Robert J. Casanas, MD, 4810 Bay Heron Pl., #1012, Tampa, FL, ph 813-390-3037

33702, Ray C. Wunderlich, Jr., MD, Ph.D., 8821 MLK St., North, St. Petersburg, FL, ph 727-822-3612

33703, John P. Lenhart, MD, BPCT, 6110-9th Street N., St. Petersburg, FL, ph 727-526-0600

33755, American College of Nutrition, 300 S. Duncan Ave. #225, Clearwater, FL, ph 727-446-6086

33755, Susan Player, DC, 1433 Gulf-to-Bay Blvd., Clearwater, FL, ph 813-449-0210

33756, Cheryl Jones-Jaye, MD, 301 Turner Rd., Clearwater, FL, ph 727-466-6789

33756, David Minkoff, MD, 301 Turner Street, Clearwater, FL, ph 727-442-5612

33756, LifeWorks Wellness Center, 301 Turner Rd., Clearwater, FL, ph 727-466-6789

33756, Lisa Nikel, ARNP, 301 Turner Rd., Clearwater, FL, ph 727-466-6789

33760, Florida Institute of Health, 4908-A Creekside Dr., Clearwater, FL, ph 813-832-3220

33760, Marilyn Somers, ARNP, 4908 Creekside Dr. Ste. A, Clearwater, FL, ph 727-573-3775

33760, Mitchell Ghen, DO, Ph.D., 4908-A Creekside Dr., Clearwater, FL, ph 813-832-3220

33760, Stephen Holt, MD, 4908-A Creekside Dr., Clearwater, FL, ph 813-832-3220

33761, David M. Wall, MD, 3023 Eastland Blvd. Ste. H113, Clearwater, FL, ph 727-791-3830

33762, Colin Chan, MD, 2685 Ulmerton Rd., #101, Clearwater, FL, ph 727-571-1688

33765, Marguerite Gerger, DC, 326-A N. Belcher Road, Clearwater, FL, ph 727-441-8110

33767, David Schenk, DO, 37 Baymont St., Clearwater, FL, ph 727-461-4644

33771, Scott M. Baker, DC, 1000 South Belcher Road, Suite 12, Largo, FL, ph 727-538-2273

33803, Harold Robinson, MD, 4406 S. Florida Ave., Ste. 27, Lakeland, FL, ph 941-646-5088

33803, S. Todd Robinson, MD, APCT, 4406 S. Florida Ave., Ste. 30, Lakeland, FL, ph 941-646-5088

33903, Robert A. DiDonato, MD, 3443 Hancock Bridge Pkwy., #301, Ft. Myers, FL, ph 239-997-8800

33912, Gary L. Pynckel, DO, APCT, 3840 Colonial Blvd., #1, Fort Myers, FL, ph 941-278-3377

33951, James Coy, MD, BPCT, 310 Nesbit St., Punta Gorda, FL, ph 941-575-8080

33990, Joan Craft, DC, 1928 Del Prado Blvd., Cape Coral, FL, ph 941-574-3533

34102, David Perlmutter, MD, 800 Goodlette Rd. N., #270, Naples, FL, ph 239-649-7400

34135, Dean R. Silver, MD, 9240 Bonita Beach Rd., #2215, Bonita Springs, FL, ph 239-949-0101

34145, Frank R. Recker, DDS, JD, 267 N. Collier Blvd., #202, Marco Island, FL, ph 800-224-3529

34145, Richard Saitta, MD, 1010 N. Barfield Dr., Marco Island, FL, ph 941-642-8488

34205, Irving Hall, MD, 712 39th W., Bradenton, FL, ph 941-748-4602

34210, Eteri Melnikov, MD, APCT, 4216 Cortez Rd. W., Bradenton, FL, ph 941-739-2225

34210, Jenny Yoshida, MD, 4216 Cortez Rd. W, Bradenton, FL, ph 941-739-2225

34236, Rebecca Roberts, DO, 1521 Dolphin St., #101, Sarasota, FL, ph 941-365-6273

34236, Ronald E. Wheeler, MD, 1819 Main St., Ste 401, Sarasota, FL, ph 941-957-0007

34239, Alan Sault, MD, 2000 S. Tamiami Trail, Sarasota, FL, ph 941-955-5579

34239, W. Frederic Harvey, MD, 3982 Bee Ridge Rd., Bldg. H, #J, Sarasota, FL, ph 941-929-9355

34285, Matthew Burks, MD, 420 Nokomis Ave., So., Venice, FL, ph 941-488-8112

34293, Arlene Martone, MD, 4140 Woodmere Park Blvd., #2, Venice, FL, ph 941-408-9838

34429, Michael Bennet, DC, 375 NE 10th Ave, Crystal River, FL, ph 352-563-6471

34461, Azael P. Borromeo, MD, APCT, 2653 N. Lecanto Hwy., Lecanto, FL, ph 352-527-9555

34471, John Podlaski, DC, 2721 SE 23rd Ave., Ocala, FL, ph 352-867-1015

34474, Nelson Karucak, MD, FAAFP, 1731 SW 2nd Ave., Ocala, FL, ph 352-694-0022

34607, Calin V. Pop, MD, 4215 Rachel Blvd., Spring Hill, FL, ph 352-597-2240

34609, Nabil Habib, MD, BPCT, 3300 Josef Ave., Spring Hill, FL, ph 352-683-1166

34683, Janice M. Piro, DC, 971-B Virginia Ave., Palm Harbor, FL, ph 727-789-4020

34684, C. Randall Harrell, MD, 34162 US 19 N., Palm Harbor, FL, ph 727-781-0818

34684, Carlos M. Garcia, MD, APCT, 36555 U.S. Hwy. 19 North, Palm Harbor, FL, ph 727-771-9669

34691, Robert Hannum III, DO, 2216 US 19, Holiday, FL, ph 727-937-6428

34741, Carmelita Bamba-Dagani, MD, 500 North John Young Pkwy., Kissimmee, FL, ph 407-935-1060

34741, Dale Barnes, DC, 316 Church Street, Kissimee, FL, ph 407-847-8254

34952, Steven T. Everett, MD, 1837 SE Port St. Lucie Blvd., Port St. Lucie, FL, ph 561-398-8884

34994, Neil Abner, MD, APCT, 705 North Federal Hwy., Stuart, FL, 772-692-9200

34997, Sherri W. Pinsley, DO, 7000 SE Federal Hwy., #302, Stuart, FL, ph 561-220-1697

35007, Elizabeth Ann Lowenthal, DO, 240 7th Ave. NE, #B, Alabaster, AL, ph 205-664-4051

35209, Lymon Fritz, MD, 3401 Independence Dr., #241, Birmingham, AL, ph 205-877-8585

35209, Michael S. Vaughn, MD, 1 Lakeshore Dr., #100, Birmingham, AL, ph 205-930-2950

35404, Elliott Rampulla, MD, 535 Jack Warner Pkwy. NW, Tuscaloosa, AL, ph 205-462-0969

35901, Andrew M. Brown, MD, 515 South 3rd St., Gadsden, AL, ph 256-547-4971

35950, John T. Wallace, DC, 3314 U.S. Highway 431, Albertville, AL, ph 256-593-9083

36117, Scott Bell, MD, 7020 Sydney Curve, Montgomery, AL, ph 334-277-5363

36117, Teresa D. Allen, DO, APCT, 7047 Halcyon Park Dr., Montgomery, AL, ph 334-273-0904

36203, Jose Oblena, MD, 1720 Hwy. 78 East, #11, Oxford, AL, ph 256-835-2366

36264, Gus J. Prosch Jr., MD, P.O. Box 427, Heflin, AL, ph 205-222-0960

36526, Glen Wilcoxson, MD DPL, P.O. Box 1347, Daphne, AL, ph 334-447-0333

36532, Charles Runels Jr., MD, 82 Plantation Pointe, Fairhope, AL, ph 334-625-2612

36532, E. Derry Hubbard, MD, 761-A Middle Avenue, Fairthorpe, AL, ph 251-990-0662

36547, Gregory S. Funk, DO, BPCT, 2103 W. 1st Street, Gulf Shores, AL, ph 251-968-2441

37087, William T. Strauss, DC, 115 Castle Heights Ave. N, Ste. 104, Lebanon, TN, ph 615-444-5335

37137, Norman Saliba, MD, 1630 S. Church St., #203, Murfreesboro, TN, ph 615-848-0113

37138, Russell Hunt, MD, 1415 Robinson Road, Old Hickory, TN, ph 615-541-0400

37215, Stephen L. Reisman, MD, 2325 Crestmoor Rd., #P-150, Nashville, TN, ph 615-298-2820

60659, Razvan Rentea, MD, 3525 W. Peterson, Ste. 611, Chicago, IL, ph 773-583-7793

37303, H. Joseph Holliday, MD, APCT, 1005 W. Madison Ave., Athens, TN, ph 423-744-7540

37311, Charles C. Adams, MD, BPCT, 2600 Executive Park Dr. NW, Cleveland, TN, ph 423-473-7080

37355, David Florence, DO, 1912 McArthur Drive, Manchester, TN, ph 931-728-5522

37402, Charles C. Adams, MD, 600 W. Main Street, Chattanooga, TN, ph 706-861-7377

37601, Robert C. Allen, MD, 1416 S. Roan St., Johnson City, TN, ph 423-979-6257

37604, David Livingston, MD, BPCT, 1567 N. Eastman Rd., #4, Kingsport, TN, ph 423-245-6671

37660, Pickens Gantt, MD, #307 – 2204 Paviliaon Dr., Kingsport, TN, ph 423-392-6053

37816, Donald Thompson, MD, 1121 W. First North St., Morristown, TN, ph 423-581-6367

37863, Larry Davenport, MD, 1981 Parkway, Pigeon Forge, TN, ph 865-453-1122

37919, Janet S. McNiel, MD, 5612 Kingston Pike, Knoxville, TN, ph 865-584-3565

37923, Joseph E. Rich, MD, MPH, MMM, 9217 Parkwest Blvd. E-1, Knoxville, TN, ph 865-694-9553

37924, Janet S. McNiel, MD, 5917 Rutledge Pike, Knoxville, TN, ph 865-525-2121

38104, Charles R. Wallace, Jr., MD, FICS, 1325 Eastmoreland Ave. #425, ph 901-272-3200

38119, Roy Page, MD, 6005 Park Ave., #828B, Memphis, TN, ph 901-763-3664

38317, John Smothers, ND, 5575 Poplar Avenue, Suite 112, Memphis, TN, ph 901-683-2777

38618, Pravin P. Patel, MD, P.O. Box 1060, Coldwater, MS, ph 601-622-7011

38834, Arnold Smith, MD, 1401 River Rd., Greenwood, MS, ph 800-720-8933

39135, Stephen Kaskie, MD, #2100 – 3501 Health Center Blvd., Bonita Springs, FL, ph 941-948-2000

39466, Thomas Purser III, MD, 1911 Read Rd., Picayune, MS, ph 601-798-0535

39564, James H. Waddell, MD, 1520 Government Street, Ocean Springs, MS, ph 228-875-5505

39701, Jacob Skiwski, MD, BPCT, 3491 Bluecutt Rd., Columbus, MS, ph 601=329-2955

40014, Steven Johnson, DO, 8909 Hwy 329, Crestwood, KY, ph 800-624-7080, www.foxhollow.com

40403, Edward K. Atkinson, MD, P.O. Box 57, Berea, KY, ph 859-925-2252

40503, Carol Perkins, ND, 509 Southland Dr., Lexington, KY, ph 859-277-5255

42160, Ray H. Houchin, DC, P.O. Box 69, Park City, KY, ph 502-749-2141

42503, Stephen S. Kiteck, MD, 600 Bogle St., Somerset, KY, ph 606-677-0459

43065, Richard R. Mason, DO, NMD, 10034 Brewster Lane, Powell, OH, ph 614-761-0555

43065, William D. Mitchell, DO, APCT, 10034 Brewster Ln., Powell, OH, ph 614-761-0555

43130, Jacqueline S. Chan, DO, 3484 Cincinnati-Zanesville Rd., Lancaster, OH, ph 740-653-0017

43130, Rene V. Blaha, MD, 3484 Cincinnati-Zanesville Rd., Lancaster, OH, ph 740-653-0017

43205, Bruce A. Massau, DO, 1492 E. Broad St., #1203, Columbus, OH, ph 614-252-1500

43235, Larry S. Everhart, MD, 730 Mt. Airyshire Blvd., Ste. A, Columbus, OH, ph 614-848-2600

43537, Elizabeth Chen Christenson, MD, 219 W. Wayne St., Maumee, OH, ph 419-893-8438

43623, James C. Roberts, MD, 4607 Sylvania Ave. #200, Toledo, OH, ph 419-882-9620

44001, Rosemary I. Moroni, MD, 530 N. Leavitt Road, Amherst, OH, ph 440-985-1800

44041, Daniel Duffy, DC, 1953 S. Broadway, Geneva, OH, ph 440-466-1186

44041, John M. Heidrich, DC, 1953 S. Broadway, Geneva, OH, ph 440-466-1186

44057, Richard Krabill, DO, 6231 N. Ridge W, Madison, OH, ph 440-428-2141

44106, Erin Holston, ND, BA, 2460 Fairmount Blvd., #219, Cleveland Heights, OH, ph 216-707-9137

44111, David A. Velasquez, MD, 3429 W. Boulevard-DN, Cleveland, OH, ph 216-861-6200

44129, Radha Baishnab, MD, 5599 Pearl Rd., Cleveland, OH, ph 440-781-5100

44131, John Baron, DO DPL, 4807 Rockside Rd. #100, Cleveland, OH, ph 216-642-0082

44136, Sherri Tenpenny, DO, 13550 Falling Water Rd. #202, Strongsville, OH, ph 440-268-0897

44143, Ronald Casselberry, MD, 27155 Chardon Rd., #102, Richmond Heights, OH, ph 440-943-3830
44145, Derrick Lonsdale, MD, APCT, 24700 Center Ridge Rd., Cleveland, OH, ph 440-835-0104
44145, James P. Frackelton, MD, APCT, 24700 Center Ridge Rd., Cleveland, OH, ph 440-835-0104
44145, Stan Gardner, MD, APCT, CNS, 24700 Center Ridge Rd., Cleveland, OH, ph 440-835-0104
44256, Douglas Weeks, 3985 Medina Rd., Medina, OH, ph 419-716-1708
44308, Leon Neiman, MD, 120 W. Bowery Street, Akron, OH, ph 330-535-3101
44313, Josephine Aronica, MD, 1867 W. Market St., Akron, OH, ph 330-867-7361
44313, Nicholas Parasson, ND, 1680 Akron Peninsula Rd., #103, Akron, OH, ph 330-928-6685
44511, James Ventresco, DO, 3848 Tippecanoe Rd., Youngstown, OH, ph 330-792-2349
44641, Joseph R. Andrejcik, DC, 908 West Main Street, Louisville, OH, ph 330-875-3400
44718, Jack Slingluff, DO, 5850 Fulton Rd. NW, Canton, OH, ph 330-494-8641
44811, Edward J. Hemeyer, MD, 521 N. Sandusky Street, Ste. B, Bellevue, OH, ph 419-483-6267
44857, Charles S. Resseger, DO, 853 S. Norwalk Rd., Norwalk, OH, ph 419-668-9615
44870, Douglas Weeks, MD, APCT, 3703 Columbus Avenue, Sandusky, OH, ph 419-625-8085
44905, Robert J. Gilbert, DC, 953 Park Ave. East, Mansfield, OH, ph 419-589-6470
45069, James E. Smith, DO DPL, 4889 Smith Rd., West Chester, OH, ph 513-765-7546
45213, Maureen Pelletier, MD, 5400 Kennedy Ave., Cincinnati, OH, ph 513-924-5049
45219, Henry Heimlich, MD, 31 Straight St., Cincinnati, OH, ph 513-559-2391
45238, Michael W. Broughton, DC, 5082 Glencrossing Way, Cincinnati, OH, ph 513-451-8000
45239, William Westendorf, DDS, 2818 Blue Rock Rd., Cincinnati, OH, ph 513-923-3839
45241, Ted Cole, MA, DO, NMD, 11974 Lebanon Rd., Ste. 228, Cincinnati, OH, ph 513-563-4321
45246, Leonid Macheret, MD, 375 Glensprings Dr., #400, Cincinnati, OH, ph 513-851-8790
45251, Craig Maxwell, DO, BPCT, 3553 Springdale Rd., Cincinnati, OH, ph 513-741-4404
45251, Kaushal K. Bhardwaj, MD, 9019 Colerain Ave., Cincinnati, OH, ph 513-385-8100
45429, Van Merckle, DC, 5761 Far Hills, Dayton, OH, ph 937-433-3241
45459, John H. Boyles, Jr., MD, 7076 Corporate Way, Centerville, OH, ph 937-434-0555
45701, Mark McAdoo, DC, 476 Richland Ave., Athens, OH, ph 614-592-6362
45817, L. Terry Chappell, MD, APCT, 122 Thurman St., Bluffton, OH, ph 419-358-4627
45817, Marian Bursten, MD, Ph.D., 122 Thurman, Bluffton, OH, ph 419-358-4627
45817, Robert Angus, ND, B.Sc., 122 Thurman St., Bluffton, OH, ph 419-358-4627
45879, Don K. Snyder, MD, 1030 West Wayne St., Paulding, OH, ph 419-399-2045
46032, Kevin Logan, MD, 13431 Old Meridian St., Carmel, IN, ph 317-582-8843
46158, Richard N. Halstead, DO, 17 Moore Street, Mooresville, IN, ph 317-831-0853
46219, Robert Prather, DC, 8716 E. 21st Street, Indianapolis, IN, ph 317-897-3121
46240, L. Dale Guyer, MD, 836 East 86th St., Indianapolis, IN, ph 317-580-9355
46256, David Darbro, MD, 8202 Clearvista Pkwy #7A, Indianpolia, IN, ph 317-913-3000
46256, Samia Merco, MD, 11216 Fall Creek Rd., Indianapolis, IN, ph 317-595-8823
46260, David R. Decatur, MD, 8925 N. Meridian, #150, Indianapolis, IN, ph 317-818-8925
46260, Gary Moore, MD DPL, 9302 N. Meridian #251, Indianpolis, IN, ph 317-705-0909
46260, Robert M. Armer, MD, 2020 W. 86th St., Ste. 306, Indianapolis, IN, ph 317-228-0992
46383, Brian McGuckin, DC, 3201 North Calumet, Valparaisio, IN, ph 219-531-1234
46385, Myrna D. Trowbridge, DO, 450-C Marsh St., Valparaiso, IN, ph 219-462-3377
46517, Larry W. Banyash, MD, 23631 US 33 S., Elkhart, IN, ph 574-875-1446
46526, Marcia Prenguber, ND, 200 High Park Ave., Goshen, IN, ph 574-535-2961
46601, Keim T. Houser, MD, 515 N. Lafayette Blvd., South Bend, IN, ph 219-232-2037
46617, Frances Dwyer, MD, 919 E. Jefferson Blvd. #107, South Bend, IN, ph 219-232-5892
46750, Thomas J. Ringenberg, DO, BPCT, 941 Etna Avenue, Huntington, IN, ph 260-356-9400
46962, Marvin D. Dziabis, MD, 107 West 7th Street, No. Manchester, IN, ph 260-982-1400
47129, Edna B. Pretila, MD, 647 Eastern Blvd., Clarksville, IN, ph 812-282-4309
47129, George Wolverton, MD, APCT, 647 Eastern BVlvd., Clarksville, IN, ph 812-282-4309
47130, H. Wayne Mayhue, MD, 207 Sparks Ave., #301, Jeffersonville, IN, ph 812-288-7169
47368, Oscar I. Ordonez, MD, 218 S. Main Street, Parker City, IN, ph 765-468-6337
47421, John D. Lockenour, DC, 3525 Mitchell Road, Bedford, IN, ph 812-275-4419
47501, Anne L. Kempf, DO, RR3, Box 357 Bedford Rd., Washington, IN, ph 812-254-5868
47909, Charles Turner, MD, BPCT, 2433 S. 9th Street, Lafayette, IN, ph 765-471-1100
47933, Tracy A. Clark, MD, 601 S. Mill, Crawfordsville, IN, ph 765-362-7600
48034, Mark Hertzberg, MD, 25865 W. 12 Mile Rd., #104, Southfield, MI, ph 248-357-3220
48065, James Ziobron, DO, 71441 Van Dyke, Romeo, MI, ph 810-336-3700

48071, Rodney Moret, MD, 1400 East 12 Mile Road, Madison Heights, MI, ph 248-547-2223
48094, Gerald D. Keyte, DO, 58024 Van Dyke, Washington, MI, ph 486-781-5535
48103, Amy L. Dean, 1955 Pauline Blvd., Ste. 100D, Ann Arbor, MI, ph 734-213-4901
48103, James Around-Thomas, MD, 220 Collingwood St., Ann Arbor, MI, ph 734-995-4999
48103, Paula G. Davey, MD, 1677 Stadium Ct., Ann Arbor, MI, ph 734-662-6492
48104, Molly F. McMullen-Laird, MD, 2385 S. Huron Parkway, Ann Arbor, MI, ph 734-677-7990
48104, Quentin R. McMullen, MD, 2385 S. Huron Parkway, Ann Arbor, MI, ph 734-677-7990
48114 Margaret Paris, 7269 Grand River, Brighton, MI, ph 810-229-2312
48116, F. R. Kazangy, MD, 8609 W. Grand River #203, Brighton, MI, ph 810-227-6107
48176, John G. Ghuneim, MD, BPCT, 1235 S. Industrial Dr., #6, Saline, MI, ph 734-429-2581
48185, Clinton L. Greenstone, MD, 36555 Warren Rd., Westland, MI, ph 734-404-9004
48197, Kyle Morgan, DO, 3020 Packard Rd., Ypsilanti, MI, ph 734-434-3300
48236, Cynthia Browne, MD, Ph.D., 19229 mack Ave., Grosse Pointe, MI, ph 313-647-3100
48236, R. B. Fahim, MD, BPCT, 20825 Mack Ave., Grosse Pointe, MI, ph 313-640-9730
48322, David Brownstein, MD, 5821 W. Maple Rd. #192, W. Bloomfield, MI, ph 248-851-1600
48322, David Brownstein, MD, 5821 W. Maple Rd., #192, West Bloomfield, MI, ph 248-851-1600
48322, Jeffrey Nusbaum, MD, 5821 W. Maple Rd. #192, Bloomfield, MI, ph 248-851-1600
48322, Richard Ng, MD, 5821 W. Maple Rd., #192, W. Bloomfield, MI, ph 248-851-1600
48331, Albert Scarchilli, DO DPL, 30160 Fox Club Dr., Farmington Hills, MI, ph 248-626-7544
48331, Paul Parente, DO DPL, 38263 French Pond, Farmington Hills, MI, ph 248-489-0263
48334, Helen Lee, MD, 30275 W. 13 Mile Rd., Farmington Hills, MI, ph 248-626-7544
48342, Vahagn Agbabian, DO, 28 N. Saginaw St., #1105, Pontiac, MI, ph 248-334-2424
48346, Nedra Downing, DO, MS, BPCT, 5639 Sashabaw Rd., Clarkston, MI, ph 248-625-6677
48446, Paul D. Lepor, DO, BPCT, 1254 North Main St., Lapeer, MI, ph 810-664-4531
48462, David Regiani, DDS, 101 South Street, Ortonville, MI, ph 248-627-4934
48502, Ann Behling, ND, BA, 601 S. Saginaw Street, Suite 315, Flint, MI, ph 248-318-5798
48503, Gerald D. Natzke, DO, 2284 S. Ballenger Hwy., Flint, MI, ph 810-223-5211
48503, William M. Bernard, DO, BPCT, 2284 S. Ballenger Hwy. #H, Flint, MI, ph 810-233-5211
48532, Janice Shimoda, DO, BPCT, 1044 Gilbert Street, Flint, MI, ph 810-233-5211
48532, Kenneth Ganapini, DO, BPCT, 1044 Gilbert Street, Flint, MI, ph 810-233-5211
48651, Daniel McGregor, DC, 1223 W. Houghton Lake Drive, Pridenville, MI, ph 517-366-4646
48706, Parveen A. Malik, MD, 808 N. Euclid Ave., Bay City, MI, ph 989-686-3760
48764, Michael D. Papenfuse, DO, 200 Hemlock Rd., Tawas City, MI, ph 517-362-9229
48912, Douglas F. Wacker, MD, 1323 E. Michigan Ave., Lansing, MI, ph 517-484-9788
48917, David Nebbling, DO, 424 Elmwood, Lansing, MI, ph 517-323-1833
49004, Eric Born, DO, APCT, 2350 East G Ave., Parchment, MI, ph 616-344-6183
49085, Jagir Judge, MD, 2550 Niles Rd., St. Joseph, MI, ph 616-429-1085
49201, Jack T. Hinkle, DO, 300 W. Washington #150, Jackson, MI, ph 517-783-4664
49341, Mary Vanderwal, NP, 350 Northland Dr. NE, Rockford, MI, ph 616-866-4474
49444, Ruth Walkotten, DO, 433 W. Seminole, Muskegon, MI, ph 231-733-1989
49464, Gary Coller, DO DPL, 300 South State St. #5, Zeeland, MI, ph 616-772-0700
49512, Ann M. Auburn, DO, 3700 52nd St. SE, Grand Rapids, MI, ph 616-656-3700
49512, Ashely E. Kepler, PA-C, 3700 52nd St. SE, Grand Rapids, MI, ph 616-656-3700
49512, Tammy Born, DO, APCT, 3700 – 52nd Street SE, Grand Rapids, MI, ph 616-656-3700
49546, Robert A. DeJonge, DO, BPCT, 2251 East Paris, Grand Rapids, MI, ph 616-956-6090
49677, Howard Mahabeer, MD, 225 N. State St., Reed City, MI, ph 616-832-2456
49686, Douglas J. Wigton, DO, 1028 Hannah Ave., Traverse City, MI, ph 231-946-7360
49709, Leo Modzinski, DO DPL, 12394 State St., Atlanta, MI, ph 989-785-4254
49870, F. Michael Saigh, MD, 411 Murray Rd. West U.S. 2, Norway, MI, ph 906-563-9600
50401, Robert Friedrichs, DC, 940 N. Tyler, Mason City, IA, ph 515-424-5415
51503, Denna J. Rogge, DC, 103 North Avenue, Suite 4, Council Bluffs, IA, ph 712-322-8504
52157, Gary Bowden, DC, 30674 Eagle Dr., McGregor, IA, ph 319-873-3404
52729, Maria Anderson, DC, 2210 160th Ave, Calamus, IA, ph 563-246-2129
52748, Anita Wubbena, DC, 18 Lincoln Avenue, Parkview, IA, ph 319-285-8453
52772, Darlene Ehlers, DC, 200 W. South Street, Tipton, IA, ph 319-886-2090
53018, Carol Uebelacker, MD, 700 Milwaukee St., Delafield, WI, ph 262-646-4600
53095, Gregory B. Gamache, DC, 1624 Clarence Court, West Bend, WI, ph 262-334-4847
53104, Jeffery Bergin, DC, 21012 107th St., Bristol, WI, ph 262-857-2781

53154, Carol Brown, DO, 147 W. Ryan Rd., Oak Creek, WI, ph 414-764-0920

53186, Glenn A. Toth, MD, 403 North Grande Ave., Waukesha, WI, ph 262-547-3055

53186, Wayne H. Konetzki, MD, 403 North Grand Ave., Waukesha, WI, ph 262-547-3055

53212, Anne Maedke, DC, 715 E. Locust Street, Milwaukee, WI, ph 414-263-7066

53217, Ken Edington, DC, 8675 N. Port Washington Road, Rox Point, WI, ph 414-351-8120

53218, William Faber, DO, 6529 W. Fond du Lac Ave., Milwaukee, WI, ph 414-464-7246

53223, Mary Lou Ballweg, 8585 North 76th Pl., Milwaukee, WI, ph 414-355-2200

53226, J. Allan Robertson, Jr., DO, 1011 N. Mayfair Rd., #301, Milwaukee, WI, ph 414-302-1011

53226, Jerry N. Yee, DO, 11803 W. North Avenue, Wauwatosa, WI, ph 414-258-6282

53516, Gina Schultz, DC, 210 S. Main Street, Blanchardville, WI, ph 608-523-4612

53516, Gina Steinmann, DC, 210 S. Main Street, Blanchardville, WI, ph 608-523-4612

53705, Timoteo Galvez, MD, 2705 Marshall Ct., Madison, WI, ph 608-238-3831

53716, Leslie Best, DC, 5217 Spaanem Ave., Madison, WI, ph 608-249-2378

53965, Robert S. Waters, MD DPL, 320 Race Street, Wisconsin Dells, WI, ph 608-254-7178

54220, Dean A. Wilhite, DC, 3713 Calumet Ave., Manitowoc, WI, ph 920-682-6680

54304, Cheryl Metzler, DC, 1804 S. Ashland, Green Bay, WI, ph 920-432-7774

54311, Eleazar M. Kadile, MD, APCT, 1538 Bellevue St., Green Bay, WI, ph 920-468-9442

54401, Barbara Bradley, DC, 2003 Robin Lane, Wausau, WI, ph 715-845-3775

54521, Kevin Branham, DC, 5680 Cloverland Drive, Eagle River, WI, ph 715-479-9066

54601, David L. Morris, MD, 615 S. 10th St., La Crosse, WI, ph 608-782-2027

54601, Patrick J. Scott, MD, 3454 Losey Blvd. South, La Crosse, WI, ph. 608-785-0038

54602, George F. Kroker, MD, 615 S. 10th St., La Crosse, WI, ph 608-782-2027

54602, Vijay K. Sabnis, MD, 615 S. 10th St., La Crosse, WI, ph 608-782-2027

54759, Bernie Finch, DC, W9410 Cedar Drive, Pepin, WI, ph 715-442-2016

54806, Craig Gilbaugh, DC, 1022 Lake Shore Drive, East, Ashland, WI, ph 715-682-5333

54868, David Sommerfeld, DC, 6 W. St. Patrick Street, Rice Lake, WI, ph 715-234-4222

54935, Steven Meress, MD, Fox Valley Wellness Ctr, Fond du Lac, WI, ph 920-922-5433

55006, Paul Bergley, DC, 105 W. Central Drive, PO Box 328, Braham, MN, ph 320-396-3375

55076, Jonathan C. Williams, DC, 3603 71st Street, Inver Going Hts., MN, ph 651-455-7048

55082, Sandra Spore, DC, 1530 Frontage, Stillwater MN, ph 651-439-1013

55102, Russel C. Des Marais, DC, 569 Selby Ave., St. Paul, MN, ph 651-291-7772

55104, Leslie Stewart, DC, 1885 University Ave., Ste. 100, St. Paul, MN, ph 651-644-8242

55109, Brenwyn Paddycoart, DC, 2599 White Bear Ave., Maplewood, MN, ph 651-770-8424

55113, G. T. Lalla, DC, 2353 Rice Street, Ste. 200, Roseville, MN, ph 651-484-8521

55128, William Lyden, DC, 1401 Helmo Ave., Oakdale, MN, ph 651-731-7588

55305, Jean R. Eckerly, MD DPL, 13911 Ridgedale Dr. #350, Minnetonka, MN, ph 952-593-9458

55316, Timothy Bertsch, DC, 12217 Champlin Dr., Champlin, MN, ph 763-323-1492

55317, Joel Eichers, DC, 340 Lake Drive E., Chanhassen, MN, ph 852-949-2507

55337, Terry Franks, DC, 1601 E. Highway 13, #209, Burnsville, MN, ph 612-890-5888

55407, Diaa Osmon, ND, 1527 East Lake Street, Minneapolis, MN, ph 952-926-1143

55414, Barry Bicanich, DC, 3404 University SE, Minneapolis, MN, ph 612-331-4529

55416, Charles L. Strauman, DC, 2900 Thomas Ave. S. Suite 350, Minneapolis, MN, ph 612-928-7894

55416, Miahcel A. Dole, MD, APCT, 3408 Dakota Ave. S, St. Louis Park, MN, ph 952-924-1053

55431, George Kramer, MD, 10564 France Ave., South, Bloomington, MN, ph 612-706-1418

55431, Kevin T. Wand, DO, 10564 France Ave. S, Bloomington, MN, ph 952-942-9303

55433, Thomas W. Miller, DC, 11413 Hanson Blvd., Coon Rapids, MN, ph 612-754-1482

55439, Jeffrey P. Anderson, DC, 7001 Cahill Rd, Suite #23, Edina, MN, ph 952-943-1170

55441, Jean R. Eckerly, MD, APCT, 13911 Ridgedale Dr., #350, Minnetonka, MN, ph 952-593-9458

55802, Robert Maki, ND, 31 S. Superior Street, Duluth, MN, ph 218-310-0081

56007, Niles Shoff, DC, 139 South Broadway, Albert Lea, MN, ph 507-373-7085

56172, Joseph H. Muldoon, DC, 2710 Broadway Avenue, Slayton, MN, ph 507-839-8971

56172, MaeBeth Lindstrom, DC, 2002 Broadway, Slayton, MN, ph 507-836-8911

56377, Tom Sult, MD, BPCT, 100 2nd Street S., Sortell, MN, ph 320-251-2600

57006, Roger Bommersbach, DC, 1611 6th Street, Brookings, SD, ph 605-692-7888

57301, Roger Prill, Jr., DC, 1501 North Main Street, Mitchell, SD, ph 605-996-7288

57701, Brett Sutton, DC, 315 E. St. Patrick, Suite A, Rapid City, SD, ph 605-341-7330

57702, David Schwietert, DC, 3936 Jackson Blvd., Rapid City, SD, ph 605-342-3861

57730, Dennis R. Wicks, MD, 1 Holiday Trail, HCR 83, Box 21, Custer, SD, ph 605-673-2689

58201, Richard H. Leigh, MD, APCT, 2600 Demers Ave., #108, Grand Forks, ND, ph 701-772-7696
58701, Brian Briggs, MD, 718 SW 6th St., Minot, ND, ph 701-838-6011
58701, Brian E. Briggs, MD, 718 – 6th St. SW, Minot, ND, ph 701-838-6011
59101, David C. Healow, MD, 2501 – 4th Ave. North, #C, Billings, MT, ph 406-252-6674
59101, Nirala Jacobi, ND, 720 N. 30th St., Billings, MT, ph 406-259-5096
59405, Nancy Patterson, ND, 2517 7th Ave. S, Ste. B-3, Great Falls, MT, ph 406-727-5778
59405, Shelley Cerasaro, ND, 1301 12th Ave. S, Ste. 203, Great Falls, MT, ph 406-727-6680
59405, Stephany Porter, ND, 1708 9th Ave. South, Great Falls, MT, ph 406-771-7114
59714, Curt G. Kurtz, MD, 8707 Jackrabbit Ln., Ste. C, Belgrade, MT, ph 406-587-5561
59715, Breana Hauskins-McElgunn, ND, 317 E. Medenhall St., Ste. B, Bozeman, MT, ph 406-587-0858
59840, Jonathan Psenka, ND, 1201 Westwood Dr., Ste. D, Hamilton, MT, ph 800-217-1629
59840, Mark Kelley, ND, Lac, 173 Blodgett Camp Road, Hamilton, MT, ph 406-363-4041
59840, Timothy Binder, ND, DC, Lac, 173 Blodgett Camp Rd., Hamilton, MT, ph 406-363-4041
60004, William J. Mauer, DO, 3401 N. Kennicott Ave., Arlington Heights, IL, ph 847-255-8988
60005, Mikaharu Hayashi, DC, 2010 S. Arlington Hts. Rd #42, Arlington Heights, IL, ph 847-593-3330
60007, Zofia Szymanska, MD, 850 Biesterfield Rd., #4006, Elk Grove Village, IL, ph 847-437-4418
60014, Gary R. Oberg, MD, 31 North Virginia St., Crystal Lake, IL, ph 815-455-1990
60014, James E. McGinn, Jr., DC, 318 Memorial Sr., Ste. 200, Crystal Lake, IL, ph 815-455-1910
60031, Mark E. Fredrick, DC, 3930 Washington Street, Suite B, Gurnee, IL, ph 847-662-1600
60045, Julie Martin, ND, 430 East Frost Place, Lake Forest, IL, ph 847-615-1224
60048, Adam Maddox, 121 West Austin Ave., Libertyville, IL, ph 847-370-6264
60050, Frederick Hult, DC, 306 N. Front St., McHenry, IL, ph 815-344-0900
60062, Jin Hwan Park, ND, MSOM, Lac, CH, 3111 Dundee Rd., Northbrook, IL, ph 847-562-0840
60062, Lisa Lotte Schuster, DC, 1535 Lake Cook Road, Ste. 312, Northbrook, IL, ph 847-509-9067
60103, Michael E. Camerer, DC, 158 Bartlett Plaza, Bartlett, IL, ph 630-830-2121
60108, Alex Zwan III, DC, 109 S. First St., Flr #1, Ste. A, Bloomingdale, IL, ph 630-539-5822
60108, William L. Epperly, MD, 245 S. Gary Ave., Ste. 105, Bloomingdale, IL, ph 630-893-9661
60123, Lester H. Holze, Jr., DC, 2000 Larkin Ave., Suite 200, Elgin, IL, ph 847-888-4770
60134, Richard E. Hrdlicka, MD, 302 Randall Rd., #206, Geneva, IL, ph 630-232-1900
60137, Caitlin Morrisroe, DC, 50 Finley Rd. # 2C, Glen Ellyn, IL, ph 630-202-2883
60137, Christena V. Nicholson, DC, 3 S. 250 Cypress Drive, Glen Ellyn, IL, ph 630-858-2262
60142, Philip Sukel, DDS, 11952 Oak Creek Parkway, Huntley, IL, ph 847-659-8500
60143, Joseph Riggio, DC, 921 W. Irving Park Road, Itasca, IL, ph 630-250-9200
60145, Marty Moegling, DC, 312 S. Sandra, Kingston, IL, ph 630-893-8556
60148, David Wickes, DC, 200 E. Roosevelt Road, Lombard, IL, ph 630-629-2000
60148, Grant Iannelli, DC, 200 E. Roosevelt Road, Lombard, IL, ph 630-889-6836
60148, James Winterstein, DC, 200 E. Roosevelt Road, Lombard, IL, ph 630-885-6604
60148, William J. Hogan, DC, 233 S. Craig Pl., Lombard, IL, ph 630-889-6522
60172, Christine Cosgrove, DC, 980 W. Lake Street, Roselle, IL, ph 630-893-8556
60181, Stephen Boudro, DC, 644 S. Comell, Villa Park, IL, ph 630-833-0236
60187, Frank Strehl, DC, 111 E. Cole Ave., Wheaton, IL, ph 630-653-5755
60187, Fred J. Schultz, MD, 2150 Manchester Rd., Wheaton, IL, ph 630-933-9722
60187, Margaret Dempster, DC, 520 W. Roosevelt, #10, Wheaton, IL, ph 630-588-9300
60187, Romeo Augusto Lucas, DC, 823 Pick Street, Wheaton, IL, ph 630-682-9865
60187, William Shelton, DC, 1600 N. Main Street, Wheaton, IL, ph 630-510-7749
60194, Anthony Pantanella, DC, 1175 N. Barrington Road, Hoffman Estates, IL, ph 847-885-1131
60195, Marsha L. Vetter, Ph.D., MD, 2500 W. Higgins Rd., Hoffman Estates, IL, ph 847-519-7772
60195, Susan Busse, MD, 2260 W. Higgins Rd., #202, Hoffman Estates, IL, ph 847-781-7500
60301, Carlos M. Reynes, MD, 1140 Westgate, Oak Park, IL, ph 708-358-0111
60301, Paul J. Dunn, MD, 1140 Westgate, Oak Park, IL, ph 708-358-0111
60301, Ross Hauser, MD, 715 Lake St. #600, Oak Park, IL, ph 708-848-7789
60408, Bernard G. Milton, MD, 233 E. Reed St., Braidwood, IL, ph 815-458-6700
60429, Prakash G. Sane, MD, BPCT, 17680 South Kedzie Ave., Hazel Crest, IL, ph 708-799-2499
60457, Linda L. Ehlers, DC, 8700 W. 95th Street, Hickory Hills, IL, ph 708-598-9010
60462, Cindy M. Howard, DC, 7714 W. 159th Street, Orland Park, IL, ph 708-429-5800
60462, Steven Zaeske, DC, 7714 W. 159th Street, Orland Park, IL, ph 708-429-5800
60465, Robert Pyne, DC, 10413 S. Roberts Road, Palos Hills, IL, ph 708-599-9585
60504, Tim Leasenby, DC, 4260 Westbrook Drive, Ste. 106, Aurora, IL, ph 630-851-9222

60521, Steven G. Ayre, MD, S.C., 322 Burr Ridge Pkwy, Burr Ridge, IL, ph 630-321-9010
60532, Delilah Anderson, DC, 2045 Burlington Ave, Lisle, IL, ph 630-960-9355
60559, Alvin C. Graun, DC, 6428 S. Cass Ave., Westmont, IL, ph 630-969-4240
60602, Alan F. Bain, DO, 111 N. Wabash Ave., Ste. 1005, Chicago, IL, ph 312-236-7010
60611, Judy Fulop, ND, MS, 680 N. Lake Shore Dr., #815, Chicago, IL, ph 312-926-DOCS
60612, Theodore Johnson, DC, 1615 West Warren Blvd., Chicago, IL, ph 312-773-6940
60614, David Edelberg, MD, 2522 N. Lincoln Ave., Chicago, IL, ph 773-296-6700
60614, Michelle Rogers, ND, 2300 Children's Plaza, Box 73, Chicago, IL, ph 773-327-9810
60623, Nicolas Martinez, DC, 3714 W. 26th Street, Chicago, IL, ph 773-277-2225
60641, Richard J. Dietzen, DC, 5545 W. Montrose Ave., Chicago, IL, ph 773-282-6648
60643, Hugh Jenkins, ND, DC, 9948 South Western Ave., Chicago, IL, ph 773-445-6800
60643, Jifunza Wright, MD, 1647 W. 105th Pl., Chicago, IL, ph 773-881-7191
60647, Rebecca Miki, ND, NSON, Lac, 1733 N. Milwaukee Ave., Chicago, IL, ph 773-278-8494
60914, Douglas Stam, DC, 396 N. Belle Aire, Bourvonnais, IL, ph 815-933-7391
60946, Thomas Stone, MD, 1374 E. 3700 N. Rd., Kempton, IL, ph 815-253-6332
61008, Oscar I. Ordonez, MD, 6413 Logan Ave., #104, Belvedere, IL, ph 815-547-8187
61021, Patricia Petrie, DC, 315 S. Peoria Ave., Dixon, IL, ph 815-288-3614
61073, Andrew Kong, DC, 5257 Swanson Rd., Ste. 2, Roscoe, IL, ph 815-397-8500
61073, Christopher Chalk, DC, 7505 Joy Lane, Roscoe, IL, ph 815-623-2690
61081, Harry W. Jensen, DC, 2002 East Fifth Street, Sterling, IL, ph 815-626-0270
61081, Thomas W. Jensen, DC, 2002 East Fifth Street, Sterling, IL, ph 815-626-0270
61252, Terry W. Love, DO, APCT, 2610-41st Street, Moline, IL, ph 309-764-2900
61548, Robert E. Thompson, MD, 205 S. Englewood Drive, Metamora, IL, ph 309-367-2321
61704, Chris Hoelscher, DC, 220 North Eldarado Road, Ste. B, Bloomington, IL, ph 309-662-8418
61832, W. Robert Elghammer, MD, 723 N. Logan Ave., Danville, IL, ph 217-446-3259
62301, Walter Barnes, MD, 3701 East Lake Centre Dr., #1, Quincy, IL, ph 217-224-3757
62450, Thomas E. Benson, MD, 1200 N. East St., Olney, IL, ph 618-395-5222
62650, Dennis Doyle, DC, 1521 D. West Walnut, Jacksonville, IL, ph 217-243-4333
62656, David Hepler, DC, P.O. Box 507, Lincoln, IL, ph 217-735-4451
62821, Rhonda J. Button, DC, 4 Smith St., Carmel, IL, ph 630-221-0881
63017, George A. Goodman, DC, 1851 Schoettler Road, Chesterfield, MO, ph 314-227-2100
63017, Mark Addante, DC, 936 Chesterfield Parkway East, Chesterfield, MO, ph 636-537-0564
63021, Duane Marquart, DC, 201 Enchanted Parkway, Manchester, MO, ph 314-227-4151
63033, Tipu Sultan, MD, 11585 West Florissant Ave., Florissant, MO, ph 314-921-5600
63040, Tracy Edelmann, DC, 16841 Manchester Road, Grover, MO, ph 636-658-9334
63127, Octavio R. Chirino, MD, 9701 Landmark Pkwy. Dr., #207, St. Louis, MO, ph 314-842-4802
63131, Katherine Conable, DC, 608 N. McKnight Road, St. Louis, MO, ph 314-991-5655
63132, Bert T. Hanicke, DC, 608 N. McKnight Road, St. Louis, MO, ph 314-991-5655
63132, Sandra G. Levy, DC, 608 N. McKnight Road, St. Louis, MO, ph 314-991-5655
63141, Lena R. Capapas, MD, BPCT, 522 N. New Ballas Rd., #334, St. Louis, MO, ph 314-995-9713
63141, Simon Yu, MD DPL, 11710 Old Ballas Rd. #205, St. Louis, MO, ph 314-432-7802
63143, Duane Lowe, DC, 7390 Flora Ave., Maplewood, MO, ph 618-256-7610
63146, Varsha Rathod, MD, 1977 Schuetz Rd., St. Louis, MO, ph 314-997-5403
63367, Jeffrey S. Ware, DC, 903 Locksley Manor Dr., Lake St. Louis, MO, ph 636-561-8302
63901, Carl E. Bosley, MD, Ph.D., 2503 Lucy Lee Pkwy., Poplar Bluff, MO, ph 573-785-5544
63901, Kimberly Wiseman, ND, 4807 West Blvd., Poplar Bluff, MO, ph 573-785-6177
64052, Bruce Stayton, MD, 2116 S. Sterling, Independence, MO, ph 816-836-5010
64052, Terry J. Nelson, DC, 10700 East Westport Rd., Ste. 300, Independence, MO, ph 816-933-1188
64055, Ray Vasquesz, DC, 19401 E. 40 Hwy #200, Independence, MO, ph 816-792-6633
64068, James W. Willoughby II, DO, 24 S. Main St., Liberty, MO, ph 816-781-0902
64068, James W. Willoughby, II, DO, 24 South Main St., Liberty, MO, ph 816-781-0902
64068, Mable M. Leckrone, DC, 257 W. Mill, Liberty, MO, ph 816-781-8810
64111, James L. Filberth, DC, 3626 Main Street, Kansas City, MO, ph 816-561-4444
64119, Charles Rudolph, DO, Ph.D., 2800-A Kendallwood Pkwy., Kansas City, MO, ph 816-453-5940
64119, Edward McDonagh, DO, 2800-A Kendallwood Pkwy., Kansas City, MO, ph 816-453-5940
65203, Bonnie Friehling, MD, 1511 Chapel Hill Road, Columbia, MO, ph 573-445-0100
65203, J. Scott Hays, DC, 1 East Broadway, Ste C-1, Columbia, MO, ph 573-443-7755
65233, Marcea Wiggins, ND, 2400 Boonslick Dr., Boonville, MO, ph 680-882-9840

65251, Raymond Ferre, DC, 760 South Franklin, Decatur, IL, ph 217-422-1097
65401, Jack Kessinger, DC, 1210 Hwy 72E, Rolla, MO, ph 573-341-8292
65775, Robert Wiehe, DC, 10734 CR 8070, West Plaines, MO, ph 417-256-2151
65803, Neil Nathan, MD, 2828 N. National, #D, Springfield, MO, ph 417-869-7583
65803, William Sunderwirth, DO, 2828 N. National Springfield, MO, ph 417-837-4158
65810, Wesley Delport, ND, 4323 S. National Avenue, Springfield, MO, ph 417-890-7400
66049, Deena Beneda-Khosh, ND, 4824 Quail Crest Pl., Lawrence, KS, ph 785-749-2255
66049, Farhang Khosh, ND, Lac, 4824 Quail Crest Place, Lawrence, KS, ph 787-749-2255
66049, Mehdi Khosh, ND, 4824 Quail Crest Place, Lawrence, KS, ph 787-749-2255
66062, Richard Snow, DC, 15370 S. Constance, Olathe, KS, ph 913-393-3711
66160, Jeanne A. Drisko, MD, BPCT, 3901 Rainbow Blvd., Kansas City, KS, ph 913-588-6208
66202, Mehdi Khosh, ND, 5509 Foxridge Dr., Mission, KS, ph 913-384-2284
66208, Stephanie Rasmussen, DC, 1900 W. 75th Street, Ste. 210, Prairie Village, KS, ph 913-677-4224
66214, David Dowling, DDS, 11644 W. 75th, #101, Shawnee, KS, ph 913-268-7077
66226, Michael Brown, NMD, 25707 W. 67th St., Shawnee, KS, ph 913-579-4437
66604, John Toth, MD, APCT, 2115 SW 10th, Topeka, KS, ph 785-232-3330
67203, Mark Alders, DC, 3305 West Central, Wichita, KS, ph 316-941-4555
67207, American Academy of Environmental Medicine, 7701 E. Kellogg, Ste. 625, Wichita, KS
67208, David Jernigan, DC, 545 N. Woodlan, Wichita, KS, ph 316-686-5900
67219, Janie Pimer, DC, 425 E. 61st N., Wichita, KS, ph 316-744-2001
67226, Melody J. Shubert, DC, 3101 North Roack Road, Ste. 100, Wichita, KS, ph 316-636-4444
67601, Roy N. Neil, MD, 105 West 13th, Hays, KS, ph 913-628-8341
67846, Terry Hunsberger, DO, 603 N. 5th Street, Garden City, KS, ph 316-275-3760
67864, H. M. Chalker, DC, 234 East Carthage, Box 757, Meade, KS, ph 316-873-2888
67901, Bob Sager, MD, 2330 N. Kansas Ave., Liberal, KS, ph 620-626-7080
68114, Jeffrey Passer, MD, 9300 Underwood Ave., Ste. 520, Omaha, NE, ph 402-398-1200
68124, James Murphy, DO, 8031 W. Center Rd., Ste. 221, Omaha, NE, ph 402-343-7963
68144, Eugene C. Oliveto, MD, 10804 Prairie Hills Dr., Omaha, NE, ph 402-392-0233
68713, Robert Randall, MD, P.O. Box 458, Atkinson, NE, ph 402-925-2811
68739, Steve Vlach, MD, 405 W. Darlene St., Hartington, NE, ph 402-254-3935
69101, Loretta Baca, MD, 302 s. Jeffers St., North Platte, NE, ph 877-534-6687
70001, Janet Perez-Chiesa, MD, BPCT, 4532 W. Napoleon Ave., #210, Metairie, LA, ph 504-456-7539
70002, Charles Mary, Jr., MD, 3813 N. Causeway Blvd., Ste. 200, Metairie, LA, ph 504-833-4338
70002, James Carter, MD DPL, 3501 Severn, Metairie, LA, ph 504-779-6363
70037, Lawrence A. Giambelluca, MD, 8200 Hwy. 23, Belle Chasse, LA, ph 504-398-1100
70043, Saroj T. Tampira, MD, 9000 Patricia St., Ste. 118, Chalmette, LA, ph 504-277-8991
70115, James P. Carter, MD, APCT, 2134 Napoleon Ave., New Orleans, LA, ph 504-779-6363
70123, Kashmir K. Rai, MD, BPCT, 824 Elmwood Park Blvd., #210, Harahan, LA, ph 504-818-2525
70461, James Fambro, MD, 303 Leeds Drive, Slidell, LA, ph 985-781-8248
70503, Sydney Crackower, MD, 701 Robley Dr., #100, Lafayette, LA, ph 337-988-4116
70506, Norman Dykes, MD, 501 W. Saint Mary Blvd., #308, Lafayette, LA, ph 337-234-1119
70508, Sangeeta Shah, MD, 211 E. Kaliste Saloom, Lafayette, LA, ph 337-235-1166
70809, Mark Cotter, MD, 5207 Essen Lane, Baton Rouge, LA, ph 225-766-3171
70810, Stephanie F. Cave, MD, BPCT, 10562 S. Glenstone Pl., Baton Rouge, LA, ph 225-767-7433
70835, Robert W. Smith, DC, P.O. Box 40362, Baton Rouge, LA, ph 225-272-7400
71303, James W. Welch, MD, 4300 Parliament Dr., Alexandria, LA, ph 318-448-0221
71913, Rheeta M. Stecker, MD, 2605 Albert Pike, Hot Springs, AR, ph 501-767-1144
71913, William L. Schmidt, DC, 316 St. Louis, Hot Springs, AR, ph 501-321-9081
72201, Norbert J. Becquet, MD, FACAM, APCT, 613 Main St., Little Rock, AR, ph 501-375-4419
72201, Richard Riley, DC, 1100 West 3rd Street, Little Rock, AR, ph 501-371-0022
72645, Melissa Taliaferro, MD DPL, 101 Cherry St., Leslie, AR, ph 870-447-2599
72745, G. Doty Murphy, MD, 326 N. Bloomington, Lowell, AR, ph 501-659-0111
72762, Jeffrey R. Baker, MD, 900 Dorman St., #E, Springdale, AR, ph 479-756-3251
73109, Richard B. Dawson, MD, FACS, 4805 S. Western Ave., Oklahoma City, OK, ph 405-636-1506
73112, Adam Merchant, MD, 3535 NW 58th Street, Oklahoma City, OK, ph 405-942-8346
73112, John Lee David, III, MD, 5701 N. Portland, Ste. 301, Oklahoma City, OK, ph 405-949-6484
73118, Charles D. Taylor, MD, APCT, 4409 Classen Blvd., Oklahoma City, OK, ph 405-525-7751
73160, Richard Santelli, DC, 1227 North Santa Fe, Moore, OK, ph 405-799-4436

74014, R. Jeff Wright, DO, 5050 E. Kenosha, Broken Arrow, OK, ph 918-496-5444
74037, Gerald Wootan, DO, BPCT, M.Ed., 715 W. Main St., #S, Jenks, OK, ph 918-299-9447
74037, Kent R. Bartell, DC, 121 South 2nd St., Jenks, OK, ph 918-298-8810
74037, Michael Leu, ND, R.Ph., 401 E. A Street, Jenks, OK, ph 918-298-9300
74135, Donald M. Dushay, DO, 4444 S. Harvard Ave., #100, Tulsa, OK, ph 918-744-0228
74135, Gerry D. Langston, DC, 4503 S. Harvard, Tulsa, OK, ph 918-747-5555
74135, Michael K. Taylor, DC, 3808 E. 51st Street, Tulsa, OK, ph 918-749-4657
74344, George Cole, DO, 240 East 3rd St., Grove, OK, ph 718-786-8746
74764, Ray E. Zimmer, DO, 602 N. Dalton, Valliant, OK, ph 580-933-4235
75032, Robert Gilbard, MD, 1604 Mariah Bay Circle, Heath, TX, ph 972-463-1744
75038, Frances J. Rose, MD, 1701 W. Walnut Hill, #200, Irving, TX, ph 972-594-1111
75056, Janie Duke, DC, 7204 Main St., #100, The Colony, TX, ph 469-384-5544
75057, Smart Idemudia, MD, Ph.D., 560 W. Main Street, #205, Lewisville, TX, ph 972-420-6777
75060, Ralph Burton, DC, 111 Delaware Street, Irving, TX, ph 972-438-9355
75075, Don Dunlap, DO, 5115 Teakwood Lane, #250, Plano, TX, ph 866-244-7246
75080, Alfred R. Johnson, DO, 101 S. Coit Road, Ste. 317, Richardson, TX, ph 972-479-0400
75086, Janie Dulce, DC, P.O. Box 860395, Plano, TX, ph 972-424-2225
75088, Robert J. Gilbard, MD, FACOG, 5429 Lakeview Pkwy., Rowlett, TX, ph 972-463-1744
75092, Danny Doty, DC, 2114 Jason Circle, Sherman, TX, ph 903-868-3829
75103, J. W. Dailey, MD, P.O. Drawer 788, Canton, TX, ph 903-567-1910
75201, Manuel Griego, Jr., DO, 700 N. Pearl, Ste. N-208, Dallas, TX, ph 214-999-9355
75225, Marina Johnson, MD, 8201 Preston Rd., #570, Dallas, TX, ph 214-739-2345
75229, Edward V. Brown, DC, 2500 Walnut Hill Lane, Dallas, TX, ph 214-352-7332
75230, June Maymand, DACBN, DC, 5925 Forest Lane, Ste. 126, Dallas, TX, ph 888-653-7229
75231, Richard G. Jaeckle, MD, 8220 Walnut Hill Lane, Ste. 404, Dallas, TX, ph 214-696-0964
75231, William J. Rea, MC, 8345 Walnut Hill Lane, Ste. 220, Dallas, TX, ph 214-368-4132
75231, Wm. Marcus Spurlock, MD, 8345 Walnut Hill Lane, Ste. 220, Dallas, TX, ph 214-368-4132
75244, George Cole, DO, 4141 Blue Lake Circle, #200, Dallas, TX, ph 972-851-0111
75244, Kenneth O'Neal, MD, 13612 Midway Rd., Suite 480, Dallas, TX, ph 972-661-8436
75460, Ballard Boren, DC, 3305 NE Loop 286, Paris, TX, ph 903-784-2111
75460, Gaylen Hayes, DO, 520 North Collegiate Dr., Paris, TX, ph 903-784-1608
75605, Patricia Sanders, MD, 472 E. Loop 281, Ste. B, Longview, TX, ph 903-236-0033
75956, John L. Sessions, DO, APCT, 1609 South Margaret, Kirbyville, TX, ph 409-423-2166
76012, R. E. Liverman, DO, 801 W. Road to Six Flags, #147, Arlington, TX, ph 817-461-7774
76017, Charles Hamel, MD, 4412 Matlock #300, Arlington, TX, ph 817-468-7755
76017, Virginia M. Thompson, DC, 5731 Champion Court, Arlington, TX, ph 214-350-1620
76021, Ken Cooper, DC, 2520 Harwood Road, Suite 200, Bedford, TX, ph 817-267-6222
76022, Howard J. Lang, DO, FAAEM, 1404 Brown Trail, Ste. D, Bedford, TX, ph 817-268-1171
76051, Constantine A. Kotsanis, MD, CCN, 1600 W. College, #260, Grapevine, TX, ph 817-481-6342
76054, Mary Ann Block, DO, 1750 Norwood Drive, Hurst, TX, ph 817-280-9933
76104, Gerald Harris, DO, BPCT, 1550 W. Rosedale St., #714, Fort Worth, TX, ph 817-336-4810
76104, Joseph F. McWherter, MD, BPCT, 1307 8th Ave., #207, Fort Worth, TX, ph 817-926-2511
76107, Barry L. Beaty, DO, 4455 Camp Bowie, #211, Fort Worth, TX, ph 817-737-6464
76107, Charles R. Hamel, MD, 4412 Matlock Rd., #300, Arlington, TX, ph 817-468-7755
76111, Ricardo Tan, MD, 3220 North Freeway, #106, Fort Worth, TX, ph 817-626-1993
76132, Karen Birdy, DO, 6431 Southwest Blvd., Fort Worth, TX, ph 817-737-3331
76308, Thomas Roger Humphrey, MD, 2400 Rushing, Wichita Falls, TX, ph 940-766-4329
76903, Benjamin Thurman, MD, 610 S. Abe Street, #A, San Angelo, TX, ph 915-481-0596
77005, Joe W. Lindley, DC, 3400 Bissonnet, Suite 220, Houston, TX, ph 713-660-0644
77005, R. G. Tannerya, MD, 2472 Bolsover, #363, Houston, TX, ph 713-807-8008
77027, Marina M. Pearsall, MD, Ph.D., 4126 Southwest Fwy., #1620, Houston, TX, ph 713-522-4037
77036, Alex Vasquex, DC, ND, 7211 Regency Square, Ste. 200, Houston, TX, ph 713-520-8765
77036, Gilbert Manso, MD, 7211 Regency Square Blvd., #200, Houston, TX, ph 713-840-9355
77055, Jerome L. Borochoff, MD, 8830 Long Point Rd., #504, Houston, TX, ph 713-461-7517
77055, Robert Battle, MD DPL, 9910 Long Point Rd., Houston, TX, ph 713-932-0552
77055, Robert M. Battle, MD, 9910 Long Point Road, Houston, TX, ph 713-932-0552
77057, Moe Kakvan, MD, APCT, 2909 Hillcroft, Ste. 250B, Houston, TX, ph 713-780-7019
77058, Dorothy Merritt, MD, 429 Bay Area Blvd., #429, Clear Lake, TX, ph 281-218-6700

77071, Stephen Joel Weiss, MD, 7907 Oakington Drive, Houston, TX, ph 713-691-0737
77089, Tim McCullough, DC, 11003 Resource Parkway, #103, Houston, TX, ph 281-481-9299
77090, William Glaros, DDS, 17222 Red Oak #101, Houston, TX, ph 281-440-1190
77338, John Trowbridge, MD DPL, 9816 Memorial Blvd., Humble, TX, ph 281-540-2329
77340, Frank O. McGehee, Jr., MD, BPCT, 1909-22nd Street, Huntsville, TX, ph 936-291-3351
77493, Stephanie Clay, 14015 Roland Road, Katy, TX, ph 281-371-0334
77536, Nikolas Hedberg, DC, 401 W. Pasadena Blvd. #824, Deer Park, TX, ph 281-478-5171
77581, Dorothy Merritt, MD, 3710 Broadway, Pearland, TX, ph 800-360-3382
77598, Donald E. Sprague, MD, MPH, 3 Professional Park Dr., Webster, TX, ph 281-554-8848
77904, Charles R. Mabray, MD, 115 Medical Drive, Ste. 202, Victoria, TX, ph 361-574-9697
77904, Rolando Arafiles, MD, 202 James Coleman Dr. #4, Victoria, TX, ph 361-570-3641
78028, Frank O. McGehee, Jr., MD, BPCT, 723 Hill Country Drive, Kerrville, TX, ph 830-896-0550
78064, Gerald Phillips, MD, 218 W. Goodwin Street, Pleasanton, TX, ph 210-569-2118
78217, Linda L. Welch, DO, 11312 Perrin Beitel, San Antonio, TX, ph 210-946-5633
78232, Doreen Lewis, DC, 1006 Central Parkway South, San Antonio, TX, ph 210-490-9169
78501, Michael R. Kilgore, MD, BPCT, 3600 N. 23rd, #201, McAllen, TX, ph 956-687-6196
78550, Robert R. Somerville, MD, 720 N. 77 Sunshine Strip, Harlingen, TX, ph 956-428-0757
78624, Dor W. Brown, MD, 205 West Windcrest, Ste. 340, Fredericksburg, TX, ph 830-997-2115
78746, Amy Neuzil, ND, 5524 Bee Caves Road, Ste. B-1, Austin, TX, ph 512-306-7344
78746, Ted Edwards, Jr., MD, 4201 Bee Caves Rd., #B-112, Austin, TX, ph 512-327-4886
78757, Vladimir Rizov, MD, BPCT, 911 W. Anderson Lane, #205, Austin, TX, ph 512-451-8149
78759, Robert R. Thoreson, DO, 11410 Jollyville Road, Ste. 3101, Austin, TX, ph 512-346-3634
79106, George Cole, DO, 2300 Bell Street, #20, Amarillo, TX, ph 806-379-7770
79109, Gerald Parker, DO, 4714 S. Western St., Amarillo, TX, ph 806-355-8263
79109, John T. Taylor, DO, 4714 S. Western, Amarillo, TX, ph 806-355-8263
79410, Rodney Franklin, MD, 3802 22nd Street #C, Lubbock, TX, ph 806-793-8963
79410, Sanford T. Ward, DO, 3719 22nd Street, Lubbock, TX, ph 806-795-4336
79413, Jim Reed, MD, 6400 Quaker Ave., Ste. B, Lubbock, TX, ph 806-792-8444
79720, Bruce E. Cox, MD, 710 S. Gregg St. #100, Big Spring, TX, ph 915-267-7411
79912, Francisco R. Soto, MD, 5862 Cromo Dr., Ste. 100, El Paso, TX, ph 800-621-8924
80014, Terry Grossman, MD, MD(H), APCT, 3150 S. Peoria St., #H, Aurora, CO, ph 303-338-1323
80026, Mary Louder, DO, 1000 W. South Boulder Rd. #226, Lafayette, CO, ph 303-604-4696
80030, Ron Rosedale, MD, APCT, P.O. Box 6278, Broomfield, CO, ph 303-530-5555
80033, Lee Patton, DC, 6650 West 44th Avenue, Wheatridge, CO, ph 303-422-2441
80110, Brian K. Wilson, DC, 3601 S. Broadway, Englewood, CO, ph 303-761-8349
80110, Cathlynn Nelson, DC, 3464 S. Downing St., Englewood, CO, ph 303-762-0626
80110, John Baer, DC, 3765 South Broadway, Engelwood, CO, ph 303-781-7825
80111, Susanna S. Choi, MD, 8200 E. Belleview, #240E, Greenwood Village, CO, ph 303-721-8117
80116, Reiner G. Kremer, DC, 7601 E. Burning Tree Dr. Ste. 100, Franktown, CO, ph 303-688-1111
80203, Brian A. Voytecek, DC, 3102 S. Parker Road, Unit A-3, Aurora, CO, ph 303-369-6555
80206, Kendall A. Gerdes, MD, Two Steel Street #200, Denver, CO, ph 303-377-8837
80209, James Rouse, ND, 3773 Cherry Creek Dr. N, Ste 760, Denver, CO, ph 303-322-9294
80212, Jenny Demeaux, RNC, ND, 3441 Tennyson St., Denver, CO, ph 303-433-5006
80224, Paula Dechert, DC, 2121 S. Oneida #626, Denver, CO, ph 303-756-5501
80231, Jacob Schor, ND, 1181 S. Parker Rd., Ste. 101, Denver, CO, ph 303-337-4884
80232, Lewis Holm, DC, 7596 West Jewell, Suite 302, Lakewood, CO, ph 303-980-1270
80301, JoHannah Reilly, ND, Lac, 2760 29th St., Suite 2E, Boulder, CO, ph 303-541-9600
80301, Kelly Parcell, ND, 2500 30th St., Ste. 200, Boulder, CO, ph 303-884-7557
80301, Mary Shackelton, ND, MPH, 2975 Valmont Rd., Ste. 100, Boulder, CO, ph 303-449-3777
80303, Michael Vamaria, DC, 2885 E. Aurora Ave., #28, Boulder, CO, ph 303-422-1656
80303, Robert Rountree, MD,d 4150 Darley Ave. #1, Boulder, CO, ph 303-499-9224
80303, Thomas Turner, DC, 4730 Table Mesa Drive, Ste. K, Boulder, CO, ph 303-494-1977
80304, Michael A. Zeligs, MD, BPCT, 1000 Alpine, #211, Boulder, CO, ph 303-442-5492
80304, Nancy Rao, ND, Rac, 1455 Yarmouth Ave., Ste. 112, Boulder, CO, ph 303-545-2021
80304, Timothy Binder, ND, DC, Lac, 875 Alpine Ave. #1, Boulder, CO, ph 303-440-6928
80308, Linda Li, DC, P.O. Box 20990, Boulder, CO, ph 303-443-1342
80401, Stephen Parcell, ND, 2801 Youngfield St., #117, Lakewood, CO, ph 303-233-4247
80401, Terry Grossman, MD, MD(H), APCT, 2801 Youngfield St., #117, Denver, CO, ph 303-233-4247

80503, Darryl Hobson, DC, 6644 Birdcliff Way, Niwot, CO, ph 303-652-6475
80503, Deborah Belote, DC, 6644 BirdCliff Way, Longmont, CO, ph 303-652-6475
80513, William Kleber, DC, 907 Mountain Ave., Berthoud, CO, ph 970-532-2755
80522, Melanie Pisarek-Tiahrt, DC, P.O. Box 1267, Fort Collins, CO, ph 303-756-5501
80522, Melanie Tiahrt, DC, P.O. Box 1267, Fort Collins, CO, ph 970-472-6263
80524, Robert M. Conlon, MD, 1032 Luke Street, Fort Collins, CO, ph 970-484-8686
80524, Roger Billica, MD, 1020 Luke Street, #A, Fort Collins, CO, ph 970-495-0999
80525, Mark Kelley, 209 East Swallow Rd., Fort Collins, CO, ph 970-223-7425
80903, Deborah J. Riekman, DC, 213 E. Cache La Poudre, Colorado Springs, CO, ph 719-630-7335
80903, Steven L. Lokken, DC, 815 East Platte Ave., Colorado Springs, CO, ph 719-633-8112
80904, Mark Cooper, ND, Lac, 1420 S. 21st St., Colorado Springs, CO, ph 719-471-8411
80909, Terry P. Collinson, DC, 2590 Palmer Park Blvd., Colorado Springs, CO, ph 719-475-2345
80917, George Juetersonke, DO, APCT, 3525 American Dr., Colorado Springs, CO, ph 719-597-6075
80918, Joel Klein, MD, 5455 N. Union Blvd., #201, Colorado Springs, CO, ph 719-457-0330
81006, David Walters, DO, 2403 Santa Fe Dr., #7, Pueblo, CO, ph 719-543-7894
81082, Lawrence Low, DC, 165 East First Street, Trinidad, CO, ph 719-846-4990
81301, Ronald E. Wheeler, MD, 2901 Main Ave., Durango CO, ph 970-259-4081
81401, Judith Boice, ND, Lac, 1008 West Oak Grove Rd., Montrose, CO, ph 970-252-0985
81501, Joseph M. Wezensky, MD, 2650 North Ave., Ste. 101, Grand Junction, CO, ph 970-263-4660
81611, Rob Krakovitz, MD, 430 W. Main Street, Aspen, CO, ph 970-927-4394
82601, Dennis Wicks, MD, 802 South Durbin St., Casper, WY, ph 307-234-4444
82718, Rebecca Painter, MD, APCT, 201 West Lakeway, Ste. 300, Gillette, WY, ph 307-682-0330
82901, A. L. Barrier, MD, FAAO-HNS, 430 Broadway, Rock Springs, WY, ph 307-362-8221
83001, Monique Lai, ND, 280 E. Broadway, #802, Jackson, WY, 83001, ph 307-734-6644
83638, Uma Mulnick, DC, P.O. Box 1005, McCall, ID, ph 208-634-8129
83651, Stephen Thornburgh, Do, APCT, 824 – 17th Ave. So., Nampa, ID, ph 208-466-3517
83864, Douglas Mackay, ND, 515 Pine St., Ste. H, Sandpoint, ID, ph 208-263-2399
83864, Gabrielle Duebendorfer, ND, 120 E. Lake Str., Ste. 201, Sandpoint, ID, ph 208-265-2213
83864, Keri Marshall, ND, 515 Pine St., Ste. H, Sandpoint, ID, ph 208-263-2399
84004, Dianne Farley-Jones, MD, 70 E. Red Pine Drive, Alpine, UT, ph 801-756-9444
84020, Dennis Harper, DO, BPCT, 12226 S. 1000 East, #10, Draper, UT, ph 801-501-9797
84065, William J. Mauer, DO DPL, 1733 W. 12600 S., #418, Riverton, UT, ph 801-509-2384
84604, Dennis W. Remington, MD, 1675 N. Freedom Blvd., Ste. 11E, Provo, UT, ph 801-373-8500
85012, Julie Gorman, NMD, Lac, 219 E. Lexington Ave., Phoenix, AZ, ph 602-265-1774
85014, Dana Keaton, ND, 5333 N. 7th St., Ste. 221, Phoenix, AZ, ph 602-266-4670
85015, Edward C. Kondrot, MD, 2001 W. Camelback Rd., #150, Phoenix, AZ, ph 602-347-7950
85018, Geoffrey Radoff, MD(H), 2525 W. Greenway Rd., #210, Phoenix, AZ, ph 602-993-0200
85018, Stanley R. Olsztyn, MD(H), 4350 E. Camelback Rd., #B-220, Phoenix, AZ, ph 602-840-8424
85022, Bruce H. Shelton, MD(H), BPCT, 14231 N. 7th Street, #A2, Phoenix, AZ, ph 602-504-1000
85028, Envita Natural Medical Centers of America, 4614 E. Sheat Blvd. #D160, Phoeniz, AZ 85028
85032, Jonathan Psenka, ND, 13832 N. 32nd St., Suite 12, Phoenix, AZ, ph 602-493-2273
85032, Konrad Kail, ND, PA-C, 13832 N. 32nd St., C2-4, Phoenix, AZ, ph 602-493-2273
85032, Warren M. Levin, 13832 N. 32nd St., Ste. 126, Phoenix, AZ, ph 602-493-2273
85202, Eric Hampton, NMD, 2058 S. Dobson Road, #11-A, Mesa, AZ, ph 480-831-7970
85203, Charles D. Schwengel, DO, MD(H), 1215 E. Brown Road, #12, Mesa, AZ, ph 480-668-1448
85206, Thomas J. Grade, MD, 6309 E. Baywood Ave., Mesa, AZ, ph 480-325-3801
85206, William W. Halcomb, Do, MD, 4323 E. Broadway, #109, Mesa, AZ, ph 602-832-3014
85224, Jeffrey Kush, DC, 1200 North Arizona Ave. #3, Chanler, AZ, ph 602-899-8836
85233, Gladys Ceballos-Logan, ND, 1757 E. Baseline Rd. Bldg. 9, Gilbert, AZ, ph 480-503-4325
85253, Alan K. Ketover, MD, 10595 N. Tatum Blvd., #E-146, Paradise Valley, AZ, ph 602-381-0800
85258, Cheryl Deroin, NMD, 8390 E. Vie De Ventura, Ste. F-11, Scottsdale, AZ, ph 480-951-0111
85258, Sam J. Walters, NMD, Ph.D., 8070 E. Morgan Trail, #125, Scottsdale, AZ, ph 480-946-9222
85260, Alan Christianson, NMD, 9200 East Raintree Ste. 100, Scottsdale, AZ, ph 480-657-0003
85260, Gordon H. Josephs, DO, MD(H), APCT, 7315 E. Evans Rd., Scottsdale, AZ, ph 480-998-9232
85260, Stuart Z. Lanson, MD, MD(H), 8406 E. Shea Blvd. #100, Scottsdale, AZ, ph 480-994-9512
85282, Paul Conyette, NMD, 226-2035 Elm St. South, Tempe, AZ, ph 480-968-7323
85282, Stephen Messer, ND, DHANP, 2140 E. Broadway Rd., Tempe, AZ, ph 480-858-9100
85308, Lloyd Arnold, DO, MD(H), APCT, 7200 W. Bell Rd., G-103, Glendale, AZ, ph 623-939-8916

85321, Patrick Mulcahy, DO, 410 N. Malacate, Ajo AZ, ph 520-387-5706
85331, Frank W. George, DO, MD(H), 6748 E. Lone Mountain Rd., Cave Creek, AZ, ph 480-595-5508
85344, Jeff A. Baird, DO, BPCT, 1413 – 16th St., Parker, AZ, ph 928-669-9229
85364, Ellis Browning, MD, 1150 W. 24th St., Yuma, AZ, ph 520-782-3819
85382, Timothy Gerhart, DC, 26427 IV 88th Ave., Peoria, AZ, ph 623-229-3919
85383, Kellie M. Gray, DC, 24022 North 79th Drive, Peoria, AZ, ph 602-439-4056
85541, Garry F. Gordon, MD, DO, 708 E. Hwy., 260, Bldg. C-1, #F, Payson, AZ, ph 928-472-4263
85614, Bryan T. McConnell, ND, 170 N. La Canada #90, Green Valley, AZ, ph 520-399-9212
85701, Gayle M. Randall, MD, 428 S. 3rd Ave., Tucson, AZ, ph 888-294-2528
85704, Bruce Sadilek, ND, 268 East River Rd., Ste. 130, Tucson, AZ, ph 520-297-9664
85704, David C. Rupley, Jr., MD, 5813 N. Oracle Rd., Tucson, AZ, ph 520-293-3751
85712, Dennis D. Best, NMD, 3956 E. Pima Street, Tucson, AZ, ph 520-326-7566
85716, Jorge Cochran, ND, 1601 North Tuscan Blvd., Ste. 37, Tucson, AZ, ph 520-322-8122
85716, Lance Morris, ND, BA, 1601 N. Tucson Blvd., Ste. 37, Tucson, AZ, ph 520-322-8122
85737, R. Michael Cessna, DC, 13401 N. Rancho Vistoso Blvd., Tucson, AZ, ph 520-544-7636
85749, Michael Stone, DC, 9100 E. Tanque Verde Road #140, Tucson, AZ, ph 520-749-2929
85750, Alexander P. Cadoux, MD(H), APCT, 6884 E. Sunrise Dr. #160, Tucson, AZ, ph 520-529-9665
85901, William W. Halcomb, DO, MD, 2000 N. 16th Ave., Show Low, AZ, ph 602-832-3014
86001, Marnie Vail, MD, BPCT, 702 North Beaver St., Flagstaff, AZ, ph 928-214-9774
86305, Robert Zieve, MD, 1000 Ainsworth Dr. #C-310, Prescott, AZ, ph 928-778-3500
86336, Annemarie S. Welch, MD, 2301 W. Hwy 89A, #104, Sedona, AZ, ph 928-282-0609
86336, Lester Adler, MD, 40 Soldiers Pass Rd., #12, Sedona, AZ, ph 928-282-2520
86336, Mark E. Laursen, MD, 150 Thunderbird Drive, Sedona, AZ, ph 520-204-0023
86403, M. Murray, ND, MA, MST, 1960-D Mesquite Ave., Lake Havasu City, AZ, ph 928-854-8448
87108, Regina De Pelichy, DC, 615 Ortiz Dr. NE, Albuquerque, NM, ph 505-266-0297
87112, Ralph J. Luciani, DO, 10601 Lomas Blvd. NE #103, Albuquerque, NM, ph 505-298-5995
87501, W. A. Shreader, Jr., MD, 141 Paseo de Peralta, Santa Fe, NM, ph 505-983-8890
33907, Dean Silver, MD, 4650 South Cleveland Ave., #e-A, Fort Myers, FL, ph 239-939-4700
87501, W.A. Shrader, Jr., MD, 141 Paseo de Peralta, Ste. A, Santa Fe, NM, ph 505-983-8890
87504, Shirley B. Scott, MD, P.O. Box 2670, Santa Fe, NM, ph 505-986-9960
87507, Erica M. Elliott, MD, 2300 W. Alameda, Ste. A2, Santa Fe, NM, ph 505-471-8531
87544, Jacqueline A. Krohn, MD, MPH, 3917 West Rd., Ste. 136, Los Alamos, NM, ph 505-662-9620
87701, Catherine Stauber, ND, DHANP, 2002 Hot Springs Blvd., Las Vegas, NM, ph 505-454-9525
88011, Burton M. Berkson, MD, Ph.D., 1155-C Commerce Dr., Las Cruces, NM, ph 505-524-3720
88012, Wolfgang Haese, MD, DTM, 2465 Bataan Memorial West, Las Cruces, NM, ph 505-373-8415
88801, Eddie L. Gaines, MD, 2100 Triviz Dr., Ste. A, Las Cruces, NM, ph 505-522-6500
89014, Dan F. Royal, DO, 2501 N. Green Valley Pkwy., #D-132, Henderson, NV, ph 702-433-8800
89102, Steven G. Holper, MD, 3233 W. Charleston, #202, Las Vegas, NV, ph 702-878-3510
89104, Adelaida Resuello, MD, 1300 S. Maryland Pkwy., Las Vegas, NV, ph 702-385-2691
89106, Robert D. Milne, MD, 2110 Pinto Lane, Las Vegas, NV, ph 702-385-1393
89108, Carol L. Barlow, MD, HMD, M.S., 3280 N. Rainbow Blvd., Las Vegas, NV, ph 702-731-3117
89121, F. Fuller Royal, MD, 3663 Pecos McLeod, Las Vegas, NV, ph 702-732-1400
89451, Christina Campbell, ND, DC, 889 Alder Ave., Ste. 202, Incline Village, NV, ph 775-831-3200
89500, Corazon I. Ibarra, MD, 6490 S. McCarran Blvd. D-41, Reno, NV, ph 775-827-6696
89509, David A. Edwards, MD, HMD, 6490 S. McCarran Blvd., Reno, NV, ph 775-828-4055
89509, Katrina Tang, MD, 380 Brinkby Ave., Reno, NV, ph 775-826-9500
89509, Michael L. Gerber, MD, APCT, 3670 Grant Dr., #101, Reno, NV, ph 775-826-1900
89509, W. Douglas Brodie, MD, HMD, 6110 Plumas St. #B, Reno, NV, ph 775-829-1009
89511, David A. Edwards, MD, APCT, 615 Sierra Rose Drive, #3, Reno, NV, ph 775-828-4055
89703, Frank Shallenberger, MD, HMD, 896 W. Nye Lane, #103, Carson City, NV, ph 775-884-3990
90025, Michael Galitzer, MD, 12381 Wilshire Blvd., #102, Los Angeles, CA, ph 310-820-6042
90028, James Julian, MD, 1654 Cahuenga Blvd., Hollywood, CA, ph 323-467-5555
90046, Victoria Batsian, Ph.D., CCN, 7315 W. Sunset Blvd. A-1, Los Angeles, CA, ph 323-512-0100
90064, Hans D. Gruenn, MD, BPCT, 2211 Corinth Ave., #204, Los Angeles, CA, ph 310-966-9194
90064, Huy Hoang, MD, 11695 National Blvd., Los Angeles, CA, ph 310-479-2266
90064, Murray Susser, MD, APCT, 2211 Corinth Ave. #204, Los Angeles, CA, ph 310-966-9194
90066, Karima Hirani, MD, 12732-B W. Washington Blvd., Los Angeles, CA, ph 310-577-0753
90211, Cathie-Ann Lippman, MD, 291 S. La Cienega Bl., Ste. 207, Beverly Hills, CA, ph 310-289-8430

90265, Deborah Banker, MD, 23852 Pacific Coast Hwy., Malibu, CA, ph 310-317-2119
90265, William Rader, MD, 22619 Pacific Coast Hwy. #125, Malibu, CA, ph 310-455-5300
90403, Joseph Sciabbarrasi, MD, 1821 Wilshire Blvd., #400, Santa Monica, CA, ph 310-828-4175
90403, Keith De Orio, MD, 1821 Wilshire Blvd., Suite 100, Santa Monica, CA, ph 310-828-4480
90405, Marianna Fisher, ND, 2210 Main St., Ste. 100, Santa Monica, CA, ph 310-890-0980
90501, Arlan Cage, ND, M.S., 2204 Torrence Blvd., 104B, Torrence, CA, ph 310-803-8803
90501, Suzanne M. Skinner, Ph.D., 2215 Torrance Blvd., #203, Torrance CA, ph 310-320-1381
90804, H. Richard Casdorph, MD, Ph.D., 1703 Termino Ave., #201, Long Beach, CA, ph 562-597-8716
91010, Paddy Jim Baggot, MD, 931 Buena Vista #301, Duarte, CA, ph 626-358-8045
91101, Ayad Alanizi, MD, FRCS, 127 N. Madison #106, Pasadena, CA, ph 626-766-9018
91101, Kathleen Power, DC, 151 So. El Molina Ave., Ste. 301, Pasadena, CA, ph 626-793-7161
91105, Maria Sulindro, MD, BPCT, 1017 S. Fair Oaks Ave., Pasadena, CA, ph 626-4093-9000
91201, Abraham Maissian, MD, BPCT, 1737 W. Glenoaks Blvd., Glendale, CA, ph 818-243-1186
91204, Jung-Sook Sue Johnson, MD, FCCP, 1510 S. Central Ave., Glendale, CA, ph 818-244-0112
91316, Ilona Abraham, MD, APCT, 17815 Ventura Blvd. Ste. 111, 113, Encino, CA, ph 818-345-8721
91320, Jay Dhawan, ND, 3533 Old Conejo Rd., Newbury Park, CA, ph 805-446-6184
91320, Jeff Sherman, MH, 3525 Old Conejo Rd., Ste. 119, Newbury Park, CA, ph 877-437-2757
91345, Sion Nobel, MD, 10306 N. Sepulveda Blvd., Mission Hills, CA, ph 818-361-0115
91361, Melissa Metcalfe, ND, 870 E. Hampshire Rd., Suite E, Westlake Village, CA, ph 805-374-7363
91364, Dean Bowman, DC, 19963 Ventura Blvd., Woodland Hills, CA, ph 818-340-8950
91501, Maxwell Cotter, MD, 500 E. Olive Ave., #102, Burbank, CA, ph 818-843-2415
91505, Douglas Hunt, MD, 3808 Riverside Dr., #510, Burbank, CA, ph 818-566-9889
91505, Nancy T. Mullan, MD, 2829 West Burbank Blvd., #202, Burbank, CA, ph 818-954-9267
91506, David J. Edwards, MD, 2202 W. Magnolia, Burbank, CA, ph 818-842-4184
91602, Salvacion Lee, MD, 11336 Camarillo St., #305, West Toluca Lake, CA, ph 818-505-1574
91604, Charles Law, Jr., MD, 3959 Laurel Canyon Blvd., Ste. I, Studio City, CA, ph 818-761-1661
91605, Christine Daniel, MD, 12650 Sherman Way, #4, N. Hollywood, CA, ph 818-982-8062
91702, William C. Bryce, MD, DO, Ph.D., 400 N. San Gabriel Ave., Azusa, CA, ph 626-334-1407
91723, James Privitera, MD, 256 W. San Bernardino Ave., Covina, CA, ph 626-966-1618
91741, N. Rowan Richards, DC, 242 S. Glendora Ave., Glendora, CA, ph 626-963-1678
91765, Hitendra Shah, MD, 23341 Golden Springs Dr., #208, Diamond Bar, CA, ph 909-860-2610
91786, Bryan P. Chan, MD, BPCT, 1148 San Bernardino Rd., #E-102, Upland, CA, ph 909-920-3578
91935, David Getoff, CCN, CNC, Box 803, Jamul, CA, ph 619-468-6846
92021, David A. Howe, MD, BPCT, 505 N. Mollison Ave., #103, El Cajon, CA, ph 619-440-3838
92021, Neil W. Hirschenbein, MD, Ph.D., 1685 E. Main St., #301, El Cajon, CA, ph 619-579-8681
92024, Mark Drucker, MD, 4403 Manchester Ave., #107, Encinitas, CA, ph 760-632-9042
92025, Aline Fournier, DO, 307 S. Ivy, Escondido, CA, ph 760-746-1133
92025, Ratibor Pantovich, DO, 560 E. Valley Pkwy., Escondido, CA, ph 760-480-2880
92037, Charles Moss, MD, BPCT, 8950 Villa La Jolla, #A217, La Jolla, CA, ph 858-457-1314
92083, Les Breitman, MD, BPCT, 2023 W. Vista Way, Ste. F, Vista, CA, ph 760-414-9955
92101, Antonio Jimenez, MD, Ave. del Pacifico #650, San Diego, CA, ph 619-572-5119
92109, James Novak, MD, 4440 Lamont Street, San Diego, CA, ph 858-272-0022
92122, Neil W. Hirschenbein, MD, Ph.D., 9339 Genesee Ave., #150, San Diego, CA, ph 858-713-9401
92128, Tracy Tranchitella, ND, 11770 Bernardo Plaza Ct., #206, San Diego, CA, ph 866-222-2838
92201, Robert Harmon, MD, 41-800 Washington St., #110, Indio, CA, ph 619-345-2696
92211, Robert Neal Rouzier, MD, 77564B Country Club Dr., #320, Palm Desert, CA, ph 760-772-8883
92262, Neal Rouzier, MD, 2825 Tahquitz Canyon Way, Palm Springs, CA 92262, ph 760-320-4292
92262, Priscilla A. Slagle, MD, 946 Avenida Palos Verdes, Palm Springs, CA, ph 760-323-4259
92262, Robert Neal Rouzier, MD, 2825 Tahquitz Canyon, Ste. 200, Palm Springs, CA, ph 760-320-4292
92374, Felix Prakasam, MD, 2048 Orange Tree Lane, Redlands, CA, ph 909-798-1614
92504, Andrew Lucas, DC, 5893 Grand Ave., Riverside, CA, ph 909-683-0809
92583, Hitendra Shah, MD, 229 West 7th Street, Hemet, CA, ph 909-487-2550
92618, Allan E. Sosin, MD, APCT, 16100 Sand Canyon Ave., #240, Irvine, CA, ph 949-753-8889
92618, Ronald Wempen, MD, BPCT, 14795 Jeffrey Rd., Ste. 101, Irvine, CA, ph 949-551-8751
92627, Andrea Purcell, ND, 1831 Orange Ave., B, Costa Mesa, CA, ph 949-903-0904
92630, Michael Grossman, MD, 24432 Muirlands Blvd., #111, Lake Forest, CA, ph 949-770-7301
92646, Francis Foo, MD, 10188 Adams Ave., Huntington Beach, CA, ph 714-968-3266
92653, Robert Abell, ND, Lac, 24953 Paseo De Valencia, 16C, Laguna Hills, CA, ph 949-206-9090

92660, Julian Whitaker, MD, APCT, 4321 Birch St., Ste. 100, Newport Beach, CA, ph 949-851-1550
92677, Joseph A. Ferreira, MD, 23 Redondo, Laguna Niguel, CA, ph 949-249-2058
92691, Duke D. Kim, MD, 27800 Medical Center Rd., Ste. 116, Mission Viejo, CA, ph 949-364-6040
92705, Catherine Arvantely, MD, 1820 E. Garry, #116, Santa Ana, CA, ph 949-660-1399
92708, Allen Green, MD, 18153 Brookhurst St., Fountain Valley, CA, ph 714-378-5656
92708, Rosemarie Melchor, MD, 11190 Warner Ave., Ste. 411, Fountain Valley, CA, ph 714-751-5800
92780, Allan Harvey Lane, MD, BPCT, 12581 Newport Ave., Ste. B, Tustin, CA, ph 714-544-9544
92780, Leigh Erin Connealy, MD, 14642 Newport Ave., #200, Tustin, CA, ph 714-669-4446
92780, Stephanie Mason, MD, 14642 Newport Ave., #200, Tustin, CA, ph 714-669-4446
92866, Gary Peralta Ruelas, DO, 1509 East Chapman Ave., Orange, CA, ph 714-771-2880
93018, James L. Kwako, MD, 1805-D East Cabrillo Blvd., Santa Barbara, CA, ph 805-565-3959
93101, Lisa Stanich, ND, Lac, 34 East Sola St., Santa Barbara, CA, ph 805-452-2908
93103, Bob Young, MD, BPCT, 119 North Milpas, Santa Barbara, CA, ph 805-963-1824
93105, Kenneth J. Frank, MD, 3463 State St. #263, Santa Barbara, CA, ph 805-683-1248
93309, Shivinder S. Deol, MD, 4000 Stockdale Hwy., Ste. D, Bakersfield, CA, ph 661-325-7452
93401, Peter Muran, MD, MBA, 1241 Johnson Ave., Ste. 354, San Luis Obispo, CA, ph 888-315-4777
93401, Zoe Wells, ND, 1439 Marsh St., San Luis Obispo, CA, ph 805-541-2614
93422, Carmelo A. Plateroti, DO, BPCT, 6895 Morro Road, Atascadero, CA, ph 805 462-2262
93465, Richard A. Hendricks, MD, 1050 Las Tablas Rd., Templeton, CA, ph 805-434-1836
93611, John Nelson, MD, 684 Medical Center Dr. E, #106, Clovis, CA, ph 559-299-0224
93720, Patrick A. Golden, MD, APCT, 1187 E. Herndon, #101, Fresno, CA, ph 559-432-0716
93727, David J. Edwards, MD, 360 S. Clovis Ave., Fresno, CA, ph 559-251-5066
93901, Vanessa da Silva, 11 Maple St., Ste. A, Salinas, CA, ph 831-262-4972
93923, Denise Mark, MD, APCT, 26335 Carmel Rancho Blvd., #8, Carmel, CA, ph 831-625-9999
93923, Gerald Wyker, MD, 25530 Rio Vista Dr., Carmel, CA, ph 831-625-0911
93924, Howard Press, MD, 13748 Center St. #B, Carmel Valley< CA, ph 831-659-5373
93933, Olga McVay, ND, 350 Reservation Rd., Marina, CA, ph 831-277-9856
93940, Audra Foster, ND, 1010 Cass St., Ste. D8, Monterey, CA, ph 831-373-0141
93940, Howard Press, MD, 172 Eldorado Street, Monterey, CA, ph 831-373-1551
94022, D. Graeme Shaw, MD, 5050 El Camino Real, #110, Los Altos, CA, ph 650-964-6700
94022, F. T. Guilford, MD, 5050 El Camino Real, #110, Los Altos, CA, ph 650-964-6700
94022, Raj Patel, MD, 5050 El Camino Real, #110, Los Altos, CA, ph 650-964-6700
94022, Robert F. Cathcart III, MD, 127 Second St., Ste. 4, Los Altos, CA, ph 650-949-2822
94024, Deborah A. Metzger, MD, Ph.D., 851 Fremont Ave. #104, Los Altos, CA, ph 650-229-1010
94040, William M. Buchholz, MD, 1174 Castro St., Ste. 275, Mountain View, CA, ph 650-988-8011
94102, Gary Ross, MD, 500 Sutter, #300, San Francisco, CA, ph 415-398-0555
94107, Carl Hangee-Bauer, ND, Lac, 1615 20th St., San Francisco, CA, ph 415-643-6600
94127, Joel F. Lopez, MD, ND, 345 W. Portal Ave. 2nd Fl., San Francisco, CA, ph 415-566-1000
94127, Paul Lynn, MD, APCT, 345 W. Portal Ave., 2nd Fl., San Francisco, CA, ph 415-566-1000
94133, Wai-Man Ma, MD, BPCT, 728 Pacific Ave., #611, San Francisco, CA, ph 415-397-3888
94301, Bryan Skinner, 359 Middlefield Rd., Palo Alto, CA, ph 650-323-7345
94301, Destia Skinner, ND, 359 Middlefield Rd., Palo Alto, CA, ph 650-323-7345
94306, Connie Hernandez, ND, 4153-B El Camino Way, Palo Alto, CA, ph 650-857-0226
94401, Kimberly Burke, Lac, OMD, 53 N. San Mateo Dr., B, San Mateo, CA, ph 650-348-2764
94401, Nicholas J. All, DC, 53 N. San Mateo Dr., B, San Mateo, CA, ph 650-348-2764
94404, Bruce Wapen, MD, 969-G Edgewater Blvd., #807, Foster City, CA, ph 650-577-8635
94520, John Toth, MD, APCT, 2299 Bacon St., #10, Concord, CA, ph 925-687-9447
94520, Tara Levy, ND, 2342 Almond Ave., Concord, CA, ph 925-602-0582
94526, Kirk Youngman, DMD, 520 Lagonda Way, #103, Danville, CA, ph 925-837-3101
94550, Geraldine P. Donaldson, MD, 1548 Holmes St. Bldg. D, Livermore, CA, ph 925-443-8282
94558, Eleanor Hynote, MD, 935 Trancas Street, Ste. 1A, Napa, CA, ph 707-255-4172
94558, Moses Goldberg, 935 Trancas St., Ste. 1A, Napa, CA, ph 707-255-4172
94583, Richard Gracer, MD, 5401 Norris Canyon Rd., #102, San Ramon, CA, ph 925-277-1100
94588, Lynne Mielke, MD, 4463 Stoneridge Dr., #A, Pleasanton, CA, ph 925-846-6300
94588, Mason Shen, Ph.D., LAC, OMD, 3510-D Old Santa Rita Rd., Pleasanton, CA, ph 925-847-8889
94609, Dennid D. Lee, Lac, 411-30th St., #302, Oakland, CA, ph 510-832-4372
94901, Jeffrey I. Friedman, DC, 711 D Street, Suite 104, San Rafael, CA, ph 415-459-4646
95008, Denise Tarasuk, ND, BSN, 51 E. Campbell Ave., Campbell, CA, ph 408-370-5291

95032, Andrew Scott Cook, MD, 15055 Los Gatos Blvd., Ste. 250, Los Gatos, CA, ph 408-358-2511

95032, Phillip Lee Miller, MD, 15215 National Ave., #103, Los Gatos, CA, ph 408-358-8855

95032, Tanya Baldwin, ND, 777 Knowles Dr., Suite 6B, Los Gatos, CA, ph 408-379-7397

95050, Cathy A. Joseph, DC, 1265 El Camino Real, Ste. 101, Santa Clara, CA, ph 408-248-8392

95050, W. Richard Kidd, DC, 1265 El Camino Real, Ste. 101, Santa Clara, CA, ph 408-248-8392

95060, Ruth Bar-Shalom, ND, Lac, 406 Mission Street, Santa Cruz, CA, ph 831-423-4300

95062, Ileana Tecchio, ND, 526 Soquel Ave., Ste. A, Santa Cruz, CA, ph 831-566-5712

95070, John C. Wakefield, MD, 18988 Cox Ave. Ste. D, Saratoga, CA, ph 408-366-0660

95124, Judy Lee, ND, 3880 S. Bascom Ave., Ste. 113, San Jose, CA, ph 408-377-9555

95139, Effie Mae Buckley, RN, 7174 Santa Teresa Blvd., Ste. A-6, San Jose, CA, ph 408-363-1498

95350, Christine G. Tazewell, MD, 1524 McHenry Ave., #310, Modesto, CA, ph 209-575-4700

95403, Moses Goldberg, ND, 175 Concourse Blvd., Santa Rosa, CA, ph 707-284-9200

95403, Terri Su, MD, 2200 County Center Dr., Ste. H, Santa Rosa, CA, ph 707-571-7560

95404, Robert Rowen, MD, 95 Montgomery Dr. #220, Santa Rosa, CA, ph 707-571-7560

95472, Norman Zucker, MD, 2405 Burnside Rd., Sebastopol, CA, ph 707-823-6116

95482, Lawrence G. Foster, MD, 230 Hospital Drive, #B, Ukiah, CA, ph 707-463-3502

95519, Evonne Barret Phillips, DC, 2720 Central Ave. Suite F, McKinleyville, CA, ph 707-839-7753

95521, Jan Dooley, DC, 912 Tenth Street, Arcata, CA, ph 707-822-9177

95608, Bernard McGinity, MD, 6945 Fair Oaks Blvd., Carmichael, CA, ph 916-485-4556

95608, Philip J. Reilly, MD, 4800 Manzanita Ave., #17, Carmichael, CA, ph 916-488-9524

95657, Donald Ray Whitaker, DO, 210 E. Elizabeth St., Jefferson, TX, ph 903-665-7781

95816, Ernest Johnson, MD, 3810 J St., Sacramento, CA, ph 916-736-3399

95825, Michael Kwiker, DO, 3301 Alta Arden, Ste. 3, Sacramento, CA, ph 916-489-4400

96013, Charles K. Dahlgren, MD, 37491 Enterprise Dr., #C, Burney, CA, ph 530-335-3833

96727, Connie Hernandez, ND, P.O. Box 510, Honokaa, HI, ph 808-775-1505

96740, Michael Traub, ND, 75-5759 Kuakini Hwy. #202, Kailua-Kona, HI, ph 808-329-2114

96741, Thomas R. Yarema, MD, BPCT, 4504 Kukui St., #13, Kapaa, Kauai, HI, ph 808-823-0994

96750, Clif Arrington, MD, P.O. Box 649, Kealakekua, HI, ph 808-322-9400

96755, Alan D. Thal, MD, P.O. Box 879, Kapaau, HI, ph 808-889-0770

96795, Jack Burke, ND, DHANP, Lac, 41-044 Aloiloi St., Waimanalo, HI, ph 808-259-6889

96813, Federick Lam, MD, APCT, 1270 Queen Emma St., #501, Honolulu, HI, ph 808-537-3311

96813, Pritam Tapryal, MD, 1270 Queen Emma St., #501, Honolulu, HI, ph 808-537-3311

96814, Kevin Gibson, ND, Lac, 1481 S. King St., Ste. 312, Honolulu, HI, ph 808-955-9556

96822, Lori Kimata, ND, 1843 Vancouver Place, Honolulu, HI, ph 808-949-4938

96822, Ye Nguyen, ND, 1843 Vancouver Place, Honolulu, HI, ph 808-949-4938

97005, Judy Neall, ND, 12270 SW 2nd Street, Beaverton, OR, ph 503-520-8859

97005, Thomas Richards, DC, 4085 SW 109th Suite 200, Beaverton, OR, ph 503-526-8600

97007, Marnie Loomis, ND, 3835 SW 185th Ave., Ste 200, Aloha, OR, ph 503-591-8855

97015, Kimberley Horner, ND, MS, 13110 SE Sunnyside Rd., Ste. B, Clackamas, OR, ph 503-698-5866

97019, Joyce Young, ND, 39514 SE Gordon Creek Rd., Corbett, OR, ph 503-695-2495

97030, Rose Martin, ND, 119 NE 3rd Street, Gresham, OR, ph 503-665-3888

97030, Steve Lumsden, DC, 657 NE Hood Ave., Gresham, OR, ph 503-661-7811

97034, Naina Sachdev, MD, 121 C Avenue, Lake Oswego, OR, ph 503-636-2550

97045, John A. Green, III, MD, 516 High Street, Oregon City, OR, ph 503-722-4270

97045, John Green, MD, 516 High Street, Oregon City, OR, ph 503-722-4270

97045, Kathleen Galligan, DC, 18996 S. Rose Road, Oregon City, OR, ph 503-656-5832

97055, Victoria Larson, ND, 38706 Pioneer Blvd., Sandy, OR, ph 503-668-1181

97062, David Braman, DC, 18847 SW 84th Street, Tualatin, OR, ph 503-692-5260

97128, Bruce Dickson, ND, DHANP, 119 NE 3rd St., McMinnville, OR, ph 503-434-6515

97128, Larry Herdener, ND, 340 NE Evans St., McMinnville, OR, ph 503-434-6170

97202, Daniel Beeson, DC, 7215 Southeast 13th Ave, Portland, OR, ph 503-238-7205

97205, Greg Nigh, ND, Lac, 1020 SW Taylor, Ste. 330, Portland, OR, ph 503-287-4970

97205, Gregory Eckel, ND, 1020 SW Taylor, Ste. 330, Portland, OR, ph 503-287-4970

97205, Rose Paisley, ND, 1020 SW Taylor, Ste. 330, Portland, OR, ph 503-287-4970

97209, Adam Maddox, ND, 811 NW 19th Ave., Ste 104, Portland, OR, ph 503-241-3579

97209, Allen Knecht, DC, 1809 NW David, Portland, OR, ph 503-226-8010

97209, Tori Hudson, ND, 2067 NW Lovejoy, Portland, OR, ph 503-222-2322

97210, Steven Bailey, ND, 2606 NW Vaughn, Portland, OR, ph 503-224-8083

97212, Jessica Nesseler-Cass, ND, 2244 NE 17th Ave., Portland, OR, ph 503-281-3226
97214, Gary Weiner, ND, DHANP, 1616 SE Ankeny Street, Portland, OR, ph 503-230-8973
97215, Loch Chandler, ND, MSOM, Lac, 1834 SE 49th Ave., Portland, OR, ph 503-231-1213
97219, Jay H. Mead, MD, 4444 SW Corbett Avenue, Portland, OR, ph 503-224-4003
97220, David J. Ogle, MD, 177 NE 102nd Ave., Bldg. V, Portland, OR, ph 503-261-0966
97220, Jeffrey Tyler, MD, 10529 NE Halsey Street, Portland, OR, ph 503-255-4256
97220, Lorraine Ginter, DC, 2155 NE 112th, Portland, OR, ph 503-251-5827
97220, Rita Bettenburg, ND, 10360 NE Wasco St., Portland, OR, ph 503-252-8125
97222, Ken Weizer, ND, 6501 SE King Road, Portland, OR, ph 503-771-0805
97223, Renee Schwartz, ND, 11930 SW Greenburg Rd., Tigard, OR, ph 503-639-1712
97223, Virginia Osborne, ND, 11930 SW Greenburg Rd., Tigard, OR, ph 503-639-1712
97232, Suzanne Scopes, ND, 316 NE 28th Ave., Portland, OR, ph 503-230-0812
97239, Alison McAllister, ND, 6105 SW Macadam Ave., Ste 150, Portland, OR, ph 503-402-4579
97304, Terence H. Young, MD, 1205 Wallace Rd. NW, Salem, OR, ph 503-371-1558
97333, Usha D. Honeyman, DC, 760 SW Madison Ave., Ste. 104, Corvallis, OR, ph 541-754-6323
97365, K. Edmisten, ND, Lac, 344 SW 7th, Ste. B, Newport, OR, ph 541-265-6378
97401, Miriam Mazure-Mitchell, ND, MS, 74 E. 18th Ave., Ste 12, Eugene, OR, ph 541-686-3399
97411, Donald Canavan, MSW, ND, 88937 Two Mile Lane, Bandon, OR, ph 541-347-5656
97415, Scott S. Northrup, DC, P.O. Box 1120, Brookings, OR, ph 541-469-4200
97417, Jim Siegel, DC, P.O. Box 375, Canyonville, OR, ph 541-839-4421
97420, Joseph T. Morgan, MD, 1750 Thompson Road, Coos Bay, OR, ph 541-269-0333
97424, Mark Thomas, DC, 500 Whiteaker Ave., Cottage Frove, OR, ph 541-942-5024
97448, John Gambee, MD, 93244 Hwy. 99 S., Junction City, OR, ph 541-998-0111
97470, Jane Birchard, ND, 2126 Del Rio Road, Roseburg, OR, ph 541-677-6300
97477, S. Kathleen Hirtz, MD, 1800 Centennial Blvd., #6, Springfield, OR, ph 541-726-1865
97504, Edward M. Geller, DC, 1744 E. McAndrews Road, Suite A, Medford, OR, ph 541-772-2787
97504, Helen Trew, MD, 2921 Doctor's Park Dr., Medford, OR, ph 541-770-1143
97520, Dwight McKee, MD, 525 E. Main St., Ashland, OR, ph 541-488-4370
97520, Franklin H. Ross, Jr., MD, 565 A Street, Ashland, OR, ph 541-482-7007
97520, Joy Craddick, MD, 525 E. Main St., Ashland, OR, ph 541-488-4370
97601, Donald Vradenburg, DC, 733 East Main Street, Klamath Falls, OR, ph 541-883-3011
97603, Robert P. Beaman, MD, 1903 Austin St. #B, Klamath Falls, OR, ph 541-885-9989
97701, Azure Karli, ND, 409 NE Greenwood Ave., Bend, OR, ph 541-385-6249
97701, Chris Hatlestad, MD, 2195 NE Professional Ct., Bend, OR, ph 541-388-3804
97838, Kristopher Peterson, DC, P.O. Box 211, 1002 WW Elm, Hermiston, OR, ph 541-567-6277
98003, George Koss, DO, 1014 South 320th Street, Federal Way, WA, ph 253-839-4100
98003, Patric J. Darby, MD, MS, 2505 S. 320th Street, #100, Federal Way, WA, ph 253-529-3050
98003, Thomas A. Dorman, MD, 2505 S. 320th St. #100, Federal Way, WA, ph 253-529-3050
98033, Andrei Mousasticoshvily, ND, 13112 NE 70th Pl., Kirkland, WA, ph 425-828-7288
98034, Jonathan Collin, MD, APCT, 12911 120th Ave. NE, #A-50, Kirkland, WA, ph 425-820-0547
98036, Cheryl Wood, ND, 19031 33rd Ave. W, Ste. 301, Lynwood, WA, ph 425-778-5673
98036, David Wood, ND, 19031 33rd Ave. W, Ste. 301, Lynnwood, WA, ph 425-778-5673
98036, Jianli Wang, ND, Lac, 5017 196th St. SW, Ste. 206, Lynnwood, WA, ph 425-672-2838
98038, Ralph Capone, ND, 13390 Byers Road, SE, Maple Valley, WA, ph 425-432-2226
98043, John Catanzaro, ND, 5603 230th Street SW, Mountlake Terrace, WA, ph 425-697-6112
98055, Davis Lamson, MS, ND, 801 SW 16th St., Ste 121, Renton, WA, ph 206-729-6654
98055, Jonathan V. Wright, MD, 801 SW 16th St., #121, Renton, WA, ph 425-264-0059
98055, Jonathan Wright, MD, 801 SW 16th Street, Renton, WA, ph 426-264-0059
98072, Kimberly Otis, ND, 16818 140th Ave. NE, Woodinville, WA, ph 425-486-2729
98103, Sevar Kroesen, DC, 4511 Densmore Ave. North, Seattle, WA, ph 206-547-2992
98105, Cathy Rogers, ND, 5502 34th Ave. NE, Seattle, WA, ph 206-525-3557
98105, Laurie Mischley, ND, 5322 Roosevelt Way, NE, Seattle, WA, ph 206-525-8012
98108, John F. Ruhland, ND, 4002 25th Ave. South, Seattle, WA, ph 206-723-4891
98109, Rebecca Wynsome, ND, 150 Nickerson St., Ste. 211, Seattle, WA, ph 206-283-1383
98112, Paul Reilly, ND, 122 16th Ave. East, Seattle, WA, ph 206-292-2277
98115, Ralph Golan, MD, 7522 – 20th Ave. NE, Seattle, WA, ph 206-524-8966
98115, Steven Milkis, ND, 1307 N. 45th Street, Ste 200, Seattle, WA, ph 206-834-4100
98225, Andrew Pauli, MD, 1116 Key Street, #200, Bellingham, WA, ph 360-527-9785

98225, Angela London, ND, 1903 D Street, Bellingham, WA, ph 360-734-9500
98225, Mark Steinberg, ND, 2505 Cedarwood Ave., Ste 5, Bellingham, WA, ph 360-738-3230
98258, Philip D. Ranheim, MD, 9407 Fourth Street NE, Bldg. A, Lake Stevens, WA, ph 425-334-1773
98312, Cathy Rogers, ND, 6670 Chico Way, NW, Bremerton, WA, ph 360-692-5554
98335, Steven Davis, ND, 5603 38th Ave. NW, Gig Harbor, WA, ph 253-857-5544
98342, Marleen Haverty, ND, P.O. Box 425, Indianola, WA, ph 360-297-2975
98368, J. Douwe Rienstra, MD, BPCT, 242 Monroe Street, Port Townsend, WA, ph 360-385-5658
98368, Jonathan Collin, MD, APCT, 911 Tyler Street, Port Townsend, WA, ph 360-385-4555
98405, Andrew Iverson, ND, 2303 South Union Ave. #C30, Tacoma, WA, ph 503-458-5885
98466, Eleanor Dubey, DC, 4103 Bridgeport Way W., Suite B, University Place, WA, ph 253-564-844
98506, Suzanne Adams, ND, 3627 Ensign Rd., Ste B, Olympia, WA, ph 360-459-9082
98516, Patricia Hastings, ND, 4324 Martin Way, Ste. B, Olympia, WA, ph 360-438-2882
98596, David Ellis, MD, P.O. Box 567, Winlock, WA, ph 360-785-0300
98597, Elmer M. Cranton, MD, APCT, 503 First St. South, Yelm, WA, ph 360-458-1061
98597, Stephen Olmstead, MD, 503 First St. South, Ste. 1, Yelm, WA, ph 360-458-1061
98601, David G. Young, ND, 42208 NE Munch Rd., Amboy, WA, ph 360-263-4770
98664, Cynthia Bye, ND, 2106 NE 104th Ave., Vancouver, WA, ph 360-281-6928
98683, Steve Kennedy, MD, BPCT, 615 SE Chkalov, #14, Vancouver, WA, ph 360-256-4566
98685, Jared Zeff, ND, Lac, 508 NE 139th Street, Vancouver, WA, ph 360-823-8121
98901, Richard S. Wilkinson, MD, 302 S. 12th Ave., Yakima, WA, ph 509-453-5506
99009, Stanley B. Covert, MD, BPCT, 42207 N. Sylvan Road, Elk, WA, ph 509-292-2748
99203, William Corell, MD, 3424 Grand Blvd. South, Spokane, WA, ph 509-838-5800
99205, H. Earl Moore, DC, 711 West Joseph Avenue, Spokane, WA, ph 509-328-0579
99206, Burton B. Hart, DO, 12104 E. Main Street, Spokane, WA, ph 509-927-9922
99326, Jon R. Mundall, MD, 111 North Columbia Ave., Connell, WA, ph 509-234-7766
99397, Geoffrey S. Ames, MD, 750 Swift Blvd., #1, Richland, WA, ph 509-943-3934
99503, Sandra Denton, MD, APCT, 3333 Denali Street #100, Anchorage, AK, ph 907-563-6200
99503, Torrey Smith, ND, 3330 Eagle St., Anchorage, AK, ph 907-561-2230
99504, Conradine Zarndt, ND, 4341 TiKishla St., Anchorage, AK, ph 503-780-4284
99507, David Mulholland, DC, 2020 Abbott Rd. #2, Anchorage, AK, ph 907-770-5700
99508, Stan R. Throckmorton, DC, 2006 E. Northern Lights Blvd., Anchorage, AK, ph 907-248-2848
99518, Renae Blanton, ANP, 615 E. 82nd Ave. #300, Anchorage, AK, ph 907-344-7775
99615, Ronald Brockman, DO, P.O. Box 95, Kodiak, AK, ph 907-563-9166
99669, Robert G. Thompson, MD, BPCT, 161 N. Binkley St., #201, Soldotna, AK, ph 907-260-6914
99701, Ruth Bar-Shalom, Lac, ND, 222 Front St., Fairbanks, AK, ph 907-451-7100
Australia, E. Varipatis, MB, BS, APCT, 2 Brady St., Mosman, NSW, ph 61-29-9604133
Australia, Glen McCabe, MB, BS, 127 Nerang St., Ste. 7, Southport, Queensland, ph 61-7-5911866
Australia, Mumtaz Vishal, MB, B.S., 9 Bennett St., Drysdale, VIC 3222, ph 0352512200
Australia, Robert Hanner, MB, BS, BPCT, 273 Camberwell Rd., Level 2, Camberwell, Victoria
Belgium 2600, Rudy Proesmans, MD, Jos Ratineckx Straat 5, Antwerpen, ph 32-3-449-7024
Belgium 9000, Michel De Meyer, MD, Nekkersberglaan 11, Gent, ph 32-9-222-33-42
Belgium B-9100, Antony de Bruyne, MD, Ankerstraat 134, St. Niklaas, ph 32-3-777-4150
Brazil 00-22290-160, Jorge Aguiar, MD, Ph.D., Rua Lauro Muller 116, Botafogo, Rio de Janeiro
Brazil, CEP 22299-900, Sergio Puppin, MD, Rua Lauro Muller 116, Rio de Janeiro, 00 Botafogo
British West Indies, Page Edgar, MD, P.O. Box 717, Anguilla, OO BWI, ph. 264-497-4166
Canada K1H 5K9, Edward Ragan, MD, 150 Billings Ave., Ottawa, ON, ph 613-737-3939
Canada K2H 5A8, Jennifer Armstrong, MD, B.Sc., 3364 Carling Ave., Ottawa, Ontario, ph 6137219800
Canada K7R1B1, Peter Hawley, DC, 8433 County Road 2, Napanee, Ontario, ph 613-354-4646
Canada L3P 1V8, John Gannage, MD, 300 Main Street North, Markham, ON, ph 905-294-2335
Canada L5A 2X4, Marian Zazula, MD, 3301 Cawthra Rd., Mississauga, Ontario, ph 9052767754
Canada L5N 1A6, Jozef Krop, MD, 6517 A Mississauga Rd., Mississauga, Ontario, ph 9058169657
Canada M4K 3T1, Paul Jaconello, MD, 751 Pape Ave. #201, Toronto, Ontario, ph 416-463-2911
Canada M4S 1C8, Anthony Maurantonio, DO, 1513 – 221 Balliol St., Toronto, Ont., ph 416-488-7364
Canada M5R 2A7, Riina I. Bray, MD, 1240 Bay Street, Toronto, Ontario, ph 4169729000
Canada M5S 1B2, Lynn M. Marshall, MD, 76 Grenville St., Toronto, ON, ph 4163513764
Canada T2L 1V9, W. James Mayhew, MD, #200 – 3604-52 Ave. NW, Calgary, AB, ph 403-284-2261
Canada T3A 2N1, Richard Johnson, MD, 222-4935 – 40th Ave NW, Calgary, Alberta, ph 403-202-0724
Canada T3A 2NA, Jeanette Soriano, MD, #110, 4935 – 40th Ave. NW, Calgary, AB, ph 403-202-0003

Canada T3B 0M3, W. James Mayhew, MD, 202 – 4411 16th Ave. NW, Calgary, AB, ph 403-286-7311
Canada T3H 3C4, Victor Karpenko, MD, 137 Sierra Vista Terr. SW, Calgary, AB, ph 403-228-3356
Canada V2T 2X9, Robert J. Ewing, ND, 2431 Clearbook Rd., Abbotsford, BC, ph 604-504-1978
Canada V6E 1M7, David Wikenheiser, ND, 408-1033 Davie St., Vancouver, BC, ph 604-681-2260
Canada, Angelica Fargas-Babjak, MD, 1200 Main St. W, Hamilton, ON, ph 905-521-2100
Canada, Bruce Hoffman, MB CHB, 1133 – 17th Ave. NW, Calgary, AB, ph 406-206-2333
Canada, Clare Minielly, MD, BPCT, 33 Williams Street E., Smiths Falls, ON, ph 613-283-7703
Canada, Dietrich Wittel, MD, APCT, 2902-31 Avenue, Vernon, BC, ph 250-542-2663
Canada, E.M. Nykiforuk, MD, APCT, 201 – 149 Pacific Ave. N, Saskatoon, Sask, ph 306-652-2620
Canada, Erik T. Paterson, MB, ChB, BPCT, 12-1000 NW Blvd., Creston, BC, ph 250-428-7887
Canada, Francesco Anello, MD, 401 Laurel St., Cambridge, ON, ph 519-653-3731
Canada, Fred Hui, MD, APCT, 566 Bryne Drive #C2, Barrie, ON, ph 705-721-1969
Canada, Godwin O. Okolo, MD, APCT, 9535 – 135 Ave., Edmonton, AB, ph 780-476-3344
Canada, J. W. LaValley, MD, 227 Central Street, Chester, N.S., ph 902-275-4555
Canada, James Hii, MD, BPCT, #401 – 1750 E. 10th Ave., Vancouver, BC, ph 604-873-2688
Canada, Jean Aubry, MD, APCT, 1209 Cassells Street, North Bay, ON, ph 705-840-1212
Canada, Johann G. Strobele, MD, BPCT, 3155 Harvester Rd., Burlington, ON, ph 905-634-6000
Canada, Jozef Krop, MD, 6517 Missisauga Road, Mississauga, ON, ph 905-816-9657
Canada, Kim Wilmot, MD, BPCT, #202, 4411 – 16 Ave. NW, Calgary, AB, ph 403-286-7311
Canada, Maria Schleifer, MD, BPCT, 3101 Bloor St. W, #305, Toronto, ON, ph 416-236-8788
Canada, N0L 1R0, Robert A. Beattie, MD, 22425-9 Jefferies Rd., Komoka, ON, ph 519-473-2600
Canada, P.V. Edwards, MD, Box 449, High Prairie, AL, ph 780-523-4501
Canada, Paul Cutler, MD, APCT, 3910 Bathurst St., North York, ON, ph 716-284-5140
Canada, R. Ross Mickelson, MD, BPCT, 2197 Riverside Dr. #506, Ottawa, ON, ph 613-523-0108
Canada, Richard Johnson, MD, 222, 4935 – 40 Ave. NW, Calgary, AB, ph 403-202-0724
Canada, Robert I. Harper, MD, #D261, 1600-90 Ave. SW, Calgary, AB, ph 403-252-8855
Canada, Ronald Young, MD, BPCT, #3-300 Central Ave. N., Swift Current, Sask, ph 306-773-9393
Canada, Samuel Bergman, MD, APCT, 1670 DufferiN St., #205, Toronto, ON, ph 416-652-9862
Canada, Thomas Wolder, MD, 17 Frank Street, Strathroy, ON, ph 519-245-1609
Canada, Tris Trethart, MD, APCT, 10303 – 65th Ave., Edmonton, AB, ph 780-433-7401
Canada, Yellepeddy Nataraj, B.Sc., MD, 533, 5th Street NE, Box 910, Wadena, Sask, ph 306-338-2598
Cyprus, Constantinos Xydas, MD, 252 Strovolos Ave., 1st Fl., Strovolos, 2048, ph 011357-22456777
Denmark 8260, Bruce P. Kyle, MD, Stavtrupvej 7A, Viby, ph 45-8628-9688
Denmark DK-7100, Knut T. Flytlie, MD, Gludsmindevej 39, Vejle, ph 45-75-72-60-90
Denmark DK-9480, Gunner Odum, MD, Kostervej 11, Lokken, ph 45-98990499
Denmark, Claus Hancke, MD, Lyngby Hovedgade 37, Copenhagen, Lyngb, ph 45-45-88-09-00
England LE12 9TA, Patrick J. Kingsley, MD, 72 Main St, Osgathorpe, Leicestershire, ph 441530223622
England NE9 7DD, Joseph Chikelue Obi, MMBS, 61 Aycliffe Crescent, Gateshead
England RG17 0E4, James R. Colthurst, MB, 3 Charnham Ln., Hungerford, Berks., ph 44-1488-669007
England TN4 9LT, F. Schellander, MD, Turnbridge Wells, 8 Chilston Rd., Kent, ph 44-1892-543535
England W1G 8YP, Wayne Perry, MB, 57a Wimpole Street, London, ph 0207-486-1095
England, Tarsem Lal Garg, MD, Prospect House, 32 Bolton Rd., Atherton, Manch., ph 1942-886644
England, Wendy Denning, MB, 43 New Cavendish St., London, ph 44-207-224-2423
France 06000, Marc Bouchoucha, MD, 18 Rue Massena, Nice, ph 33-04-93-876301
France 75008, Elie Attias, MD, 28 Ave. Hoche, Paris, ph 33-142-892286
France 75015, Christian Champion, MD, 50 Ave. de la Motte-Picquet, Paris, ph 33-1-40650505
Germany 65185, Heinz Mastall, MD, Bahnhofstrasse, 39, Wiesbaden, ph 011-49-611-301-215
Germany D-57072, Ilie Urlea-Schoen, MD, Ypern Str. 89, Siegen, ph 49-271-312070
Germany D-59368, Jens-Ruediger Collatz, MD, Fuerstenhof 2, Fuerstenhofklinik, Werne
Germany D-77933, Karin Loeprich, ND, Karlstrasse 5, Lahr, Black Forest, 00, ph 497821-41854
Germany D-79098, Joachim W. Picht, MD, Erasmusstrasse, 16, Freiburg, ph 49-761-3839801
Greece GR 54640, Ioannis Liapis, MD, 26-B Georgiou, Thessaloniki, ph 301-839705
Greece, Spyridon V. Joannides, MD, 164 Kifissias Ave., 115 25 Psychico, Athens, ph 301-6890100
Hungary 1116, Judit Szalontai, MD, Kondorosi Ut. 15, Budapest, ph 36-1-208-2154
Ireland, Paschal Carmody, MB, The East Clinic, Killaloe, Co. Clare, ph 353-61-376349
Ireland, T.E. Gabriel Stewart, MB, 29 Hawthorn Lodge, Castleknock, Dublin 15, ph 353-1-8212540
Italy 90139, Michele Ballo, MD, Via Ruggero Settimo, 55, Palermo, ph 39-091-580301
Italy, Sandro Mandolesi, MD, Via Firenze 47, Rome, ph 39-6-4873984

Japan 158-0085, Satoshi Ishikawa, MD, Ph.D., 1-6-14 Tamagawa Denenchofu, Setagaya-ku, Tokyo
Mexico, Carlos Lopez Moreno, MD, Col. Toreon; Jardin, Tulipanes 475, Torreon, Coahu
Mexico, Gregorio Gonzalez Nunez, MD, Reforma #21, Parras, Coah, ph 01152-842-4220591
Mexico, Humberto Berlanga Reyes, MD, Ave. de Montes 2118, Col. San Felipe, Chihu
Mexico, Jesus Gonzalez Nunez, MD, Tapia #435 Oriente, Monterey, Nuevo, ph 011-52-818-3753264
Mexico, Jesus R. Medina, MD, Ave. Mariano Ma Lee #150, Los Algodones, BC, 21970
Mexico, Jorge G. Cochran, MD, Av.B y Calle 2da, Algodones, BC, 21970, ph 658-517-7740
Mexico, Jose L. Diaz, Calle 2da. #10, Los Algodones, B.C., CP, 21970, ph 52-651-77783
Mexico, Josefina Corona Aguilar, MD, S. Diaz Miron, #167, Delegacion, Cuahtemoc, 06400
Mexico, Rodrigo Rodriguez, MD, Frac. Del Prado, Azucenas 15, Tijuana, B.C., ph 52-66-813171
Netherlands 3723 MB, Eduard Schweden, MD, Prof. Bronkhorstlaan 10, Bilthoven, ph 31-10-251114
Netherlands, 00, Lydia S. Boeken, MD, Reigersbos 100, 1107 ES Amsterdam, 00 Amsterdam
Netherlands, 00, Peter Vanderschaar, MD, 2 Penheide, Leende 559847, ph 31-495-592-232
Netherlands, 00, Raymond Pahlplatz, MD, 2 Penheide, Leende 559847, ph 31-495-592-232
Norway 0165, Anna Kathrine Ljogodt, MD, Munchsgate 7, Oslo
Norway 0484, Roald Strand, MD, Kilden Helse, Gjerddrumsv. 17A, Oslo
Norway 1523, Arild Abrahamsen, MD, Svindal 11, Svindal, ph 4769-286015
Norway 7500, David de Clive-Lowe, MB, Hognesaunvegen 23, St. Tordal, ph 0047-7482-5797
Puerto Rico, Hector R. Stella, MD, 421 Munoz Rivera Ave., San Juan, 00966, ph 787-754-0145
Puerto Rico, Manuel Marcano, MD, P.O. Box 4035, Ste. 457, Arecibo, ph 787-878-3151
Spain 28016, Felix Pedrero Ramallo, MD, Pza. Valparaiso, 7-Esc. Izda 2do B, Madrid
Spain 46004, Antonio Marco Chover, MD, Pasaje Dr. Serra 109, Valencia, ph 34-96-3514383
Spain, Eduardo A. Recio Roura, MD, C/El Roque, 73, Portal E, 1ro IZD, Telde, Gran
Spain, Rosella Mazzuka, MD, Calle Co.#20 3E, Palma de Mallorca, Islas Baleares, ph 34-971-570-574
Switzerland 4102, Anita Baxas, MD, Haupstrasse 4, Binningen, ph 41-61-422-1292
Switzerland 4102, Joachim W. Picht, MD, Haupstrasse 4, Binningen, ph 41-61-4221292
Switzerland 6052, Martin H. Jenzer, MD, Sonnenbergstrasse 11, Hergiswil, ph 41-41-630-1681
Switzerland CH-6052, Martin H. Jenzer, MD, Seestr. 79, Hergiswil
Switzerland, Walter Blumer, MD, 8754 Netstal, Glaurus bei Zurich

ETIOLOGY FOR MOST DISEASES
pull out the weed by the root

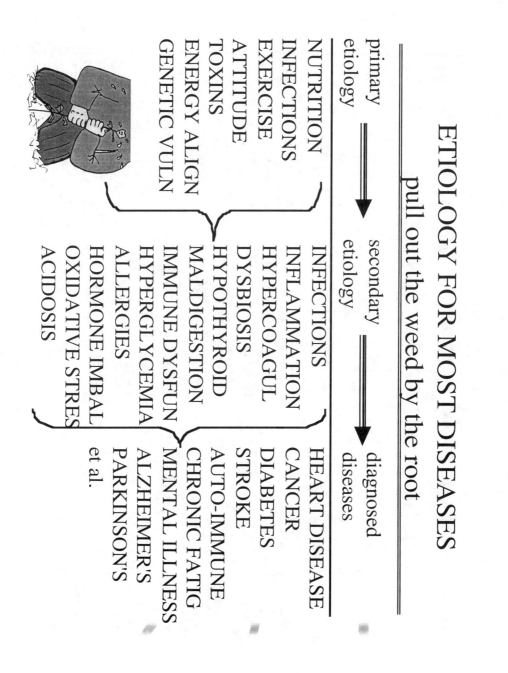

primary
etiology

NUTRITION
INFECTIONS
EXERCISE
ATTITUDE
TOXINS
ENERGY ALIGN
GENETIC VULN

secondary
etiology

INFECTIONS
INFLAMMATION
HYPERCOAGUL
DYSBIOSIS
HYPOTHYROID
MALDIGESTION
IMMUNE DYSFUN
HYPERGLYCEMIA
ALLERGIES
HORMONE IMBAL
OXIDATIVE STRES
ACIDOSIS

diagnosed
diseases

HEART DISEASE
CANCER
DIABETES
STROKE
AUTO-IMMUNE
CHRONIC FATIG
MENTAL ILLNESS
ALZHEIMER'S
PARKINSON'S
et al.

COMPREHENSIVE CANCER
TREATMENT INCLUDES:

1 →

change underlying
cause(s) of disease

NUTRITION
DETOXIFICATION
DYSBIOSIS
HORMONE BAL.
HYPERGLYCEMIA
INFECTIONS
STRESS
EXERCISE
ENERGY PATHWAYS
ETC.

2 →

restrained tumor
debulking

CHEMO?
RADIATION
SURGERY
BURZYNSKI
HYPERTHERM
PHOTO-CYTO
HERBALS
APHERESIS
LYMPH.INFUS.

3 →

symptom
management

PAIN**
NAUSEA
ANOREXIA
ANEMIA
LEUKOPENIA
DEPRESSION
CACHEXIA
HAIR LOSS